T0271343

THE EUROPEAN UNION AS A GLOBAL HEALTH ACTOR

Global Health Diplomacy
ISSN: 2010-0493

Series Editors: Thomas E. Novotny *(San Diego State University, USA)*
Ilona Kickbusch *(Graduate Institute of International and
Development Studies, Switzerland)*

Published:

Vol. 1: Innovative Health Partnerwships: The Diplomacy of Diversity
edited by Daniel Low-Beer

Vol. 2: Negotiating and Navigating Global Health: Case Studies in
Global Health Diplomacy
edited by Ellen Rosskam and Ilona Kickbusch

Vol. 3: 21st Century Global Health Diplomacy
edited by Thomas E. Novotony, Ilona Kickbusch and Michaela Todd

Vol. 4: The European Union as a Global Health Actor
edited by Thea Emmerling, Ilona Kickbusch and Michaela Told

THE EUROPEAN UNION AS A GLOBAL HEALTH ACTOR

Editors

Thea Emmerling
European Union Delegation to the United States of America, USA

Ilona Kickbusch & Michaela Told
Graduate Institute of International and Development Studies, Switzerland

W🌐 World Scientific

Published by

World Scientific Publishing Co. Pte. Ltd.
5 Toh Tuck Link, Singapore 596224
USA office: 27 Warren Street, Suite 401-402, Hackensack, NJ 07601
UK office: 57 Shelton Street, Covent Garden, London WC2H 9HE

Library of Congress Cataloging-in-Publication Data
The European Union as a global health actor / editors, Thea Emmerling, Ilona Kickbusch, Michaela Told.
    p. ; cm. -- (Global health diplomacy ; vol. 4)
    Includes bibliographical references.
    ISBN 978-9814704540 (hardcover : alk. paper) -- ISBN 9814704547 (hardcover : alk. paper)
    I. Emmerling, Thea, 1961-   , editor. II. Kickbusch, Ilona, 1950-   , editor. III. Told, Michaela, editor. IV. Series: Global health diplomacy ; v. 4.
    [DNLM: 1. European Union. 2. Global Health--Europe. 3. Health Policy--Europe.
4. Internationality--Europe. WA 530 GA1]
    RA395.E85
    362.1094--dc23

                                    2015023648

British Library Cataloguing-in-Publication Data
A catalogue record for this book is available from the British Library.

Printed in Singapore

Contents

List of Contributors

Tomas Baert
European Commission,
Directorate-General for Trade
Brussels
Belgium

Samantha Battams
Torrens University
Australia, and
Southgate Institute for Health
Society and Equity,
Flinders University
South Australia

Jorge Castilla
ECHO's Health Sector Global Coordinator
Avenue Appia
Geneva
Switzerland

Lourdes Chamorro
Delegation of the European Union to the United Nations and other
International Organisations
Geneva
Switzerland

Nicoletta Dentico
Health Innovation in Practice
Geneva
Osservatorio Italiano Salute Globale
Italy

Thea Emmerling
Health, Food Safety, and Consumer Affairs Section
Delegation of the European Union to the United States
Washigton DC
USA

Juan Garay
Head of Cooperation Section,
Delegation of the European Union in Mexico
Mexico

Annika Herbel
University of Heidelberg,
Germany

Didier Houssin
University Paris Descartes
Paris
France

Knud Erik Jørgensen
Yasar University
Izmir
Turkey

Stephen A. Matlin
Global Health Programme
Graduate Institute of International and Development Studies
Geneva, and
Institute of Global Health Innovation
Imperial College London
UK

Davide Mosca
Migration Health Department
International Organization for Migration
Geneva
Switzerland

Arne Niemann
University of Mainz
Germany

Canice Nolan
DG Health and Food Safety
European Commission
Brussels
Belgium

Andrzej Rys
Health Systems and Medical Products and Innovation
European Commission,
Health and Food Safety Directorate
Brussels
Belgium

Jean-Olivier Schmidt
Competence Centre, Health and Social Protection
Deutsche Gesellschaft für
Internationale Zusammenarbeit
Eschborn
Germany

Caroline Schultz
International Organization for Migration
Migration Health Division
Geneva
Switzerland

Yonatan Schvartzman
VIA University College,
Aarhus
Denmark

Louise van Schaik
Clingendael, Netherlands Institute of Internation Relations
The Hague
Netherlands

Remco van de Pas
Clingendael, Netherlands Institute of Internation Relations
The Hague
Netherlands

1

The EU as a Global Actor

Knud-Erik Jørgensen* and Yonatan Schvartzman**

Introduction

In order to achieve a coherent European foreign and security policy and strengthen the EU's voice in global affairs, the Lisbon Treaty established the High Representative of the Union for Foreign Affairs and Security Policy (HR). The HR, until summer 2014 Catherine Ashton, and currently Federica Mogherini, is assisted by the European External Action Service (EEAS) and is charged with ensuring consistency and coordination of the Union's external actions. The new service was meant to cover all areas of foreign policy and all questions relating to the Union's security, and to enhance the consistency between the different areas of its external action and between these and other Union policies. Member States shall support the Union's external and security policy actively and comply with the Union's actions in this area.

In several ways, however, the EU has always been an international actor. Actually, it has been possible to characterize the EU as an international actor ever since the Treaty of Rome and the establishment of the European Community. The reason for this is simple: a customs union has an internal and an external dimension. As regards the latter, relations with the external environment must be defined and subsequently cultivated.

*Yasar University, Izmir, Turkey.
**VIA University College, Aarhus, Denmark.

Moreover, an increasing number of "internal" policies have attained "external" dimensions over time and, on top of that, the Union increasingly aspired to international engagement. Today, EU involvement in global affairs can be related to many different policy fields, and objectives are being pursued through bilateral and multilateral relations. Policy areas are typically intertwined and cannot be handled in isolation, as they are more or less related to other policy fields. International health policy, for example, is related to other areas such as humanitarian aid, development, trade and agricultural policy. Directly or indirectly, each policy area has contributed to constituting the EU's role as a global actor. Strengthening this role requires the thorough coordination of often complementary but potentially also contradictory policy areas. Finally, the EU is a union of sovereign states, but each policy area is characterized by its distinct balance between "Union" and "Member States," depending on how much sovereignty was transferred to the EU level in a specific area.

This chapter examines the role of the EU as a global actor and discusses the contribution of the newly established EEAS in this context. The first part of the chapter examines the potential of the HR and the EEAS to promote a coherent European external policy and strengthen the EU's role in the world. Subsequently, we examine the EU's portfolio of international policies and those EU policies with an international dimension. The third section reviews the EU's web of bilateral and multilateral relations through which the policies are implemented while also encountering the policies of third states. We emphasize the interaction between bilateral and multilateral relations. Finally, we conclude and outline a number of broader perspectives.

Foreign Policy with the EU's Actor Characteristics

In 2010, the European Commission urged a stronger common European voice in international health policy.[1] The initiative was followed by Council Conclusions on global health, calling on EU Member States and the Commission to act together in all internal and external health policies and actions and to increase the EU's leadership in meeting global health challenges.[2] This kind of interplay between Member States and EU institutions is typical of the EU. However, the example represents only one policy area, highlighting how the task of formulating coherent international policies involves major challenges. In order to meet these and other challenges and strengthen the EU's voice in global affairs, the Lisbon Treaty established the HR, who subsequently set up the EEAS in 2011.

The development of a common foreign policy does not imply that national foreign policies are withering away.[3] The EU is a union of Member States, but each policy area is characterized by its distinct balance between "Union" and "Member States," and individual member states may obstruct common policies and decisions in different policy areas. The HR exercises, in foreign affairs, the function which so far were exercised by the six-monthly rotating Presidency, the High Representative for Common Foreign and Security Policy (CFSP) and the Commissioner for External Relations (EEAS website). In terms of a common voice, who speaks for Europe is not always obvious. In policy areas within the domain of the CFSP, the HR represents the Union, although the Member States remain the dominant *decision*-makers. In other areas, such as trade, the European Commission has exclusive competence to represent the EU in the world, such as in the WTO.

The configuration of involved institutions, their roles and their policy- and decision-making processes vary across policy areas, and it matters whether a policy is primarily internal or external. To complicate matters, this configuration changes over time and change is sometimes triggered by formal Treaty reform processes, and at other times by social or institutional learning. For outsiders, identifying a relevant negotiation partner and how large the scope for negotiation is can take some time.

The decision to create the EEAS is enshrined in the Lisbon Treaty and was driven by aspirations to strengthen the EU as a global actor and to enhance the possibility of achieving a coherent European foreign and security policy. The HR is "double-hatted": as Commission Vice President, the HR is in principle able to coordinate policy areas placed in different parts of the Commission; toward Member States, the HR chairs the Foreign Affairs Council (FAC), thus replacing the former EU Presidency in this task. The creation of the EEAS placed the EU delegations within this single hierarchical entity, a move which may strengthen the coordination between the EU and Member State delegations in third country capitals.

These aspirations clearly informed the decade-long process leading to the Constitutional Treaty, and the aspirations maintained their momentum and came to fruition in the Lisbon Treaty despite the failure of the

Constitutional Treaty. Five years after the Lisbon Treaty came into force, aspirations have been replaced by sometimes serious frustrations, especially because the EEAS seems not to have significantly strengthened the EU as a global actor or contributed to the EU's global impact. Five factors explain why this is the case.

First, the process of creating the EEAS was highly politicized and the implementation of the blueprint demonstrated that key players had significantly different ideas about what the EEAS should be like or capable of. Along the vertical axis, the balance between Member States and the new EU service had to be defined, which proved to be no plain sailing. The EEAS should support the HR in ensuring compliance with common decisions by the Member States [TEU Article 24(3)]. Member States shall support the Union's foreign policy, comply with its decisions and develop their national foreign policies in the spirit of mutual solidarity. (Ref. 4, p. 19) The EEAS must rely on informal instruments such as persuasion, leadership and the "goodwill" of Member States. Along the horizontal axis, the EEAS has an element of supranationality and an element of intergovernmentalism, as it is situated somewhere between the European Commission and the Council Secretariat — but where exactly? As Commission Vice President, the HR is tasked with coordinating the activities of fellow Commissioners on "other aspects of external action" [TEU Article 18(4)]. But the Commission is still eager to maintain the responsibility for the external dimensions of internal policies as well as for development and enlargement policies, a feature that can render the task of horizontal coordination almost impossible.[5]

Second, the EEAS is a merger of institutions employing former staff from the Commission and the Council Secretariat together with Member State diplomats. Any textbook on organizational mergers will emphasize how such merger processes tend to be difficult exercises for the management, merged units and staff alike. The processes are influenced by great uncertainty among staff, institutional inertia and different organizational cultures. Ways of doing things tend to be disrupted (sometimes intentionally), and nostalgia might trump future scenarios.[6] Creating a unified and professional organization also requires staff training. Member State diplomats must learn more about the EU, while personnel from the Commission, many with a more technical background, will require better understanding of diplomacy; however, the EEAS has no training facility that can contribute to achieving those objectives.[6]

Third, the EEAS was created on the basis of a Council Decision (2010/427/EU of 26 July 2010 establishing the organization and functioning of the European External Action Service, Article 6 para 11, OJL 201, 3 August 2010). The Commission, the Council and the European Parliament have therefore significant influence in defining the financial and human resources of the new diplomatic service. The enhancement of a strong and coherent European foreign policy requires that the EEAS gain some level of autonomy.[5] However, the emerging literature on the EEAS suggests that the Commission, the Council and the European Parliament might continue to utilize their budget control as an instrument for limiting the autonomy of the HR and the EEAS.[6]

Fourth, the implementation of the Lisbon Treaty has been marked by systematic obstruction from the UK government, not least the Conservative Party. The Conservatives failed to acknowledge the implications of the Lisbon Treaty; and when they did, they attempted to undermine them. While previous Conservative British governments frequently attacked the *acquis communautaire*, i.e. the edifice of the EU's legal order, the current UK government has targeted the EEAS and other novel bodies. The Conservative Party seems to be drifting into a position of isolationism *vis-à-vis* Europe.

Fifth, the EEAS is headed by the High Representative, previously Catherine Ashton and now Federica Mogherini. Ashton was not the first choice (but would Tony Blair have done a better job?); she was relatively inexperienced and the job description had "mission impossible" written all over it. Member States express dissatisfaction when she acts too independently — but also when she waits to see if consensus can be established among the Member States. She is supposed to fly to global hot spots and distribute ECHO food packages, but also to set out strategic directions for the EU in the EEAS headquarters at *Place Schuman* (in a triangular building first made available to the EEAS three years *after* it was supposed to function). In short, the HR/EEAS story is so dense with pros and cons that unambiguous analytical accounts are bound to suffer from a lack of credibility.

Despite the critique of the EEAS outlined above, however, it is still too early to properly assess the new body. The EEAS is still a relatively new service, and with Federica Mogherini we are only at the HR version 2.0. There is still room for learning, consolidation and new people that might drive the organization forward. With the interim Iran deal — which would not have been possible without Ashton having stayed in dialogue with Iran over several years — Ashton and the EEAS have gained in authority. Second, the extensive criticism of the EEAS is possibly the result of a lack of empirical research on the new body and how it operates. The relatively narrow literature on the EEAS has been focusing on *a priori* evaluations of organizational constraints. There has been limited empirical work on whether, when and how the EEAS and its delegations promote the implementation of coherent EU foreign policy. Thus, we still know relatively little about how the EEAS works and whether the new institution has brought changes toward more coherent EU foreign policy.

In summary, the EU can be characterized as a composite or patchwork actor — even an accidental superpower.[7] The Lisbon Treaty changed the configuration of the composite actor; specifically, entities from the European Commission (such as the former DG Relex) and the Council Secretariat have been merged and contribute significantly to the volume of the EEAS. In this fashion, the EU might appear less patchwork-like than previously, but the distribution of competence continues to vary significantly across policy areas, and the direct involvement of EU Member States staff in the EEAS has added a novel component to the composite actor.

The EU's International Policies

The EU's portfolio of international policies, i.e. policies aimed at changing the state of affairs outside the EU, has expanded considerably over time. Health policy has been one of the more recent additions to these policies. This section provides an overview of the international policies and, moreover, discusses key issues such as the EU's performance — the extent to which the EU achieves its policy objectives — and changes related to the Lisbon Treaty.

Variation is generally the name of the game. In several policy areas, e.g. trade and development, the EU is a relatively experienced player, not least because these policy areas have been handled by the EU ever since the Rome Treaty. In other policy areas, such as territorial defense, the EU is hardly a player at all. In between these two options, there is a mixed zone of arrangements. The general impact of the Lisbon Treaty is that the EU remains a composite, patchwork-like actor, now just characterized by new configurations. The EU therefore remains challenged within several policy fields. Acknowledging this diversity is very important in order to understand the EU as an international actor.

When examining the EU's international policies, it is useful to consider the origin of international policies. The rationale for some of the international policies is that they represent the international dimension of domestic EU policies. In the late 1960s, Philippe Schmitter pointed out the expectation that domestic would spill over into international and formulated the "externalization hypothesis." This externalization feature is hardly unique to the EU, as it characterizes the foreign affairs of many states around the world, demonstrated for instance by line ministries handling a range of international questions. Obviously, this is far from the classical image of the ministry of foreign affairs managing foreign interests in a manner detached from any domestic factors, but it more accurately characterizes the state of affairs at the beginning of the 21st century.

Moreover, foreign affairs also include policies aimed at shaping the environment in which the EU is operating. Enlargement policy is one example of the EU having an interest in and being able to shape its environment — indeed, successfully redefining the European order along legal, administrative and political lines. As enlargement policy has its natural limits — only European states are eligible for membership — the EU invented its neighborhood policy (ENP), aimed at reorienting states in the EU's neighborhood in a direction more compatible with the EU's own political, economic and legal arrangements.

The EU's trade policy can be seen as even more ambitious, especially because some aspects of EU trade policy aim at establishing global rules and norms for free trade. Whereas the EU previously employed mainly multilateral strategies to achieve these objectives, it now uses both multilateral (such as in the WTO context) and bilateral strategies (such as negotiating bilateral free trade agreements). The EU trade policy is one of the most important areas of EU foreign policy. Given that the EU is the world's largest trader, its policies in this area are of great significance.[8,9,10] The European Commission (DG Trade) represents the Union in trade negotiations, and the creation of the EEAS has not changed this arrangement. Since the outset, the Union's trade policy has been characterized by tensions between support for global trade regimes and the liberalization of global markets as opposed to the protection of a varying number of European producers.[10] For a long time, the EU's regime concerning trade with ACP countries was not in line with global norms and rules, a factor in explaining the EU's interest in redefining EU–ACP relations.

Finally, there is also the EU's development policy which aims at contributing to lifting poor countries out of poverty. Development policy is a key dimension of European foreign policy, demonstrated by the fact that the EU-28 is the world's largest public donor of development and humanitarian assistance, representing 51% of the world total.[9] The EU's engagement in development cooperation already began with the Treaty of Rome.[8,3] With the entrance of new members of the European adventure, including Great Britain, Spain and Portugal, development engagements also came to include Asian and Latin American countries. In 2000, the UN General Assembly adopted the Millennium Development Goals (MDG), a framework agreement for supporting developing countries (http://www.un.org/millenniumgoals/bkgd.shtml). Subsequently, the EU acknowledged its obligation to support the MDG and issued the European Consensus on Development (2006/C 46/01). The consensus identifies shared values, goals and commitments to be implemented by the Union through its development policies and defines the framework for development activities across different policy areas. Health has been identified as a policy area that could accelerate progress toward achieving the MDG (*ibid.*).

As mentioned above, health is a relatively new issue in the EU foreign policy. The EU has enjoyed institutionalized relations with the World Health Organization since 1982, but priority areas for EU–WHO cooperation were first identified in 2000, including health information, communicable diseases, research, environment and health, and sustainable health development.[11] In 2007, the external dimensions became part of the EU

Health Programme 2008–2013, which called for coherence and synergies between the program and the Community's external action (EC 1350/2007). In 2010, the Commission called on the Member States to take common global action to improve health, reduce inequalities and increase protection against global health threats.[12] The foreign ministers welcomed the call from the Commission the same year, urging the Member States to act together in all relevant internal and external policies and actions and to prioritize their support to strengthen comprehensive health systems in partner countries.[2] Despite the increasing focus on global health issues, establishing a common European policy in health still poses significant challenges. EU Member States primarily consider health policy a national affair in which Brussels should not interfere.[13,11] The EU has shared competence in common safety concerns in public health matters, but only complementary competence in other public health issues (Article 6, TFEU), and health policy has largely remained in the hands of the Member States. (EU health-related legislation such as food safety or pharma legislation is based on the internal market or the agricultural policy, but not on the health article.)

Consequently, there is no clear policy guidance for EU external health policy other than some general statements in the documents referred to above. The EU position on global health issues shifts according to topic and the ability to reach common decisions. Despite the limited mandate and vague policy, external health issues have been directly embodied in various policy areas, and this has shaped the role of the EU as a global health actor. For example, health has been a constant dimension in EU development policy.[12]

The EU in International Diplomacy: Bilateral and Multilateral Relations

The previous section examined the EU's international policies and highlighted a range of policies that the EU has adopted. However, it is when the EU cultivates its relations with third countries or international institutions that the policies might begin to acquire a certain degree of consequence. This section focuses on the bilateral and multilateral relations characterizing the EU's role as a global actor.

Bilateral Relations

The EU's network of 130-plus diplomatic delegations indicates the scope of EU engagement in international diplomacy. The Union has bilateral relations of varying range and substance with most countries and regions in the world. Five major groups of countries are in focus to provide an overview:

- Eligibility for EU enlargement
- Countries in the EU's neighborhood
- Strategic partners
- ACP countries
- Special relations

Enlargement. The EU's enlargement policy has traditionally been one of the most important dimensions of European foreign policy. In the first place, it is one of the policies that have been pursued almost since the signing of the Treaty of Rome. The UK was among the first to apply for membership, and that was soon followed by other countries. Moreover, due to the EU's soft power — the pull of attraction — enlargement policy is one of the policies that work, i.e. the EU is capable of influencing the development in the applicant countries. In terms of economic, legal and political order, most of the European continent has been transformed over the last five decades. Finally, given that less than a dozen more countries are eligible for membership, the enlargement policy is approaching an end. While it is impossible to predict when Norway, Iceland, Switzerland, Turkey, Belarus, Ukraine, Macedonia, Serbia, Albania, Montenegro and Kosovo will join the EU, it is easy to conclude that, with the exception of Turkey, they are not countries characterized by massive volume in terms of population or economy. While enlargement policy is fundamental to European foreign policy, it is not the EEAS but DG Enlargement that is in charge of policy-making.

Countries in the EU's neighborhood. At the beginning of the 21st century, when the EU entered a phase of acute enlargement fatigue, it became important for decision-makers to emphasize that enlargement is a finite process; that the number of countries eligible for membership is limited. However, a map of EU Member States and the countries eligible for membership will reveal that in the EU's neighborhood — in Russian terms, "the near abroad" — there are many countries that cannot join the EU and to them the EU's enlargement policy does not apply. This group of countries includes the states along the southern and eastern shores of the Mediterranean and Turkey's neighbors. As the EU nonetheless has a direct interest in a neighborhood characterized by peace, stability and European values in general, there is a strong rationale for creating what is now known as the EU's neighborhood policy (ENP). In contrast to the enlargement policy, the ENP's general direction is handled by the EEAS. While far from consolidated as a new service, the EEAS was catapulted into addressing the so-called Arab Spring, a basket full of difficult dilemmas and potentially contradictory objectives.

During the heyday of the Arab Spring, the EU — in concrete terms the EEAS — adopted a cautious wait-and-see policy, conducted a thorough policy review and subsequently adopted a revised policy, addressing what appeared to be a new situation. However, in contrast to the previous, largely multilateral EU policies for the Mediterranean area, including the Barcelona process, the ENP is conducted on a predominantly bilateral platform.

Strategic partners. During the last decade, the EU has established so-called strategic partnerships with an increasing number of (major) countries around the world. The EU is currently cultivating such partnerships with Brazil, China, Mexico, South Africa, India, South Korea, Russia, Canada, Japan and the United States; some of these partnerships are formal, and others are informal.

The EU has always cultivated a strategic partnership with the United States. Historically, it was the US that encouraged the integration of Western Europe and provided some of the templates for integration. Transatlantic relations have been prioritized, thereby constituting one of the backbones of the "West." This is a relationship that spans every possible issue area worth mentioning. In the sphere of political economy, the EU has traditionally been heavily involved in US-initiated trade talks, such as the Tokyo and Uruguay rounds.[14] Likewise, FDIs flow across the Atlantic in a two-way highway fashion, generating a volume that remains unmatched in any other corner of the world. In the sphere of defense, most EU members are also members of NATO, a military alliance within which the US enjoys *primus inter pares* status. EU Member States have therefore been reluctant to grant the EU a significant role concerning territorial defense, especially during the Cold War. In the 25 years since the end of the Cold War, however, the security environment has changed dramatically and both defense and security have been redefined. EU Member States have found the EU increasingly relevant to contemporary security governance, and launched the first-ever military mission under EU command in 2003.

In addition to the United States, the EU cultivates bilateral relations of strategic significance with a handful of other major countries around the world. Concerning trade, relations with both China and Japan are of key importance for the EU's foreign economic relations. Russia is the only great power with which the EU has a common border and though energy relations increase interdependence the troubled relationship seems to be a constant. Competition in the mixed zone of influence (e.g. Ukraine and Georgia) indicates the problematic nature of the difficult encounter. The general trend of emerging economies implies that two handfuls of countries have become much more relevant as EU trade partners (e.g. Brazil, Mexico, Indonesia and South Korea), and one of the consequences of the stalled multilateral Doha trade negotiations is that bilateral relations are upgraded.

ACP Countries. The EU's relations with the group of African, Caribbean and Pacific countries (ACP) began with the Rome Treaty, simply because some of the six founding members had colonies at the time. A post-colonial relationship between Europe and the former colonies had to be defined after a few years.[15,3] For years, the ACP countries constituted a privileged group within the Third World, especially concerning trade and development aid.[3,8] The Union has used trade incentives to encourage export from ACP countries, thereby improving their economic situation. Bilateral agreements include different forms of trade provisions and subsidies for export products aimed at the development of Third World countries.[20,8] From 1971, the Community's Generalized System of Preferences (GSP) granted all developing countries non-reciprocal, prudential access to EU markets. This system was reformed in 2012 and an amended GSP system will apply as of 2014. For the least developed countries (LDCs), the GSP was supplemented in 2001 with the Everything But Arms initiative, which gives all LDCs duty-free and quota-free access to the EU market for all their exports except for arms and ammunitions. In 2005, the Commission established a general strategy — Aid for Trade — to help developing countries improve their capacities for trade.

Concerning development, the EU has supported development projects in ACP countries through regional and thematic funds.[21] The EU uses these funds to directly support health system improvements in many of those countries. Indirectly, the Union supports projects for gaining access to safe food and drinking water.[16] Since 2004, more than 32 million people have gained access to improved water supplies thanks to support from the Commission.[13] Some health programs, for instance the South African HIV Programme, are entirely funded by the EU.[17,18] In other cases, EU funds empower civil societies to make effective demands on health issues, including holding leaders and governments responsible and accountable for decisions that affect the citizens' lives. One example is a project in Tanzania that recruits health workers to rural areas where health workers were once non-existent.[19] Although such examples can be viewed as unsustainable "islands" of success in a sea of failure,[17] they still represent focused projects that are important for specific areas and for inspiring further long-term development.[18]

The fifth and final way of categorizing the EU's bilateral relations is to focus on the geographical areas with which some EU countries cultivate special relations. The accession of Spain and Portugal to the EU strengthened relations with Latin American countries. The EU has ongoing negotiations with several Latin American countries, as well as Mercosur. However, relations with Latin American countries do not enjoy the institutionalized character of EU–ACP relations, and the focus is therefore broader, incorporating different political and economic issues.[9] Sweden and Finland have sponsored the so-called Northern Dimension, a bundle of transborder initiatives and policies toward Russia. With the accession of countries in Central and Eastern Europe came an increased emphasis on relations with countries to the east of Central and Eastern Europe.

Finally, it is significant that the EU's bilateral relations are characterized by what has euphemistically been referred to as "coordination problems." While the EU has exclusive competence to negotiate trade agreements with third countries or regions, Member States might want to promote their own interests in other issue areas. For example, while the EU is considered the dominant aid donor and trade partner in ACP countries (interview 1), Member States such as Sweden, Denmark and the UK prefer to pursue many of their development policies regarding Africa in parallel to the EU efforts.[22] Likewise, some Member States prefer to negotiate with the US bilaterally or in multilateral organizations such as NATO, where the EU has a weak hand.[23] The EU is therefore considered a weaker actor in transatlantic relations, at least in the areas of defense and security. Finally, some Member States have been tempted to cultivate exclusive bilateral relations with Russia. In turn, Russia has utilized its role as an energy exporter to weaken the EU's ability to speak with one voice toward Russia.[24]

Multilateral Relations

For a decade, the EU has declared its support for a largely underspecified "effective multilateralism," and the state of affairs appears somewhat unclear. For quite some time, the EU has been cultivating relations with a broad range of international institutions, and some of the policies reviewed above are pursued by means of multilateral strategies.[25] Relations are in principle two-way streets of influence. However, the degree to which such two-way streets carry asymmetrical flows of traffic remains an empirical question. The 2003 European Security Strategy is renowned for making support for international organizations one of the EU's key foreign policy objectives and EU–UN relations have been singled out as particularly important. The EU and (especially) its Member States have a considerable share of votes in UN fora and constitute the biggest financial contributor to the general UN budget, as well as many of the specialized agencies. However, the EU's ability to translate or interest in translating these assets into political ends seems rather limited.

Concerning international financial institutions — the IMF and the World Bank — the EU has stated for years an interest in strengthening its influence. The EU-28 contributes collectively about twice the amount of the single largest state. However, the EU's influence in the financial institutions has never matched the financial contribution or the share of votes. The reluctance or structural inability of the EU-28 to make use of its power is intriguing and requires further research. However, the topic has attracted little attention from scholars.[7,26,27] These two cases — the UN and the international financial institutions — are representative of a general pattern, not least because the EU-28 often has a significant presence in international institutions in terms of membership and financial contributions. Thus, the EU/EU-28 has 28 members of the OSCE's total of 55 member states.

Given the EU's considerable formal power in many international institutions, one might expect an instrumental linkage between the EU and specific organizations. What are the EU's objectives? What does the EU consider to be the key functions of specific institutions? How does the EU influence policy-making within institutions? All such question focus on the EU as an actor within international institutions. The opposite flow of influence runs from international institutions to the EU and concerns situations in which "multilateralism hits Brussels."[28]

Given the predominance of Euro-centric perspectives and the focus on European decision- or policy-making processes, the outside-in perspective is often overlooked. However, EU policies and policy-making processes may have been influenced by international organizations. Such influence should come as no surprise. Instead, it would be expected and connect to the literature on how international organizations "teach" states what states (really) want, thereby influencing the definition of national interests.[29]

Several studies demonstrate how the EU has been a newcomer in several policy fields and how policy learning has become a standard operating procedure in the processes by which European interests are defined. Examples abound and include relations between the EU and the WHO,[30] NATO (de Witte) and the World Bank.[31]

Finally, it should be added that the distinction between the two flows of influence — inside-out and outside-in — is not unproblematic. Even if the

world hangs together in very complex ways, drawing distinctions is analytically convenient if not downright necessary. It is simply impossible to
analyze everything in one go, and methods of bracketing exist and are
ready to be used. On the other hand, we should keep in mind that these
processes are possibly dynamic. Even if the EU has been an inexperienced
newcomer in one period, this is not necessarily the case in the subsequent
period and thus might reverse the direction of flows of influence. Relations
between the EU and the WHO represent an example of such role change
over time.[28] Moreover, some of the seemingly external influences might
have been initiated domestically, either by one or more EU Member States
or by parts of the European Commission seeing an advantage in taking an
issue to the international level.

In conclusion, we should take note of the serious problems and challenges that flow from attempts at assessing multilateralism from a constituent actor perspective. In their efforts to evaluate the effectiveness or
influence of a particular actor, most scholars tend to dichotomize the
international organization and the actor whose influence they want to
explore. Yet international organizations are constituted by these very
Member States. When analytically splitting off constituent parts from the
organizations, we are in some sense erasing a fundamental part of any
international organization. These problems are further complicated when
we begin analyzing the EU. While the EU is not formally a constituent
part of most international organizations, in practice it can be regarded as
a *de facto* constituent member of several IOs that have been recognized as
such by both EU Member States and other IO members.

Conclusions and Broader Perspectives

The EU has been called a composite unit and a patchwork actor, and both
labels have some merit. While the EEAS is the outcome of merged institutions, the EU remains patchwork-like, especially because the distribution
of legal competences reveals a picture of rich diversity. In many ways,
the EU is a unique global actor, characterized by distinct institutions and
policy-making processes. The conferral of sovereignty and competences
to the supranational level is at the heart of its distinctiveness and clearly
differentiates the EU from any other intergovernmental policy-making or
institutional setting.

This conferral of sovereignty, linked with a distinct separation of institutions and the ever-important balance between Member States and the Union, provides unique features. Although this assumes that other major global actors are not uniquely distinct — analysts of American, Chinese or Russian foreign policy would have an easy time emphasizing how unique and distinct their global actor is, pointing out for example American exceptionalism, Chinese relations between party and government and foreign policy with distinctly Russian characteristics — none of these players have transferred sovereignty to a new level where they decide commonly and often with a qualified majority as EU Member States have.

Patchwork or not, the EU has developed an impressive portfolio of international policies. Some of these policies have existed throughout the history of the EU, whereas other policies have been added along the integrative path, especially during the last 25 years. Some of the international policies can be seen as the extension of domestic policies — environmental policies are just one example. Other policies address the state of affairs in third countries that the EU aims at changing, such as promoting the abolishment of capital punishment throughout the world. The EEAS has thus inherited a policy catalogue, and part of the EEAS mission is to make sure that every single policy adequately represents the EU's preferences or is suitable for an ever-changing international order.

We have also demonstrated how the EU cultivates bilateral relations with most states around the world. While EU delegations obviously play a significant role in these relations, we highlight the substantive dimension of the EU's international relations. We conclude that variation is pronounced: some relations focus predominantly on development, others on economy and still others on politics. In addition to bilateral relations, the EU engages (increasingly) in relations with multilateral institutions. While strong conclusions would be premature, our preliminary conclusion is that much seems to have changed with the introduction of the EEAS and the High Representative. There is more continuity in how the EU is represented, and the potential accumulation of experience has been strengthened. Diplomats from third countries are less uncertain about who does what, when and why in the EU. Finally, we have shown that the EU is both a strong and a weak global actor. As a composite or patchwork actor, the EU has not fully understood its potential as a global actor. The prime reason is not that the EU has different priorities, but rather that the EU is in a structural state of affairs that hinders the achievement of stated objectives.

References

1. European Commission. (2010) The EU role in global health. Communication, Brussels, 31 March 2010.
2. EU Council. (2010) EU Council conclusion on the EU role in global health. 9505/10. Brussels, 7 May 2010.
3. Jørgensen KE. (2007) Overview: the European Union and the world. In: Jørgensen KE, Pollack MA, Rosamond B, *Handbook of European Union Politics*. Sage, London.
4. Paul J. (2008) EU foreign policy after Lisbon. Will the new High Representative and the External Action Service make a difference? http://edoc.vifapol.de/opus/volltexte/2009/785/ accessed 17 March 2015.
5. Furness M. (2013) Who controls the European External Action Service? Agent autonomy in EU external policy. *European Foreign Affairs Review* **18(1):** 103–127.
6. HOUSE OF LORDS. (2013) The EU's External Action Service, European Union Committee, 11th Report of Session 2012–2013, The Stationery Office Limited, London.
7. Pisani-Ferry J. (2009) The accidental player: the EU and the global economy. In: Jørgensen KE (ed.), *The European Union and International Organizations*. Routledge, London.
8. Holland M. (2002) *The European Union and the Third World*. Palgrave, New York.
9. Bretherton C, Vogler J. (2006) *The European Union as a Global Actor*. Routledge, New York.
10. Van Reisen M. (1997) European Union. In: Randel J, German T (eds.), *The Reality of Aid*. Earthscan, London, pp. 160–178.
11. Van Schaik L. (2011) The EU's performance in the World Health Organization: internal cramps after the "Lisbon Cure". *Journal of European Integration* **33:** 699–713.
12. European Council. (2010) Council conclusion on the EU role in Global Health, http://ec.europa.eu/health/eu_world/docs/ev_20100610_rd04_en.pdf, accessed 17 March 2015.

13. Greer S. (2006) Uninvited Europeanization: neofunctionalism and the EU health policy. *Journal of European Public Policy* **13:** 134–152.

14. Grieco JM. (1990) *Cooperation among Nations: Europe, America, and Non-tariff Brriers to Trade.* Cornell University Press.

15 European Commission. (2004) Taking Europe to the World: 50 years of the European commission's external service. Office for official Publication of the European Communities, Luxembourg.

16. European Commission. (2012) EU work on water and sanitation: projects and stories from the field. Available at http://ec.europa.eu/europeaid/eu-work-water-and-sanitation-projects-and-stories-field_en.

17. Schneider H, Gilson L. (1999) Small fish in a big pond? External aid and the health sector in South Africa. *Health Policy and Planning* **14:** 264–272.

18 Interview 1: David Guyader, Head of Division for Special Issues. 28 November 2012.

19 Shuma D. (2012) EU aid success story: taking action for health in Tanzania. Available at http://www.one.org/international/blog/eu-aid-success-story-taking-action-for-health-in-tanzania/

20. EU–ACP relations have been institutionalized in a convention system with clear guidance for bilateral relations; Youndé Convention I–II (1964–1975), Lomé Convention I–IV (1976–2000), Cotenau Partnership Agreement (2000–2020).

21. Development and Cooperation Instruments (DCI) and the European Development Fund (EDF).

22. Larsen H. (2005) *Analyzing the Foreign Policy of Small States in the EU: The Case of Denmark.* Palgrave, Basingstoke.

23. Shapiro J, Withney N. (2009) *Towards a Post-American Europe: A Power Audit of EU–US Relations.* ECFR, Cambridge.

24. Leonard M, Popescu N. (2007) A Power Audit of EU–Russia Relations. Policy Paper (European Council on Foreign Relations, London).

25. Jørgensen KE, Laatikainen KV. (2013) *Handbook on the European Union and International Institutions: Policy, Performance, Power.* Routledge, Abingdon.

26. Smaghi LB. (2004) A single EU seat in the IMF?. *JCMS: Journal of Common Market Studies* **42(2):** 229–248.

27. Wouters J, De Meester B. (2005) Safeguarding the coherence in global policy-making on trade and health: the EU–WHO–WTO triangle. *International Organizations Law Review* **2:** 295–335.

28. Costa O, Jørgensen KE (eds.). (2012) *The Influence of International Institutions on the EU: When Multilateralism Hits Brussels.* Palgrave Macmillan, Basingstoke.
29. Finnemore M. (1996) *National Interests in International Society.* Cornell University Press, Ithaca.
30. Guigner S. (2006) The EU's role(s) in European public health: The interdependence of roles within a saturated space of international relations. In: Elgström O, Smith M (eds.), *The European Union's Role in International Politics.* Routledge, New York.
31. Baroncelli E. (2011) The EU at the World Bank: Institutional and policy performance. *Journal of European Integration* **33(6):** 637–650.

2

The Development of EU Health Policy: Treaty Basis, Health Acquis and History

Thea Emmerling and *Andrzej Rys*[†a]

The Treaty Basis[b]

What is today the European Union has gradually evolved from the idea of stepwise economic integration. The process started with the Treaty establishing the European Coal and Steel Community (ECSC), which came into force on 18 April 1951, thus putting the coal and steel sector of the six founding members (France, Germany, Italy, The Netherlands, Belgium, Luxembourg) under a common authority and framework. A few years later, on 25 March 1957, the Treaty establishing the European Economic Community (EEC) and the Treaty establishing the European Atomic Energy Community (Euratom) were signed. They came into force on 1 January 1958. These three treaties created the European Communities,

[*]Thea Emmerling, Minister Counselor, Head of the Health, Food Safety, and Consumer Affairs Section, Delegation of the European Union to the United States, Washington DC, USA.
[†]Health Systems and Medical Products and Innovation Director European Commission, Health and Food Safety Directorate, Rue Breydel 4, 1040, Brussels, Belgium.
[a]The views expressed in this article are the personal views of the authors and in no way constitute the official views of the institution.
[b]This section is heavily based on the article "The EU as an Actor in Global Health Diplomacy," from: Emmerling T, Heydemann J (2013). In: Kickbusch I, Graham L, Told M, Drager N (eds.), *Global Health Diplomacy, Concepts, Issues, Actors, Instruments, Fora and Cases*. Springer Science and Business Media, New York, pp. 223–241.

i.e. the system of joint decision-making on coal, steel, nuclear power and other major sectors of the Member States' economies.[1]

Health was not explicitly on the agenda of the founders. It was only dealt with from the angle of occupational health, in Article 55 of the ECSC.[c] The core treaty, the EEC Treaty, aimed at creating a single market in Western Europe with free movement of goods, people, services and capital, and only mentioned public health in connection with the use of prohibitions or restrictions on the movement of goods (Article 36). However, this article, together with Articles 43, 39 and 100, made it possible to gradually set up a common veterinary policy. Free trade should not include the free spread of infectious agents and toxic substances by animals and food of animal origin, which were primarily considered as economic/market "goods."[2]

The Single European Act, which came into force in 1987, was the first major amendment of the Treaty establishing the EEC. It introduced a specific legal basis for health and safety at work, which gave a fresh impetus to EU action in this area. Otherwise it did not mention health as a distinct policy, but subsumed it as an objective of the single market. Nevertheless, several pieces of health related legislation were subsequently developed on the basis of using the treaty articles on agriculture, the single market, environmental or health and safety at work provisions.

It was the Maastricht Treaty, which came into force in November 1993, that marked the breakthrough for public health at European level. For the first time in the history of the Community, a treaty contained a separate article on public health: Article 129. This article limited Community actions to contributions to cooperation between Member States in human health protection with a focus on disease prevention, research promotion, health information and education. It did not follow a broad public health concept and could hardly be used as a basis for secondary, health-related legislation. Nevertheless, the attainment of a high level of health protection as one objective of Community activities was also enshrined in the treaty

---

[c]Health was always part of EU development policy though, but this was not explicitly mentioned in the treaties. This chapter mainly focuses on the evolution of the (public) health legal basis for internal EU policies including their external dimension, where appropriate. It also touches upon food safety and occupational health and safety, but this is not its prime focus.

Box 1. European Treaty Development and Health*

Treaty	Major Health-related Treaty Articles	Remarks
Treaty of Paris (ECSC); entry into force 23.07.1952, expiry 23.07.2002	**Article 55:** High authority to promote research on occupational safety in coal and steel industry.	Health not mentioned explicitly, only occupational safety research at the workplace.
Treaty of Rome; entry into force 01.01.1958 • **EEC Treaty**	**Article 48:** Freedom of movement for workers can be limited on public health grounds. **Article 56:** Freedom of establishment can be limited on public health grounds.	Health not mentioned in its own right; public health only mentioned as a possible limitation on the rights and freedoms of workers and the freedom of establishment.
• **Euratom Treaty**	**Article 2, b:** The Community shall establish uniform safety standards to protect the health of workers and the general public and ensure that they are applied. **Article 30:** The Community is to lay down basic standards for the protection of the health of workers and the general public against the dangers arising from ionizing radiations.	Only geared toward nuclear energy; contains a whole chapter on health and safety (Articles 30–39); establishes uniform safety standards to protect the health of workers and of the general public.
Merger Treaty; entry into force 01.07.1967		Does not mention "health" at all — pure administrative treaty which merges insitutions of the three founding treaties.

(Continued)

Box 1. (*Continued*)

Treaty	Major Health-related Treaty Articles	Remarks
Single European Act (SEA); entry into force 01.07.1987	**Article 18 supplements Article 100a of EEC Treaty:** In its proposals, the Commission will take a high level of health, safety, environmental and consumer protection as a basis. **Article 21 supplements Article 118a of EEC Treaty:** The objective is harmonization of health and safety conditions at work. **Article 25 adds Article 130r to EEC Treaty:** Community actions for the environment shall contribute to protecting human health.	Health not mentioned as a distinct policy, but subsumed as an objective of the single market. Introduction of a legal base for the harmonization of "health and safety at work."
Maastricht Treaty (EU)1,[†] entry into force 01.11.1993	**Article 3, o:** Community activities shall include contributions to attaining a high level of health protection. **Article 129:** Public Health: The Community is to: • Contribute to cooperation between Member States in human health protection, focus on disease prevention, research promotion, health information and education. • Foster cooperation with third countries and competent international organizations. • Adopt incentive measures, recommendations.	First own public health article in its own right (Article 129), but without major legislative competences. Attainment of a high level of health protection as one objective of Community activities.

(*Continued*)

Box 1. (*Continued*)

Treaty	Major Health-related Treaty Articles	Remarks
Amsterdam Treaty; entry into force 01.05.1999	**Article 129 slightly amended:** Human health protection to be ensured in the definition and implementation of all Community policies and activities. The scope for legislative measures is enlarged to quality and safety of organs and substances of human origin, blood and blood derivatives, veterinary and phytosanitary measures whose direct objective is protection of public health. The Community shall fully respect national healthcare financing and provision.	Driven by the BSE crisis, the scope for legislative measures concerning human health protection was enlarged. The Treaty specifies that the Community shall not affect national measures set out for health care financing and provision.
Nice Treaty; entry into force 01.02.2003	No change as regards health provisions; Article 129 became Article 152 in a consolidated version.	

(*Continued*)

Box 1. *(Continued)*

Treaty	Major Health-related Treaty Articles	Remarks
Lisbon Treaty; entry into force 01.12.2009	**Article 152 amended; became new Article 168:** Monitoring, early warning, combating serious cross-border threats to health enlarged; tobacco and alcohol specifically mentioned; Union can adopt measures setting high standards of quality and safety of medicinal products and devices for medical use. **Article 2C (k):** Common safety concerns in public health matters are shared competence. **Article 2E (a):** Protecting and improving human health is coordinating competence.	The health security provisions were slightly strengthened: tobacco and alcohol specifically mentioned; quality and safety of medicinal products and devices for medical use; clearer delineation between shared and coordinating competence in health.

*This table presents "health" in a narrow sense — only where health is explicitly mentioned or referred to as public health or health at the workplace, although the latter is not the focus of the table. Social security, development, assistance and provisions are left out.

†Opting out of the social policy by the UK. See: *Agreement on social policy concluded between the MS of the EC with the exception of the United Kingdom of Great Britain and Northern Ireland* (the promotion of healthy working conditions).

Box 2.   Charter Development and Health*

Charter	Health-related Articles	Remarks
European Social Charter (ESC); entry into force 26.02.1965	**Article 3:** The right to safe and healthy working conditions. **Article 11:** The right to protection of health. **Article 13:** The right to social and medical assistance.	First explicit mentioning of the effective exercise of the right to protect health and undertaking measures to promote health and to prevent epidemic, endemic and other diseases.
Revised European Social Charter; entry into force the 01.07.1999	See above.	Unchanged as regards Articles 11 and 13; rights to safe and healthy working conditions amended.
Charter of Fundamental Rights of the EU; drafted 18.12.2000 and made legally binding following the coming into force of the Lisbon Treaty. Opting-out protocols by: UK and PL from the Charter; and later by the CZ[†]. cmsUpload/cg00014.en07.pdf (TL/P/en 17–18) and http://www.consilium.europa.eu/ uedocs/cms_data/docs/pressdata/en/ ec/110889.pdf (Annex I).	**Article 31:** Every worker has the right to working conditions which respect his or her health, safety and dignity. **Article 35:** Everyone has the right to preventive health care and the right to benefit from medical treatment under the conditions established by national laws and practices. *A high level of human health protection shall be ensured in the definition and implementation of all Union policies and activities.*	Health in line with solidarity and universal coverage of health systems.

*This table presents "health" in a narrow sense — only where health is explicitly mentioned or referred to as health at the workplace. Social security, development, assistance and provisions are left out.
[†] http://www.consilium.europa.eu/uedocs/

and the Community was enabled to foster cooperation with third countries and competent international organizations in public health.

Partly driven by the BSE crisis, the Amsterdam Treaty then enlarged the scope for legislative measures concerning human health protection to quality and safety of organs and substances of human origin, blood and blood derivatives, and veterinary and phytosanitary measures whose direct objective is protection of public health. It stipulated that the Community shall fully respect national healthcare financing and provisions. The following Nice Treaty saw no changes in substance for public health, only that Article 129 became Article 152.

The Lisbon Treaty, which entered into force on 1 December 2009 and sets the present legal framework for all EU activities, clarified that today the EU shares competence with the Member States on common safety concerns in public health matters (for the aspects defined in the Treaty). The Union also has the competence to carry out actions to support, coordinate or supplement the actions of the Member States as regards the protection and improvement of human health.

The specific public health article (Article 168; see Box 3) also specifies the health provisions and stipulates that a high level of human health protection shall be ensured in the definition and implementation of all Union policies and activities. It emphasizes that the Union action shall respect the responsibilities of the Member States for the definition of their health policy and for the organization and delivery of health services and medical care and the allocation of resources assigned to them.

However, it is worth noting that even if Member States are reluctant to discuss healthcare legislation at EU level, a strong consensus and deep commitment exist across all Member States and European societies on the right to healthcare, on the overarching values of universality, access to good quality care, equity and solidarity.[d] This can also be seen in the Charter of Fundamental Rights,[3] which came into force on the same day

---

[d]Council Conclusions on Common Values and Principles in European Union Health Systems (2006), based on shared values of solidarity and equity, were adopted in 2006. See *Official Journal of the European Union, C* **146(01)**, available at http://eur-lex.europa. eu/LexUriServ/LexUriServ.do?uri=OJ:C:2006:146:0001:0003:EN:PDF (accessed on 20 August 2010).

Box 3. Lisbon Treaty — Article 168

1. A high level of human health protection shall be ensured in the definition and implementation of all Union policies and activities.

Union action, which shall complement national policies, shall be directed towards improving public health, preventing physical and mental illness and diseases, and obviating sources of danger to physical and mental health. Such action shall cover the fight against the major health scourges, by promoting research into their causes, their transmission and their prevention, as well as health information and education, and monitoring, early warning of and combating serious cross-border threats to health.

The Union shall complement the Member States' action in reducing drugs-related health damage, including information and prevention.

2. The Union shall encourage cooperation between the Member States in the areas referred to in this Article and, if necessary, lend support to their action. It shall in particular encourage cooperation between the Member States to improve the complementarity of their health services in cross-border areas.

Member States shall, in liaison with the Commission, coordinate among themselves their policies and programmes in the areas referred to in paragraph 1. The Commission may, in close contact with the Member States, take any useful initiative to promote such coordination, in particular initiatives aiming at the establishment of guidelines and indicators, the organization of exchange of best practice, and the preparation of the necessary elements for periodic monitoring and evaluation. The European Parliament shall be kept fully informed.

3. The Union and the Member States shall foster cooperation with third countries and the competent international organizations in the sphere of public health.

4. By way of derogation from Article 2(5) and Article 6(a) and in accordance with Article 4(2)(k) the European Parliament and the Council, acting in accordance with the ordinary legislative procedure and after consulting

(Continued)

Box 3. (*Continued*)

the Economic and Social Committee and the Committee of the Regions, shall contribute to the achievement of the objectives referred to in this Article through adopting in order to meet common safety concerns:

(a) measures setting high standards of quality and safety of organs and substances of human origin, blood and blood derivatives; these measures shall not prevent any Member State from maintaining or introducing more stringent protective measures;

(b) measures in the veterinary and phytosanitary fields which have as their direct objective the protection of public health;

(c) measures setting high standards of quality and safety for medicinal products and devices for medical use.

5. The European Parliament and the Council, acting in accordance with the ordinary legislative procedure and after consulting the Economic and Social Committee and the Committee of the Regions, may also adopt incentive measures designed to protect and improve human health and in particular to combat the major cross-border health scourges, measures concerning monitoring, early warning of and combating serious cross-border threats to health, and measures which have as their direct objective the protection of public health regarding tobacco and the abuse of alcohol, excluding any harmonization of the laws and regulations of the Member States.

6. The Council, on a proposal from the Commission, may also adopt recommendations for the purposes set out in this Article.

7. Union action shall respect the responsibilities of the Member States for the definition of their health policy and for the organization and delivery of health services and medical care. The responsibilities of the Member States shall include the management of health services and medical care and the allocation of the resources assigned to them. The measures referred to in paragraph 4(a) shall not affect national provisions on the donation or medical use of organs and blood.

as the Lisbon Treaty and accompanies it.[e] The Charter gives every citizen the right to social security (Article 34), the right of access to preventive healthcare and the right to benefit from medical treatment (Article 35).

---

[e] Except for the UK, Poland and the Czech Republic.

A high level of human health protection shall be ensured in the definition and implementation of all Union policies and activities (also Article 35).

In addition, European Court of Justice case law exists as regards the freedom of services in the health sector. Directive 2011/24/EU on the application of patients' rights in cross-border healthcare — with the main purpose of codifying this case law — was adopted in 2011.[f] And the European Semester, the cycle of economic policy coordination that was introduced in 2009, also includes for some countries, like Greece or Spain, health sector reforms.[4] Via the instrument of the European Semester the Commission can give policy guidance and make recommendations to governments before the national budgets are decided. In 2011, only 4 countries received country-specific recommendations (CSRs) related to healthcare, and 16 countries in 2014.

As regards EU development policy (which has always had an important social and health component), the Treaty of Rome had provided for the creation of a European Development Fund. The Maastricht Treaty formally integrated development cooperation in its Articles 177–181 and outlined its objectives: fight against poverty, enhance social and sustainable development, integrate developing countries into the world economy. The Nice Treaty introduced the potential for separate aid arrangements with pre-accession and neighboring countries, the Amsterdam Treaty stressed the need for consistency of the development policy with other external policies and the Lisbon Treaty confirmed development cooperation as an area of shared competence. It also strengthened the final objective of development cooperation, namely poverty eradication.

The Lisbon Treaty also contains the conversion of the Community into the European Union, the designation of a President of the European Council, a High Representative for Common Foreign and Security Policy and the setting up of a new European External Action Service. One key objective of the Treaty was to increase the effectiveness of European external actions by strengthening the common foreign and security policy. Since then, the different elements such as diplomacy, security, trade, development, humanitarian aid and international negotiations, have been

---

[f]EU countries had until 25 October 2013 to pass their own laws implementing the Directive. This Directive has clear linkages with the already existing coordination of social security rules under Regulation 883/2004 on the coordination of social security systems.

increasingly connected. This also puts the external aspects of EU health policy in a new light.

The Health-related Acquis Communautaire[g]

The real internal power of the EU lies in its law-making capacity. Its powers to legislate derive from the competences conferred to the EU level by the EU Member States in the treaties that form the EU. European law supersedes national law and can be enforced by using infringement procedures. In order to understand EU activities in health it is therefore useful to be aware of the health-related pieces of law that exist at EU level.

Due to the treaty developments outlined above — which show the very reluctance of EU Member States to give more competences on health to the EU level — major pieces of health-related EU legislation were developed over time on the basis of other treaty articles, mostly using the agricultural, single market, environmental or health and safety at work provisions of the treaty. These legislative provisions, although geared towards a high level of health and consumer protection, mainly pursued the objectives of the relevant policies. Although they took health concerns into account, the legislation that was set up did not follow a consistent concept of public health and thus led to a piecemeal approach to health and health-related legislation at the European level.

Ironically, it seems that a major health-related crisis was always necessary to improve the legislative health provisions at the EU level. The most important ones were the BSE crisis (which led to the development of a consistent "farm-to-fork approach" for food and feed safety, covering the whole production chain), the blood scandal (which led to EU blood safety legislation), the terrorist attacks of 11 September 2001 in the US and the H1N1 pandemic (which led to the strengthening of health security provisions and activities).

---

[g]This section is heavily based on the article "The EU as an Actor in Global Health Diplomacy" from: Emmerling T, Heydemann J (2013). In: Kickbusch I, Graham L, Told M, Drager N (eds.), *Global Health Diplomacy, Concepts, Issues, Actors, Instruments, Fora and Cases*. Springer Science and Business Media, New York, pp. 223–241.

This could now also be the case for the financial and economic crisis. Today, with an ageing population, an increase in non-communicable diseases, rising costs of technological progress and the financial and economic crisis, the sustainability of health systems in Europe is at risk — the healthcare sector contributed 10% of the EU's GDP and public spending on healthcare accounted for almost 15% of all government expenditure in 2010.[h] As part of the European Semester and budgetary consolidation, Member States have started to include health systems reform in their National Reform Programs.[i] Some Member States — Bulgaria, Estonia, Hungary, Ireland, Italy, Greece, Latvia, Romania, Portugal, Spain — have reduced their healthcare budgets.[j]

Although the Treaty explicitly stipulates that Union action shall respect the responsibilities of the Member States for the definition of their health policy and for the organization and delivery of health services and medical care, "at the EU level, the Council has recognized the need to tackle these economic and budgetary difficulties by reforming health systems, while balancing the need to provide universal healthcare and take account of their implications in all relevant fields of EU economic policy coordination."[k] In a reflection process Member States identified "effective ways of investing in health for modern, responsive and sustainable health systems," and Council conclusions were adopted in December 2013.[5] To support this work and advise on effective ways of investing in health, the Commission had set up an independent expert panel.[6]

The European Parliament, once it had acquired more power, was an immense supporter and promoter of health actions at the European

---

[h] European Commission. (2013) European Commission Staff Working Document Investing in Health, accompanying the Commission Communication "Towards Social Investment for Growth and Cohesion — Including Implementing the European Social Fund 2014–2020." SWD (2013) 43 final, p. 2. Available at http://ec.europa.eu/health/strategy/docs/swd_investing_in_health.pdf.

[i] See above, p. 6.

[j] See above, p. 3.

[k] See above, p. 4, and see Council Conclusions on the Joint Report on Health Systems in the EU, 3054th Council Meeting, Economic and Financial Affairs, 7.12.2010, available at http://www.consilium.europa.eu/uedocs/cms_Data/docs/pressdata/en/ecofin/118273.pdf.

level — be it through financial programs, public health, food safety or legislation on medicines and medical devices. Also, the European Court of Justice acted as a driver for health, mainly through case law as regards the freedom of (health) services.[1]

Another push for Community health actions came from the Council of Europe, which is a separate structure with separate objectives and has no direct link to the EU. The Council of Europe, for example, gave the impetus to launch the first Community cancer program in 1985. This program eventually led to major tobacco control activities at the EU level and subsequently tobacco control legislation, based on the single market article. The Council of Europe also worked on ethical questions, as regards tissues and cells, blood and blood derivatives, and organs, and parts of its ethical work influenced the evolving Community legislation in these fields.

The following tables give an overview of the most important pieces of existing EU legislation in public health (Table 2.1), in food safety (Table 2.2) and in animal health and welfare (Table 2.3).

Hand in hand with these developments came the attempt to gradually make a consistent whole out of the different health-related policies and pieces of legislation which had been developed over time. The first step was the White Paper on Food Safety[7] in 1999, followed by an EU Health Strategy[8] in 2007 and an Animal Health Strategy for the EU[9] in 2007. In May 2013, the Commission adopted a set of legal proposals to update and modernize its food safety legislation: the "smarter rules for safer food" package.[10] The package cuts down around 70 pieces of legislation to 5 major regulations and "provides a modernised and simplified, more risked-based approach to the protection of health and more efficient control tools to ensure the effective application of the rules guiding the operation of the food chain."[11]

EU actions in health and safety at work were outlined in the Community Strategy 2007–2012 on health and safety at work.[12] Council conclusions

---

[1]Until recently, only European Court of Justice case law existed as regards the freedom of services in the health sector. Directive 2011/24/EU on the application of patients' rights in cross-border healthcare was adopted in 2011. EU countries had until 25 October 2013 to pass their own laws implementing the Directive.

Table 2.1. EU Legislation in Public Health*

Communicable Diseases Legislation

Decision No. 2119/98/EC of the European Parliament and of the Council of 24 September 1998 setting up a network for the epidemiological surveillance and control of communicable diseases in the Community.	Network for epidemiological surveillance and control of communicable diseases in the Community.	L 268, 03/10/1998, p. 1
Commission Decision of 22 December 1999 on the early warning and response system for the prevention and control of communicable diseases under Decision No. 2119/98/EC of the European Parliament and of the Council.	Early warning and response system for the prevention and control of communicable diseases — EWRS.	L 21, 26/01/2000, p. 32
Commission Decision of 22 December 1999 on the communicable diseases to be progressively covered by the Community network under Decision No. 2119/98/EC of the European Parliament and of the Council (notified under document C (1999) 4015) (2000/96/EC).	Communicable diseases to be progressively covered by the Community network.	L 28, 03/02/2000, p. 50
Commission Decision of 19 March 2002 laying down case definitions for reporting communicable diseases to the Community network under Decision No. 2119/98/EC of the European Parliament and of the Council.	Case definitions for reporting communicable diseases to the Community network.	L 86, 03/04/2002, p. 44

(Continued)

Table 2.1　(Continued)

Commission Decision of 17 July 2003 amending Decision No. 2119/98/EC of the European Parliament and of the Council and Decision No. 2000/96/EC as regards communicable diseases listed in those decisions and amending Decision No. 2002/253/EC as regards the case definitions for communicable diseases.	Amending communicable diseases listed Decision Nos. 2119/98/EC and 2000/96/EC and case definitions for communicable diseases Decision No. 2002/253/EC.	L 184, 23/07/2003, p. 35
Commission Decision of 17 July 2003 amending Decision No. 2000/96/EC as regards the operation of dedicated surveillance networks.	Amending Decision No. 2000/96/EC re-operation of dedicated surveillance networks.	L 185, 24/07/2003, p. 55
Regulation (EC) No. 851/2004 of the European Parliament and of the Council establishing a European center for disease prevention and control.	European center for disease prevention and control.	L 142, 30/04/2004, p. 1
Commission Decision of 18 December 2007 amending Decision No. 2119/98/EC of the European Parliament and of the Council and Decision No. 2000/96/EC as regards communicable diseases listed in those decisions (notified under document number C (2007) 6355) (2007/875/EC).	Amendment — list of communicable diseases listed in earlier Decisions.	L 344, 28/12/2007, p. 48
Commission Decision of 28 April 2008 amending Decision No. 2000/57/EC as regards events to be reported within the early warning and response system for the prevention and control of communicable diseases.	Amendment — events to be reported in the early warning and response system for the prevention and control of communicable diseases.	L 117, 01/05/2008, p. 40

Commission Decision of 28 April 2008 amending Decision No. 2002/253/EC laying down case definitions for reporting communicable diseases to the Community network under Decision No. 2119/98/EC of the European Parliament and of the Council (2008/426/EC).	Amendment — case definitions for reporting communicable diseases to the Community Network.	L 159, 18/06/2008, p. 46
Commission Decision of 2 April 2009 amending Decision No. 2000/96/EC as regards dedicated surveillance networks for communicable diseases.	Amending Decision No. 2000/96/EC as regards dedicated surveillance networks for communicable diseases.	L 91/27, 03/04/2009
Commission Decision No. 2009/363/EC of 30 April 2009 amending Decision No. 2002/253/EC laying down case definitions for reporting communicable diseases to the Community network under Decision No. 2119/98/EC of the European Parliament and of the Council (OJ L 110, 1.5.2009) was adopted on 30 April.	Amending Decision No. 2002/253/EC laying down case definitions for reporting communicable diseases to the Community network.	L 110, 01/05/2009, p. 58
Commission Decision No. 2009/539/EC of 10 July 2009 amending Decision No. 2000/96/EC on communicable diseases to be progressively covered by the Community network under Decision No. 2119/98/EC of the European Parliament and of the Council.	Commission Decision No. 2009/539/EC amending Decision No. 2000/96/EC on communicable diseases to be progressively covered by the Community network.	L 180/20, 11/07/2009

(Continued)

Table 2.1   (*Continued*)

Commission Decision No. 2009/547/EC of 10 July 2009 amending Decision No. 2000/57/EC on the early warning and response system for the prevention and control of communicable diseases under Decision No. 2119/98/EC of the European Parliament and of the Council.	Commission Decision No. 2009/547/EC amending Decision No. 2000/57/EC on the early warning and response system for the prevention and control of communicable diseases.	L 181/57, 11/07/2009
Decision No. 1082/2013/EU of the European Parliament and of the Council of 22 October 2013 on serious cross-border threats to health and repealing Decision No. 2119/98/EC.	Strengthen capacities and structures for effectively responding to serious cross-border health threats.	L 293, 05/11/2013, pp. 1–15

Blood Legislation

Directive No. 2002/98/EC of the European Parliament and of the Council on setting standards of quality and safety for the collection, testing, processing, storage and distribution of human blood and blood components and amending Directive No. 2001/83/EC.	Standards of quality and safety for the collection, testing, processing, storage and distribution of human blood and blood components.	L 33, 08/02/2003, p. 30
Commission Directive No. 2004/33/EC implementing Directive No. 2002/98/EC of the European Parliament and of the Council as regards certain technical requirements for blood and blood components.	Technical requirements for blood and blood components.	L 91, 30/03/2004, p. 25

Commission Directive No. 2005/61/EC implementing Directive No. 2002/98/EC of the European Parliament and of the Council as regards traceability requirements and notification of serious adverse reactions and events.	Traceability and notification of serious adverse reaction as regards blood and blood components.	L 256, 01/10/2005, p. 32
Commission Directive No. 2005/62/EC implementing Directive No. 2002/98/EC of the European Parliament and of the Council as regards Community standards and specifications relating to a quality system for blood establishments.	Quality system for blood establishments.	L 256, 01/10/2005, p. 41
Commission implementing Directive No. 2011/38/EU amending Annex V to Directive No. 2004/33/EC with regard to maximum pH values for platelet concentrates at the end of the shelf life.	Maximum pH values for platelet concentrates at the end of the shelf life.	L 97, 11/04/2011, p. 28

Tissues, Cells and Organs Legislation

Directive No. 2002/98/EC of the European Parliament and of the Council setting standards of quality and safety for the collection, testing, processing, storage and distribution of human blood and blood components and amending Directive No. 2001/83/EC.	Standards of quality and safety of human blood and of blood components in order to ensure a high level of human health protection.	L 33/30, 08/02/2003

(Continued)

Table 2.1   *(Continued)*

Commission Directive 2004/33/EC implementing Directive No. 2002/98/EC of the European Parliament and of the Council as regards certain technical requirements for blood and blood components.	Implementation of Directive No. 2004/33/EC.	L 91/25, 30/03/2004
Commission Directive No. 2006/17/EC implementing Directive No. 2004/23/EC of the European Parliament and of the Council as regards certain technical requirements for the donation, procurement and testing of human tissues and cells.	Quality and safety of human tissues and cells — technical requirements.	L 38, 09/02/2006, p. 40
Commission Directive No. 2006/86/EC implementing Directive No. 2004/23/EC of the European Parliament and of the Council as regards traceability requirements, notification of serious adverse reactions and events and certain technical requirements for the coding, processing, preservation, storage and distribution of human tissues and cells.	Quality and safety of human tissues and cells — traceability and technical requirements.	L 294, 25/10/2006, p. 32
Commission Decision of 3 August 2010 establishing guidelines concerning the conditions of inspections and control measures, and on the training and qualification of officials, in the field of human tissues and cells provided for in Directive No. 2004/23/EC of the European Parliament and of the Council.	Guidelines concerning conditions of inspections and control measures, and on the training and qualifications of officials in the field of tissues and cells.	L 213, 13/08/2010, p. 48

Directive No. 2010/53/EU of the European Parliament and of the Council of 7 July 2010 on standards of quality and safety of human organs intended for transplantation.	Quality and safety of human organs intended for transplantation.	L 207, 06/08/2010, pp. 0014–0029
Corrigendum to Directive No. 2010/45/EU of the European Parliament and of the Council of 7 July 2010 on standards of quality and safety of human organs intended for transplantation.	Corrigendum.	L 207, 06/08/2010, p. 68

Patients' Rights in Cross-Border Healthcare Legislation

Directive No. 2011/24/EU of the European Parliament and of the Council of 9 March 2011 on the application of patients' rights in cross-border healthcare.	Application of patients' rights in cross-border healthcare.	L 88, 04/04/2011, pp. 45–65

Medical Devices

Council Directive No. 90/385/EEC on the approximation of the laws of the Member States relating to active implantable medical devices.	Ensure that the devices placed on the market and/or put into service comply with the requirements laid down in this Directive.	L 189, 20/07/1990, p. 17
Council Directive No. 93/42/EEC concerning medical devices.	Harmonization of standards relating to medical devices; products considered to meet the requirements must bear the CE mark of conformity.	L 169, 12/07/1993, p. 1

(Continued)

Table 2.1   (*Continued*)

Directive No. 98/79/EC of the European Parliament and of the Council on *in vitro* diagnostic medical devices.	Establishment of a single regulation for *in vitro* diagnostics; devices considered to meet the requirements must bear the CE mark of conformity.	L 331, 07/12/1998, p. 1
Pharmaceuticals (Selection)*		
Directive No. 2001/20/EC of the European Parliament and of the Council on the approximation of the laws, regulations and administrative provisions of the Member States relating to the implementation of good clinical practice in the conduct of clinical trials on medicinal products for human use.	Requirements for the conduct of clinical trials in the EU.	L 121, 01/05/2001, p. 34
Directive No. 2001/82/EC of the European Parliament and of the Council on the Community code relating to veterinary medicinal products.		L311/1, 28/22/2001
Directive No. 2001/83/EC of the European Parliament and of the Council on the Community code relating to medicinal products for human use.	Establishment of a Community code relating to medicinal products for human use.	L 311, 28/11/2011, p. 67
Directive No. 2011/62/EU of the European Parliament and of the Council amending Directive 2001/83/EC as regards the prevention of the entry into legal supply chain of falsified medicinal products.	Addresses falsified medicinal products.	L174/74, 1/7/2011

Regulation (EC) No. 141/2000 of teh European Parliament and of the Council on orphan medical products.		L18/1, 28/1/2000
Regulation (EC) No. 726/2004 of the European Parliament and of the Council laying down Community procedures for the authorization and supervision of medicinal products for human and veterinary use and establishing a European Medicines Agency.	Introduction of Community procedures for the authorization, supervision and pharmacovigilance of medicinal products for human and veterinary use; establishment of the European Medicines Agency.	L 136, 30/04/2004, p. 1
Regulation (EC) No. 1901/2006 of the European Parliament and of the Council on medicinal products for pediatric use.	Rules concerning the development of medicinal products for human use in order to meet the specific therapeutic needs of the pediatric population.	L 378, 27/12/2006, p. 1
Regulation (EC) No. 1394/2007 of the European Parliament and of the Council on advanced therapy medicinal products.	Rules ensuring the free movement of advanced therapy products within the EU and fostering the competitiveness of European companies in the field while guaranteeing the highest level of health protection for patients.	L 324, 10/12/2007, p. 121
Regulation (EC) No. 470/2009 on maximum residue limits of pharamcologically active substances in foodstuffs on animal origin.		L152/11, 16/6/2009

*The full pharmaceutical legislation can be found in the Compendium of EI pharmaceutical law EudraBook V. 1-May 2015, ISBN 978-92-79-44434-0.

(Continued)

Table 2.1   (*Continued*)

Regulation (EU) No. 536/2014 of the European Parliament and of the Council of 16 April 2014 on clinical trials on medicinal products for human use, and repealing Directive No. 2001/20/EC.		L 158, 27/05/2014, pp. 1–77

Tobacco Control Legislation

Directive No. 2001/37/EC of the European Parliament and of the Council on the approximation of the laws, regulations and administrative provisions of the Member States concerning the manufacture, presentation and sale of tobacco products.	Manufacture, presentation and sale of tobacco products.	L 194, 18/07/2001, p. 26
Directive No. 2003/33/EC of the European Parliament and of the Council on the approximation of the laws, regulations and administrative provisions of the Member States relating to the advertising and sponsorship of tobacco products.	Advertising and sponsorship of tobacco products.	L 152, 20/06/2003, p. 16
Commission Decision of 5 September 2003 on the use of color photographs or other illustrations as health warnings on tobacco packages.	Use of photographs and illustrations as health warnings.	L 226, 10/09/2003, p. 24
Council Decision of 2 June 2004 concerning the conclusion of the WHO Framework Convention on Tobacco Control.	EU ratification of the WHO Framework convention on Tobacco Control — (FCTC).	L 213, 15/06/2004, p. 8

Commission Decision C (2006) 1502 final amending Commission Decision C (2005) 1452 final of 26 May 2005 on the library of selected source documents containing color photographs or other illustrations for each of the additional warnings listed in Annex 1 to Directive No. 2001/37/EC of the European Parliament and of the Council.	Library containing photographs and illustrations.	
Directive No. 2010/13/EU of the European Parliament and of the Council on the coordination of certain provisions laid down by law, regulation or administrative action in Member States concerning the provision of audiovisual media services (Audiovisual Media Services Directive).	Provision of audiovisual media services that regulate, among other things, TV advertising of tobacco and alcohol products.	L 95, 15/04/2010, pp. 1–24
Commission Directive No. 2012/9/EU amending Annex I to Directive No. 2001/37/EC of the European Parliament and of the Council on the approximation of the laws, regulations and administrative provisions of the Member States concerning the manufacture, presentation and sale of tobacco products.	New set of written health warnings for tobacco products.	L 69, 07/03/2012, pp. 15–16

(Continued)

Table 2.1   *(Continued)*

Directive No. 2014/40/EU of the European Parliament and of the Council of 3 April 2014 on the approximation of the laws, regulations and administrative provisions of the Member States concerning the manufacture, presentation and sale of tobacco and related products and repealing Directive No. 2001/37/EC.	Manufacture, presentation and sale of tobacco products.	L 127, 29/04/2014, pp. 1–38

Nutrition and Labeling[†]

Council Directive No. 90/496/EEC on nutrition labeling for foodstuffs.	Nutrition labeling of foodstuffs.	L 276, 06/10/1990, pp. 0040–0044
Regulation (EU) No. 1169/2011 of the European Parliament and of the Council on the provision of food information to consumers.	Basis for ensuring a high level of consumer protection in relation to food information.	L 304/18, 22/11/2011
Directive No. 2000/13/EC of the European Parliament and of the Council on the approximation of the laws of the Member States relating to the labeling, presentation and advertising of foodstuffs.	General rules on food labeling (information on composition, manufacturer, storage methods, etc.); EU rules until 12 December 2014.	L 109, 06/05/2000, p. 29
Directive No. 2009/39/EC of the European Parliament and of the Council on foodstuffs intended for particular nutritional uses.	Principal framework regarding foodstuffs for particular nutritional uses.	L 124/21, 20/05/2009

Alcohol

Directive No. 2010/13/EU of the European Parliament and of the Council on the coordination of certain provisions laid down by law, regulation or administrative action in Member States concerning the provision of audiovisual media services.	Rules concerning criteria that television advertising of alcohol must meet.	L 95/1, 15/04/2010, pp. 1–24

eHealth

Commission implementing Decision of 22 December 2011 providing the rules for the establishment, management and functioning of the network of responsible national authorities on eHealth.	Rules for the establishment, management and functioning of the network of responsible national authorities on eHealth.	L 344, 28/12/2011, pp. 48–50

Rare Diseases: Patient Safety — Decisions and Recommendations

Commission Decision No. 2009/872/EC establishing a European Union Committee of Experts on Rare Diseases.	Establishing an EU Committee of Experts on Rare Diseases.	L 315, 02/12/2009, pp. 18–21
Commission Decision No. 2010/C 204/02 on the appointment of the members of the European Union Committee of Experts on Rare Diseases set up by Decision No. 2009/872/EC.	Appointment of members of the EU Committee of Experts on Rare Diseases.	C 204, 28/07/2010, pp. 2–5

(Continued)

Table 2.1   (*Continued*)

Health Workforce/Mobility		
Directive No. 2005/36/EC on recognition of professional qualifications.	Reform of the system of recognition of professional qualifications in order to make labor markets more flexible, further liberalize the provision of services and facilitate free movement of health professionals.	L 255, 30/09/2005, pp. 28–32

*DG Health and Consumers, http://ec.europa.eu/health/index_en.htm. Commission database on EU legislation, http://europa.eu/legislation_summaries/public_health/index_en.htm

†We can also find those acts in the table relating to the food safety legislation.

Table 2.2 Main EU Legislation on Food and Feed Safety*

Animal Nutrition and Feed Safety

Council Directive No. 90/167/EEC laying down the conditions governing the preparation, placing on the market and use of medicated feedingstuffs in the Community.	Rules governing the preparation, placing on the market and use of medicated feedingstuffs within the common market.	L 092, 07/04/1990, pp. 0042–0048
Council Directive No. 96/23/CE on measures to monitor certain substances and residues thereof in live animals and animal products.	Rules on veterinary medicines, pesticides and contaminants in food of animal origin.	L 125, 23/05/1996, pp. 0010–0032
Directive No. 2002/32/EC of the European Parliament and of the Council on undesirable substances in animal feed.	Set maximum limits for undesirable substances in animal nutrition in order to ensure that feed materials, feed additives and feedingstuffs are sound.	L 140, 30/05/2002, pp. 10–22
Regulation (EC) No. 1831/2003 of the European Parliament and of the Council on additives for use in animal nutrition.	Authorization for the placing on the market and use of feed additives, as well as rules for supervision and labeling of feed additives.	L 268/29, 18/10/2003
Regulation (EC) No. 183/2005 of the European Parliament and of the Council laying down requirements for feed hygiene.	Feed safety is considered at all stages that may have an impact on feed and food safety.	L 35/1, 08/02/2005
Regulation (EC) No. 767/2009 of the European Parliament and of the Council on the placing on the market and use of feed.	Rules governing the marketing of feed materials and compound feed.	L 229/1, 01/09/2009

(Continued)

Table 2.2   *(Continued)*

Biotechnology

Directive No. 2001/18/EC of the European Parliament and of the Council on the deliberate release into the environment of genetically modified organisms and repealing Council Directive No. 90/220/EEC.	Render the procedure for granting consent for the deliberate release and placing on the market of genetically modified organisms more efficient and more transparent.	L 106, 17/04/2001, pp. 1–39
Directive No. 2009/41/EC on contained use of genetically modified organisms.	Common measures for the contained use of GMOs.	L125, 21/5/2009, pp. 75–97
Regulation (EC) No. 1829/2003 of the European Parliament and of the Council on genetically modified food and feed.	General frameworks for regulating genetically modified (GM) food and feed in the EU.	L 268, 18/10/2003, pp. 1–23
Regulation (EC) No. 1830/2003 of the European Parliament and of the Council concerning the traceability and labeling of genetically modified organisms and the traceability of food and feed products produced from genetically modified organisms and amending Directive No. 2001/18/EC.	Traceability and labeling of GMOs and products made from these organisms throughout the food chain.	L 268, 18/10/2003
Regulation (EC) 1946/2003 on transboundary movements of GMOs.	Aims ot implement the provisions of the Cartegena Protocol on preventing biotechnological risks.	L287, 5/11/2003, pp. 1–10
Commission Regulation (EC) No. 65/2004 establishing a system for the development and assignment of unique identifiers for genetically modified organisms.	Applications for the placing on the market of GMOs shall include an identifier for each GMO concerned.	L 10/5, 16/01/2004

Legislation	Description	Official Journal
Directive No.2015/412/EU of the European Parliament and the Council amending Directive No. 2001/18/EC as regards the possibility for the Member States to restrict or prohibit the cultivation of GMOs in their territory.	Allows Member States an opt-out under certain conditions.	L68, 13/3/2015, pp.1–8

Food Safety and Biological Safety

Legislation	Description	Official Journal
Council Regulation No. 315/93/EEC laying down Community procedures for contaminants in food.	Rules which fix maximum levels of certain contaminants in food.	L 137, 13/02/1993, p. 1
Directive No. 1999/2/EC of the European Parliament and of the Council on the approximation of the laws of the Member States concerning foods and food ingredients treated with ionizing radiation.	Harmonization of analytical methods in order to detect irradiated foods.	L 66, 13/01/1999, pp. 16–23
Regulation (EC) No. 178/2002 of the European Parliament and of the Council laying down the general principles and requirements of food law, establishing the European Food Safety Authority and laying down procedures in matters of food safety.	Establishment of the European Food Safety Authority as well as introduction of common principles and definitions for national and Community food law in order to achieve free movement of food within the EU.	L 31/1, 01/02/2002
Council Directive No. 2002/99/EC laying down the animal health rules governing the production, processing, distribution and introduction of products of animal origin for human consumption.	Harmonization of veterinary public health requirements.	L 18, 23/01/2003

(Continued)

Table 2.2 (*Continued*)

Directive No. 2003/99/EC of the European Parliament and of the Council on the monitoring of zoonoses and zoonotic agents.	Minimum requirements to reinforce existing monitoring systems on feed and food (listeriosis, salmonellosis, tuberculosis, etc.).	L 325, 12/12/2003
Directive No. 2004/41/EC of the European Parliament and of the Council repealing certain Directives concerning food hygiene and health conditions for the production and placing on the market of certain products of animal origin intended for human consumption.	Repeal of certain directives concerning food hygiene and health conditions for the production and placing on the market of certain products of animal origin intended for human consumption.	L 195, 02/06/2004, pp. 0012–0015
Regulation (EC) No. 852/2004 of the European Parliament and of the Council on the hygiene of foodstuffs.	General rules for food business operators on the hygiene of foodstuffs.	L 139/1, 30/04/2004, pp. 1–54
Regulation (EC) No. 853/2004 laying down specific hygiene rules for food of animal origin.	General hygiene rules for food of animal origin.	L 139, 30/04/2004, pp. 55–205
Regulation (EC) No. 1935/2004 of the European Parliament and of the Council on materials and articles intended to come into contact with food and repealing Directives No. 80/590/EEC and No. 89/109/EEC.	General requirements for all food contact materials.	L 338/4, 13/11/2004, pp. 4–17
Regulation (EC) No. 396/2005 of the European Parliament and of the Council on maximum residue levels of pesticides in or on food and feed of plant and animal origin and amending Council Directive No. 91/414/EEC.	Introduction of the maximum quantities of pesticide residues permitted in products of animal or vegetable origin intended for human or animal consumption.	L 70, 16/03/2005

Commission Regulation (EC) No. 2073/2005 on microbiological criteria for foodstuffs.	Food safety criteria for certain important foodborne bacteria, such as *Salmonella* or *Listeria.*	L 338/1, 22/12/2005
Regulation (EC) No. 1331/2008 of the European Parliament and of the Council establishing a common authorization procedure for food additives, food enzymes and food flavorings.	EU authorization for food additives, food enzymes and food flavorings.	L 354, 31/12/2008, pp. 1–6
Regulation (EC) No. 1332/2008 of the European Parliament and of the Council on food enzymes.	EU authorization for food enzymes.	L 354, 31/12/2008, pp. 7–15
Regulation (EC) No. 1333/2008 of the European Parliament and of the Council on food additives.	EU authorization for food additives.	L 354, 31/12/2008, pp. 16–33
Regulation (EC) No. 1334/2008 of the European Parliament and of the Council on flavorings and certain food ingredients with flavoring properties for use in and on foods.	EU authorization for flavorings and certain food ingredients with flavoring properties.	L 354, 31/12/2008, pp. 34–50
Directive No. 2009/32/EC of the European Parliament and of the Council on the approximation of the laws of the Member States on extraction solvents used in the production of foodstuffs and food ingredients.	Rules governing the use of extraction solvents in the production of foodstuffs and food ingredients.	L 141, 06/06/2009, p. 3–11
Directive No. 2009/129/EC of the European Parliament and of the Council establishing a framework for Community action to achieve the sustainable use of pesticides.	Framework to achieve sustainable use of pesticides by reducing the risks and impacts of pesticide use on human health.	L 309, 24/11/2009, pp. 71–86

(Continued)

Table 2.2　(Continued)

Commission Regulation (EU) No. 1276/2011 amending Annex III to Regulation (EC) No. 853/2004 of the European Parliament and of the Council as regards the treatment to kill viable parasites in fishery products for human consumption.	Rules governing treatment to kill viable parasites in fishery products for human consumption.	L 327/39, 09/12/2011
Veterinary/Official Controls		
Council Directive No. 95/53/EC fixing the principles governing the organization of official inspections in the field of animal nutrition.	Harmonization of rules for carrying out inspections in the field of animal nutrition.	L 265 08/11/1995, pp. 17–22
Regulation (EC) No. 2160/2003 of the European Parliament and of the Council on the control of salmonella and other specified foodborne zoonotic agents.	Rules establishing controls on intra-European trade and imports with specific control methods.	L 325, 12/12/2003
Regulation (EC) No. 882/2004 of the European Parliament and of the Council on official controls performed to ensure the verification of compliance with feed and food law, animal health and animal welfare rules.	Official controls to ensure the verification of compliance with feed and food law, animal health and animal welfare rules (including EU Reference Laboratories).	L 165, 30/04/2004, pp. 1–141
Commission Regulation (EC) No. 669/2009 implementing Regulation (EC) No. 882/2004 of the European Parliament and of the Council as regards the increased level of official controls on imports of certain feed and food of non-animal origin and amending Decision No. 2006/504/EC.	Rules concerning the increase of official controls to be carried out pursuant to Article 15(5) of Regulation (EC) No. 882/2004.	L 194/13, 25/07/2009

Food and Feed Labeling

Council Directive No. 90/496/EEC on nutrition labeling for foodstuffs.	Nutrition labeling of foodstuffs.	L 276, 06/10/1990, pp. 0040–0044
Directive No. 2000/13/EC of the European Parliament and of the Council on the approximation of the laws of the Member States relating to the labeling, presentation and advertising of foodstuffs.	General rules on food labeling (information on composition, manufacturer, storage methods, etc.); EU rules until 12 December 2014.	L 109, 06/05/2000, p. 29
Commission Directive No. 2008/5/EC concerning the compulsory indication on the labeling of certain foodstuffs of particulars other than those provided for in Directive No. 200/13/EC.	Compulsory indication on the labeling of certain foodstuffs.	L 27/13, 31/01/2008
EU Regulation No. 1169/2011 of the European Parliament and of the Council on the provision of food information to consumers.	New Provision of food information to consumers; EU rules after 13 December 2014.	L 304, 22/01/2011, pp. 18–63
Regulation (EU) No. 1169/2011 of the European Parliament and of the Council on the provision of food information to consumers.	Basis for ensuring a high level of consumer protection in relation to food information.	L 304/18, 22/11/2011

Plant Health

Directive No. 91/414/EEC concerning the placing of plant protection products on the market.	Authorization, placing on the market, use and control of plant protection products within the common market.	L 230, 19/08/1991, pp. 1–32

(Continued)

Table 2.2 (*Continued*)

Directive No. 2009/128/EC of the European Parliament and of the Council establishing a framework for Community action to achieve the sustainable use of pesticides.	Member States are requested to introduce National Action Plans which set quantitative objectives, measures and timelines.	L 309/71, 24/11/2009
Regulation (EC) No. 1107/2209 of the European Parliament and of the Council concerning the placing of plant protection products on the market and repealing Council Directives No. 79/117/EC and No. 91/414/EEC.	Rules concerning the authorization of plant protection products in commercial form and their placing on the market, use and control within the Community.	L 309, 24/11/2009, pp. 1–50
Regulation (EC) No. 528/2012 of the European Parliament and of the Council concerning the making available on the market and the use of biocidal products.	Harmonization of the rules governing the making available on the market and the use of biocidal products.	L 167, 27/06/2012

*DG Health and Consumers, http://ec.europa.eu/food/food/index_en.htm.

Commission Database on EU legislation, http://europa.eu/legislation_summaries/food_safety/index_en.htm.

UK Government, Department for Environment, Food and Rural Affairs, *Animal Health, Welfare and Food Safety Review*, November 2012. https://www.gov.uk/government/uploads/system/uploads/attachment_data/file/82687/consult-eu-competence-legislation-20121127.pdf.

Table 2.3 Main EU Legislation on Animal Health and Welfare.*

Welfare of All Farm Species

Council Decision No. 78/923/EEC concerning the protection of animals kept for farming purposes.	Approval of the European Convention for the protection of animals kept for farming purposes.	L 323, 17/11/1978, pp. 0012–0013
Council Directive No. 98/58/EC concerning the conclusion of the European Convention for the protection of animals kept for farming purposes.	Minimum standards for the protection of animals bred or kept for farming purposes.	L 221, 08/08/1998, pp. 0023–0027
Council Regulation (EC) No. 834/2007 on organic production and labeling of organic products.	Minimum welfare standards for organic cattle, pig and poultry production.	L 189, 20/7/2007, p. 1
Calves		
Council Directive No. 2008/119/EC laying down minimum standards for the protection of calves.	Common minimum standards for the calves' welfare.	L 010, 15/01/2009, pp. 007–0013
Pigs		
Council Directive No. 2008/120/EC laying down minimum standards for the protection of pigs.	Common minimum standards for the pigs' welfare.	L 47, 18/02/2009, p. 5
Laying hens		
Council Directive No. 1999/74/EC laying down minimum standards for the protection of laying hens.	Common minimum standards for the laying hens' welfare.	L 203, 03/08/1999, pp. 0053–0057
Commission Directive No. 2002/4/EC on the registration of establishments keeping laying hens, covered by Council Directive No. 1999/74/EC.	Establishment of a system for registering all relevant information concerning laying hens.	L 30, 31/01/2002, pp. 0044–0046

(Continued)

Table 2.3   *(Continued)*

Chickens		
Council Directive No. 2007/43 laying down minimum rules for the protection of chickens kept for meat production.	Minimum standards for the chickens' welfare.	L 182, 12/07/2007, pp. 0019–0028
Protection of animals at the time of slaughter or killing		
Council Decision No. 80/306/EEC on the conclusion of the European Convention for the protection of animals for slaughter.	Introduction of uniform methods for sparing animals, as far as possible, suffering and stress at slaughter.	L 137, 02/06/1988, pp. 0027–0038
Council Decision No. 88/306/EEC on the conclusion of the European Convention for the protection of animals for slaughter.	Approval of the European Convention for the protection of animals for slaughter.	L 137, 02/06/1988, pp. 0025–0026
Council Directive No. 93/119/EC on the protection of animals at the time of slaughter or killing.	Rules and methods of killing animals.	L 340, 31/12/1993, pp. 0021–0034
Council Regulation (EC) No. 1099/2009 on the protection of animals at the time of killing.	Protection of animals at the time of killing.	L 303/1, 18/11/2009
Protection during transport		
Council Decision No. 2004/544/EC on the signing of the European Convention for the protection of animals during international transport.	Signature of the European Convention for animal protection and welfare during international transport.	L 241, 13/07/2004, pp. 21–21

Council Regulation (EC) No. 1/2005 on the protection of animals during transport and related operations and amending Directives No. 64/432/EEC and No. 93/119/EC and Regulation (EC) No. 1255/97.	Common minimum standards for the transport of animals.	L 3, 05/01/2005, pp. 1–44
Welfare of other animals		
Council Directive No. 1999/22/EC relating to the keeping of wild animals in zoos.	Measures to be adopted by Member States for inspection and licensing of zoos.	L 094, 09/04/1999, pp. 0024–0026
Council Decision No. 1999/575/EC concerning the conclusion by the Community of the European Convention for the protection of vertebrate animals used for experimental and other scientific purposes.	Approval of the European Convention for the protection of vertebrate animals used for experimental and other scientific purposes.	L 222/30, 24/08/1999, pp. 29–30
Directive No. 2010/63/EU of the European Parliament and of the Council on the protection of animals used for scientific purposes.	Protection of animals used for scientific purposes.	L 276, 20/10/2010, pp. 33–79
Disease Prevention		
Council Directive No. 82/894/EEC on the notification of animal diseases within the Community.	Establishment of the Animal Disease Notification System (ADNS).	L 378, 31/12/1982, pp. 58–62
Council Directive No. 88/407/EEC laying down the animal health requirements applicable to intra-Community trade in and imports of deep-frozen semen of domestic animals of the bovine species.	Rules governing trade in and imports of deep-frozen semen of bovine species.	L 194, 22/07/1988
Council Directive No. 92/35/EEC laying down control rules and measures to combat African horse sickness.	Measures to be taken once outbreaks of African horse sickness are suspected.	L 177/19, 10/06/1992

(Continued)

Table 2.3   *(Continued)*

Council Directive No. 92/66/EEC introducing Community measures for the control of Newcastle disease.	Measures to be taken once outbreaks of Newcastle disease are suspected.	L 260, 05/09/1992, pp. 1–20
Council Directive No. 2000/75/EC laying down specific provisions for the control and eradication of blue tongue.	Measures to be taken once outbreaks of blue tongue are suspected.	L 327, 22/12/2000, pp. 74–83
Regulation (EC) No. 999/2001 of the European Parliament and of the Council laying down rules for the prevention, control and eradication of certain transmissible spongiform encephalopathies.	Rules governing the production, placing on the market and in certain cases the exportation of live animals and products of animal origin.	L 147, 31/05/2001, pp. 1–40
Council Directive No. 2001/89/EC on Community measures for the control of classical swine fever.	Measures to be taken once outbreaks of classical swine fever are suspected	L 316, 01/12/2001, pp. 5–35
Council Directive No. 2002/60/EC laying down specific provisions for the control of African swine fever and amending Directive No. 92/119/EEC as regards Teschen disease and African swine fever.	Measures to be taken once outbreaks of African swine fever are suspected.	L 192/27, 20/07/2002, pp. 26–46
Council Directive No. 2003/85/EC on Community measures of the control of foot-and-mouth disease repealing Directive No. 85/511/EEC and Decisions No. 89/531/EEC and No. 91/665/EEC and amending Directive No. 92/46/EEC.	Measures to be taken once outbreaks of foot-and-mouth disease are suspected.	L 306/2, 22/11/2003

Council Directive No. 2005/94/EC on Community measures for the control of avian influenza and repealing Directive No. 92/40/EEC.	Measures to be taken once outbreaks of avian influenza are suspected.	L 10, 14/01/2006, pp. 16–65
Council Directive No. 2006/88/EC on animal health requirements for aquaculture animals and products thereof, and on the prevention and control of certain diseases in aquatic animals.	Measures to be taken once outbreaks of diseases affecting aquatic animals are suspected.	L 328/14, 24/11/2006

Further EU legislation on specific diseases (such as swine vesicular disease) can be found at the following link: http://ec.europa.eu/food/animal/diseases/controlmeasures/other_en.htm.

Veterinary/Official Controls and Imports/Intra-Eu Trade of Animals and Animal Products, Including Labeling

Council Directive No. 64/432/EEC on animal health problems affecting intra-Community trade in bovine animals and swine.	Health rules governing intra-EU trade in bovine animals or swine.	L 121, 29/07/1964, pp. 1977–2012
Council Directive No. 89/662/EEC concerning veterinary checks in intra-Community trade with a view to the completion of the internal market.	Veterinary checks on imports of products of animal origin.	L 395, 30/12/1989, pp. 13–22
Council Directive No. 90/425/EEC concerning veterinary and zootechnical checks applicable in intra-Community trade in certain live animals and products with a view to the completion of the internal market.	Checks to be applied to live animal and product of animal origin for intra-Community trade.	L 224, 18/08/1990, pp. 29–41

(Continued)

Table 2.3   (*Continued*)

Council Directive No. 91/68/EEC on animal health conditions governing intra-Community trade in ovine and caprine animals.	Animal health requirements for trade between the Member States concerning sheep and goats.	L 46, 19/02/1991, pp. 19–36
Council Directive 91/496/EEC laying down the principles governing the organization of veterinary checks on animals entering the Community from third countries and amending Directives No. 89/662/EEc, No. 90/425/EEC and No. 90/675/EEC.	Veterinary checks carried out at the EU's border inspection posts on each consignment of live animals.	L 268, 24/09/1991, pp. 56–68
Council Directive No. 92/65/EEC laying down animal health requirements governing trade in and imports into the Community of animals, semen, ova and embryos not subject to animal health requirements laid down in specific Community rules referred to in Annex A(1) to Directive No. 90/425/EEC.	Harmonization of the rules regarding trade and imports of certain live animals, sperm, ova and embryos.	L 268, 14/09/1992, pp. 54–72
Council Directive No. 92/118/EEC laying down animal health and public health requirements governing trade in and imports into the Community of products not subject to the said requirements laid down in specific Community rules referred to in Annex A(1) to Directive No. 89/662/EEC and, as regards pathogens, to Directive No. 90/425/EEC.	Health framework governing the trade in and imports of certain animal products to ensure the protection of human and animal health whilst complying with internal market rules.	L 62, 15/03/1993, pp. 49–68

Council Directive No. 97/78/EC laying down the principles governing the organization of veterinary checks on products entering the Community from third countries and repealing Directive No. 90/675/EC.	Veterinary checks on products from third countries introduced into the Community.	L 24, 20/01/1998, pp. 9–30
Regulation (EC) No. 1760/2000 of the European Parliament and of the Council establishing a system for the identification and registration of bovine animals and regarding the labeling of beef and beef products and repealing Council Regulation (EC) No. 820/97.	System establishing the identification and registration of bovine animals.	L 204, 11/08/2000, p. 1
Commission Regulation (EC) No. 1825/2000 laying down detailed rules for the application of Regulation (EC) No. 1760/2000 of the European Parliament and of the Council as regards the labeling of beef and beef products.	Beef labels that include precise information about where the animal was born and reared as well as the place of fattening, slaughtering and cutting.	L 216, 26/08/2000, p. 8
Commission Decision No. 2002/459/EC listing the units in the ANIMO computer network and repealing Decision No. 2000/287/EC.	Introduction of TRACES (Trade Control and Expert System), a trans-European network for veterinary health which notifies, certifies and monitors imports, exports and trade in animals and animal products.	L 159, 17/06/2002, pp. 27–50

(Continued)

Table 2.3   *(Continued)*

Regulation (EC) No. 998/2003 of the European Parliament and of the Council on the animal health requirements applicable to the non-commercial movement of pet animals and amending Council Directive No. 92/65/EEC.	Harmonization of health requirements concerning the pet animals.	L 146, 13/06/2003, pp. 1–9
Council Regulation (EC) No. 21/2004 establishing a system for the identification and registration of ovine and caprine animals and amending Regulation (EC) No. 1782/2003 and Directives No. 92/102/EEC and No. 64/432/EEC.	Identification and registration for traceability of sheep and goats.	L 5, 09/01/2004, pp. 8–17
Regulation (EC) No. 854/2004 of the European Parliament and of the Council laying down specific rules for the organization of official controls on products of animal origin intended for human consumption.	Community establishments and imports are subject to official controls regarding products of animal origin.	L 139, 30/04/2004, pp. 206–320
Regulation (EC) No. 882/2004 of the European Parliament of the Council on official controls performed to ensure the verification of compliance with feed and food law, animal health and animal welfare rules.	Official controls to ensure the verification of compliance with feed and food law, animal health and animal welfare rules.	L 165, 30/04/2004, pp. 1–141

Council Directive No. 2004/68/EC laying down animal health rules for the importation into and transit through the Community of certain live ungulate animals, amending Directives No. 90/426/EEC and No. 92/65/EEC and repealing Directive No. 72/462/EEC.	Health rules for the importation and transit of ungulate animals.	L 139, 30/04/2004, pp. 321–361
Commission Decision No. 2007/142/EC establishing a Community Veterinary Emergency Team to assist the Commission in supporting Member States and third countries in veterinary matters relating to certain animal diseases.	In time of crisis, animal disease experts have been called upon to support the authorities of the Member States or third countries that were affected by a disease for the first time.	L 62, 01/03/2007, pp. 27–29
Commission Regulation (EC) No. 318/2007 laying down animal health conditions for imports of certain birds into the Community and the quarantine conditions thereof.	Harmonious development of imports of certain species into the Community and preventing the risk of disease.	L 84, 24/03/2007, pp. 7–29
Council Directive No. 2008/71/EC on the identification and registration of pigs.	Identification and registration for traceability of pigs.	L 213, 08/08/2008, pp. 31–36
Council Directive No. 2009/156/EC on animal health conditions governing the movement and importation from third countries of Equidae.	Health conditions governing the movement and importations from third countries of Equidae.	L 192, 23/07/2010

(Continued)

Table 2.3 *(Continued)*

Council Directive No. 2009/158/EC on animal health conditions governing intra-Community trade in and imports from third countries of poultry and hatching eggs.	Rules governing intra-EU trade in and imports of poultry and hatching eggs; it does not apply to movements of animals within a Member State.	L 343, 22/12/2009, pp. 74–113
Others		
Commission Decision of 23 April 2007 amending Decision No. 2004/210/EC setting up Scientific Committees in the field of consumer safety, public health and the environment.	Scientific committees in the field of consumer safety, public health and the environment.	L 114, 01/05/2007, p. 14
Commission Decision of 20 June 2008 amending Decision No. 04/858/EC in order to transform the "Executive Agency for Public Health" into the "Executive Agency for Health and Consumers."	Executive Agency for Health and Consumers.	L 173, 03/07/2008, pp. 27–29

*DG Health and Consumers, http://ec.europa.eu/food/animal/index_en.htm.
Commission Database on EU legislation, http://europa.eu/legislation_summaries/food_safety/index_en.htm.
UK Government, Department for Environment, Food and Rural Affairs, *Animal Health, Welfare and Food Safety Review*, November 2012. https://www.gov.uk/government/uploads/system/uploads/attachment_data/file/82687/consult-eu-competence-legislation-20121127.pdf.

on a health in all policies approach were adopted in 2006 and 2010.[13] In 2010, the EU tried to better link the internal and external aspects of its health policy in its Communication and Council conclusions on the EU's role in global health.[14]

In areas where the EU could not legislate, it tried to unite Member States for some common health efforts by using the means of Council conclusions and Council recommendations. Therefore, the public health area is extensively working with these — more political — instruments to push health at European level.

Table 2.4 gives an overview of the major pieces of "soft acquis" in public health.

Another instrument is financial programs. They are used to promote an internal policy on public health (for more details see "The Public Health Programs" of this chapter), but also the external and development policies to, among other things, push the social and health agenda.[15] Policies on the Millennium Development Goals in general and health in particular were developed over time[16]: Article 5 of the regulation establishing the Development Cooperation Instrument stipulates that "prime attention shall be given on the supply of primary education and health." Since 2002, the EC has been fostering its policy framework to guide investments in health, HIV/AIDS and population for the achievement of the MDGs.[17] In 2005, an action program to tackle the critical shortages of health workers in developing countries (2007–2012) was adopted[18] and external policies to deal with HIV/AIDS, malaria and TB and a human and social development priorities instrument, Investing in People, was developed. Since 2000, clear investments have been deployed in the general budget to go to health and education.

The term "global health" was used for the first time in the EU Health Strategy 2008–2013 as one of four fundamental principles for EU action on health. It was defined as referring "to health issues which transcend EU and national borders and individual governments. It includes those health problems affecting citizens inside and outside the EU which need to be addressed through actions at global level."[19] Over time, global health has also gradually taken up a space in foreign policy, national health strategies, development partnerships and global public goods. Since the Lisbon Treaty came into effect, one has been able to observe efforts to better link the different external action elements together — external policy with

Table 2.4   Main "Soft Acquis" in EU Public Health*

Communicable Diseases: Recommendation

Council Recommendation No. 2009/1019/EU of 22 December 2009 on seasonal influenza.	Seasonal influenza vaccination.	L 348, 29/12/2009, pp. 71–72

Rare Diseases: Patient Safety — Recommendations

Council Recommendation No. 2009/C 151/01 on patient safety, including the prevention and control of healthcare associated infections.	Patient safety.	C 151, 03/07/2009, pp. 1–6
Council Recommendation No. 2009/C 151/02 on a European Action in the field of rare diseases.	European Action in the field of rare diseases.	C 151, 03/07/2009, pp. 7–10

Mental Health: Drug Abuse Prevention Acts

Council Resolution No. 00/86/01/EC on the promotion of mental health.	Promotion of mental health.	C 86, 24/03/2000, p. 1
Council Conclusions (Con. No. 02/06/01 EC) of 15 November 2001 on combating stress and depression-related problems.	Council Conclusions of 15 November 2001 on combating stress and depression-related problems.	C 6, 09/01/2002, p. 1
Council Conclusions (Con. No. 03/9688/1/EC) of 2 June 2003 on combating stigma and discrimination in relation to mental illness.	Combating stigma and discrimination in relation to mental illness.	C 141, 17/06/2003, p. 1
Council Recommendation No. 03/488/EC on the prevention and reduction of health-related harm associated with drug dependence.	Drug dependence prevention and reduction of health-related harm.	L 165, 03/07/2003, p. 31

Council Conclusions (Con. No. 05/9805/EC) of 3 June 2005 on a Community Mental Health Action.	Community mental health action.	Not published in *OJ*
Council Conclusions (Con. No. 11/3095/EC) on "The European Pact for Mental Health and Well-being: Results and Future Action."	"The European Pact for Mental Health and Well-being: Results and Future Action."	Not published in *OJ*
Notice No. 2008/C 326/09 from EU Institutions and Bodies: EU Drugs Action Plan for 2009–2012.	EU Drugs Action Plan for 2009–2012.	C 326, 20/12/2008, p. 7
Healthy Lifestyle, Nutrition, Health Inequalities Acts		
Council Resolution No. 00/C218/3/EC on action on health determinants.	Action on health determinants.	C 218, 31/07/2000, p. 8
Council Conclusions (Con. No. 04/C22/1/EC) on healthy lifestyles: education, information and communication.	Healthy lifestyles: education, information and communication.	C 22, 27/01/2004, p. 1
Council Conclusions (Con. No. 05/9803/EC) on obesity, nutrition and physical activity.	Obesity, nutrition and physical activity.	Not published in *OJ*
Council Conclusions (Con. No. 10/1149994/EC) on equity in health.	Equity in health.	Not published in *OJ*
Council Conclusions (Con. No. 11/122100/EC) on an EU Framework for National Roma Integration Strategies up to 2020.	EU Framework for National Roma Integration Strategies up to 2020.	Not published in *OJ*

(Continued)

Table 2.4   (*Continued*)

Council Conclusions (Con. No. 11/126542/EC) on closing health gaps within the EU through concerted action to promote healthy lifestyle behaviors.	Closing health gaps within the EU; promoting healthy lifestyles.	Not published in *OJ*
Tobacco Control: Recommendations		
Council Recommendation of 2 December 2002 on the prevention of smoking and on initiatives to improve tobacco control.	Prevention of smoking and initiatives to improve tobacco control.	L 22, 25/01/2003, p. 31
Council Recommendation of 30 November 2009 on smoke-free environments [COM (2009) 328 final].	Smoke-free environments.	C 296, 05/12/2009, pp 4–14
Alcohol Abuse Prevention		
Council Recommendation No. 01/458/EC on the drinking of alcohol by young people, in particular children and adolescents.	Alcohol consumed by young people.	L 161, 16/06/2001, p. 38
Council Conclusions (Con. No. 01/C175/EC) on a Community strategy to reduce alcohol-related harm.	Community strategy to reduce alcohol-related harm.	C 175, 20/06/2001, p. 1
Council Conclusions (Con. No. 16165/06) on EU strategy to reduce alcohol-related harm.	Supports the EU Alcohol Strategy and its priorities.	Not published in *OJ*
Council Conclusions (Con. No. 2009/C 302/07) on alcohol and health.	Invites Member States to implement the good practices identified in the EU Alcohol Strategy and the Commission to define priorities for the next phase after the end of the current strategy in 2012.	C 302, 12/12/2009, p. 15

Cancer Screenings

Council Recommendation No. 03/878/EC of 2 December 2003 on cancer screening.	Cancer screening.	L 327, 16/12/2003, p. 34
Council Conclusions on reducing the burden of cancer (10 June 2008).	Council Conclusions on reducing the burden of cancer.	Not published in *OJ*
Council Conclusions (Con. No. 13420/2/10) on action against cancer (13 September 2010).	The Council adopted conclusions set out in doc. 12667/10.	Not published in *OJ*
Council Conclusions (Con. No. 12/11) on prevention, early diagnosis and treatment of chronic respiratory diseases in children.	Prevention, early diagnosis and treatment of chronic respiratory diseases in children.	Not published in *OJ*

Healthy Environment, Including Prevention of Injury and Promotion of Safety

Council recommendation No. 99/519/EC on the limitation of exposure of the general public to electromagnetic fields (0 Hz to 300 GHz).	Limitation of exposure to electromagnetic fields.	L 199, 30/07/1999, p. 59
Council recommendation No. 07/C164 on the prevention of injury and the promotion of safety.	Prevention of injury and promotion of safety.	C 164, 18/07/2007, p. 1
European Parliament Resolution (EP 2008/2211) on health concerns associated with electromagnetic fields.	Health concerns associated with electromagnetic fields.	Not published in *OJ*

Antimicrobial Resistance

Council Recommendation on the prudent use of antimicrobial agents in human medicine.	Recommends prudent use.	L 34, 05/02/2002, pp. 13–16

(Continued)

Table 2.4   (*Continued*)

Council Conclusions on the impact of antimicrobial resistance in the human health sector and the veterinary sector — a "One Health" perspective.	Puts a "One health" perspective on the fight against antimicrobial resistance.	C 211, 18/07/2012, p. 2
Council Conclusions on antimicrobial resistance (AMR).	Beefs up efforts on antimicrobial resistance.	C 151, 3/07/2008, p.1
Council Conclusions on innovative incentives for effective antibiotics.	Focuses on incentives for effective antibiotics.	C 302, 12/12/2009, p. 10
Commission implementing Decision of 12 November 2013 on the monitoring and reporting of antimicrobial resistance in zoonotic and commensal bacteria.	Harmonizes monitoring and reporting.	L 303, 14/11/2013, pp. 26–39

eHealth

Commission Recommendation of 2 July 2008 on cross-border interoperability of electronic health record systems (notified under document number C (2008) 3282).	Cross-border interoperability of electronic health record systems.	L 190, 18/07/2008, pp. 37–43
Council Conclusions of December 2009 on Safe and efficient healthcare through eHealth.	Safe and efficient healthcare through eHealth.	Not published in *OJ*

*DG Health and Consumers, http://ec.europa.eu/health/index_en.htm.

Commission database on EU legislation, http://europa.eu/legislation_summaries/public_health/index_en.htm.

development policy, external policy with trade policy, and so on, but also to better tie the external elements of internal policies with the external policies, such as the EU's internal and external health policies.

Consequently, in 2010, the EU tried to specify these links and define action priorities in this respect in the Commission Communication and Council conclusions on the EU's role in global health.[m] With this, the EU was at the time at the forefront of efforts to achieve better policy coherence, following the example of some progressive countries in this respect.[n] The work on policy coherence is ongoing and got new impetus from the discussions on the future development agenda. In its Communication on a post-2015 development framework,[20] the Commission identified, among other topics, implementation of the Communication on the EU role in global health as one of the main current and forthcoming actions in the EU and internationally that contribute to the implementation of Rio +20.[21]

The Public Health Programs

The financial instrument for public health actions within the EU developed in the same scattered manner as the health-related EU legislation. After the Maastricht Treaty had come into effect, several Community actions were developed over several years as of the mid-1990s.[o] The

---

[m]European Commission. (2010) Communication (thereafter: The Communication) from the Commission to the Council, the European Parliament, the European Economic and Social Committee and the Committee of the Regions: The EU Role in Global Health. COM (2010) 128. European Commission, Brussels. The Communication was followed by Council Conclusions on the EU Role in Global Health at the 3011th Foreign Affairs Council meeting on 10 May 2010, in Brussels.

[n]The UK, Switzerland and Norway.

[o] — Decision No. 645/96/EC of the European Parliament and of the Council of 29 March 1996, adopting a program of Community action on health promotion, information, education and training within the framework for action in the field of public health (1996–2000);

— Decision No. 646/96/EC of the European Parliament and of the Council of 29 March 1996, adopting an action plan to combat cancer within the framework for action in the field of public health (1996 to 2000);

— Decision No. 647/96/EC of the European Parliament and of the Council of 29 March 1996, adopting a program of Community action on the prevention of AIDS and certain

Commission reviewed the public health framework in its communication of 15 April 1998 on the development of public health policy in the European Community and indicated that a new health strategy and program were needed in view of the new Treaty provisions, new challenges and experience so far. The legislator supported this view and adopted the first public health program (2003–2008) with the amount of €312 million.[22] The program was designed to support and complement the Member States' actions and measures. It had three general objectives: firstly, improving information for the development of public health; secondly,

---

other communicable diseases within the framework for action in the field of public health (1996–2000);

—Decision No. 102/97/EC of the European Parliament and of the Council of 16 December 1996, adopting a program of Community action on the prevention of drug dependence within the framework for action in the field of public health (1996–2000);

— Decision No. 1400/97/EC of the European Parliament and of the Council of 30 June 1997, adopting a program of Community action on health monitoring within the framework for action in the field of public health (1997–2001);

— Decision No. 372/1999/EC of the European Parliament and of the Council of 8 February 1999, adopting a program of Community action on injury prevention in the framework for action in the field of public health (1999–2003);

— Decision No. 1295/1999/EC of the European Parliament and of the Council of 29 April 1999, adopting a program of Community action on rare diseases within the framework for action in the field of public health (1999–2003); and

— Decision No. 1296/1999/EC of the European Parliament and of the Council of 29 April 1999, adopting a program of Community action on pollution-related diseases in the context of the framework for action in the field of public health (1999–2001).

These eight action programs were all developed in the context of the public health framework set out in the Commission communication of 24 November 1993 on the framework for action in the field of public health. Furthermore, Decision No. 2119/98/EC of the European Parliament and of the Council of 24 September 1998, on setting up a network for the epidemiological surveillance and control of communicable diseases in the Community, was adopted. Pursuant to that Decision, the Commission adopted on 22 December 1999 Decision No. 2000/57/EC, on the early warning and response system for the prevention and control of communicable diseases. Other activities in the context of the public health framework included Council Recommendation 98/463/EC of 29 June 1998, on the suitability of blood and plasma donors and the screening of donated blood in the European Community, and Recommendation 1999/519/EC of 12 July 1999, on the limitation of exposure of the general public to electromagnetic fields 0 Hz to 300 GHz.

reacting rapidly to health threats; and thirdly, tackling health determinants through health promotion and disease prevention, underpinned by inter-sectoral action. This program also already mentions cooperation with third countries and the competent international organizations in the sphere of health, such as the WHO, the Council of Europe and the OECD, not only in the field of collecting and analyzing data (including indicators) but also in the field of intersectoral health promotion.

The first public health program was followed by the second program (2008–2013) with a financial envelope of €321.5 million.[23] Like its pre-decesor, it focuses on health security, health promotion and health infor-mation. This program introduced nevertheless some new considerations, such as reminding that the health sector includes considerable potential for growth, that healthcare systems will face challenges in terms of finan-cial and social sustainability due, among other reasons, to the ageing of the population and medical advances. It mentions antimicrobial resistance and the mainstreaming of health objectives in all Community policies and activities.

Since then, the economic climate has changed. Driven by the financial and economic crisis, the EU is increasingly focusing its efforts on growth promotion. It is an uphill struggle to promote social and health themes. The third program for the Union's action in the field of health (2014–2020) was finally adopted on 11 March 2014.[25] It strengthens and empha-sizes the links between economic growth and a healthy population to a greater extent than the previous public health programs. It also looks at sustainable health systems — and, with this approach, for the first time comes closer to health aspects of the EU's development policy with its focus on health system strengthening.[p] Although this program — like its

---

[p]It focuses on four specific objectives with strong potential for economic growth through better health:

(1) To develop common tools and mechanisms at EU level to address shortages of resources, both human and financial, and to facilitate uptake of innovation in health-care in order to contribute to innovative and sustainable health systems.

(2) To increase access to medical expertise and information for specific conditions also beyond national borders and to develop shared solutions and guidelines to improve health care quality and patient safety in order to increase access to better and safer health care for EU citizens.

predecessors — covers certain aspects of global health work, such as cross-border health threats, it only mentions the term "global health" in its recital 15.[q] The term does not appear in the annex, which defines eligible actions.

Institutional Developments

Commission

The treaty developments outlined in "The Treaty Basis," of this chapter are reflected in the institutional structure of the European Commission.[r] From the 1980s until the mid-1990s, it had a Directorate on occupational health in the Social DG (Directorate-General); veterinary health was dealt with in the Agricultural DG, and food in the Enterprise DG. Following the BSE crisis and the criticism that health issues should be treated independently of commercial and economic interests, a new DG on consumer health policy was set up in 1997. The main idea behind that was to separate the elaboration of scientific advice from the legislation (which means separating risk assessment from risk management) and to introduce transparency in the process of giving advice and translating

---

(3) To identify, disseminate and promote the uptake of validated best practices for cost-effective prevention measures by addressing the key risk factors, namely smoking, abuse of alcohol and obesity, as well as HIV/AIDS, with a focus on the cross-border dimension, in order to prevent diseases and promote good health.

(4) To develop common approaches and demonstrate their value for better preparedness and coordination in health emergencies in order to protect citizens from cross-border health threats.

[q]Recital 15: "… Special efforts should be undertaken to ensure coherence and synergies between the programme and global health work carried out under other Union programmes and instruments that address, in particular, the areas of influenza, HIV/AIDS, tuberculosis and other cross-border health threats in third countries." http://eur-lex.europa.eu/legal-content/EN/TXT/PDF/?uri=CELEX:32014R0282&from=EN.

[r]This paragraph is heavily based on the article "The EU as an Actor in Global Health Diplomacy," from: Emmerling T, Heydemann J (2013). In: KickbuschI, Graham L, Told M, Drager N (eds.), *Global Health Diplomacy, Concepts, Issues, Actors, Instruments, Fora and Cases*. Springer Science and Business Media, New York, pp. 223–241.

this scientific advice into legal and political action. The DG was gradually strengthened with the relevant food and feed safety legislation, as well as public health legislation under the Prodi Commission 1999. Finally, under the Barroso II Commission at the end of 2009, the legislation on pharmaceuticals and medical devices, as well as the legislation on genetically modified organisms, came under the health roof. The Juncker Commission reorganized the services in 2014 and placed medical devices under the authority of DG GROW and consumer policy under DG Justice.

The Health and Consumer DG today therefore deals with public health (including pharmaceuticals), food, feed and plant health and safety and genetically modified organisms. E-health activities are being developed in strong collaboration with the DG for Communications Networks, Content and Technology, and health and safety at work and labor mobility remains with DG Employment. DG Research and Innovation manages the important component of health research, DG Internal Market Industry, Entrepreneurship and Small and Medium-sized Enterprises manages regulated professions (including doctors, nurses, midwives and pharmacists) and DG Development defines health in development. DG Environment deals with environmental legislation, which has a strong health dimension. An interservice group on global health exists to bind together the different strands of health-related work in the Commission.

European Agencies

In parallel with those organizational developments within the European Commission, several health-related agencies were set up that are linked today to the Health and Food Safety Department of the Commission (Directorate-General Health and Food Safety).

The European Medicines Agency (EMA; formerly the European Agency for the Evaluation of Medicinal Products) in London, set up in 1995, coordinates the evaluation and monitoring of centrally authorized products developed by pharmaceutical companies for use in the EU. Furthermore, EMA develops technical guidance and provides scientific advice.[26]

The Community Plant Variety Office (CPVO) in operation since 1995, is the EU agency responsible for implementing a system for the protection of plant varieties. Since 1997, its headquarters has been located in Angers, France.[27]

The European Food Safety Agency (EFSA), established in 2002 in Parma, Italy, provides independent scientific advice and communication on existing and emerging risks regarding food and feed safety. It supports the Commission, the European Parliament and Member States in taking risk management decisions in all matters directly or indirectly associated with the food chain, including animal health and welfare, plant protection, plant health and nutrition, and manages the scientific committees.[28]

Finally, the European Centre for Disease Prevention and Control (ECDC), set up in 2005 in Stockholm, Sweden, identifies, assesses and communicates current and emerging threats to human health posed by infectious diseases. ECDC pools Europe's health knowledge, so as to develop authoritative scientific opinions about the risks posed by current and emerging infectious diseases. It also manages disease surveillance and early warning systems.[29]

The Consumers, Health and Food Executive Agency (Chafea), located in Luxembourg, manages the public health program.

Four other health-related agencies are worth mentioning in this context as well, but they are linked to other Directorates-General in the Commission: The European Agency for Health and Safety at Work in Bilbao, Spain; the European Monitoring Centre for Drugs and Drug Addiction in Lisbon, Portugal; the European Chemicals Agency in Helsinki, Finland; and the European Environment Agency in Copenhagen, Denmark.

European Parliament

In parallel with the organizational developments in the Commission, in the European Parliament health gained more and more prominence.[30] The European Parliament set up an Environment Committee in 1973 as its 12th specialist committee. Its subsequent increase in size (from 36 to 63 members) and in power arose through extended responsibilities and co-legislation in the Union on environmental matters, as regards the single market and through greater sensitivity to environmental protection and consumer protection, and later also food safety and public health matters. The Committee was the driving force in setting up the Committee of Inquiry on the handling of mad cow disease in the Commission at the end of the 1990s — and the subsequent reorganization of the Commission. As already outlined, the European Parliament, once it had acquired more power, was mostly an immense supporter and promoter of health actions at the European level — be it through financial programs, public health, food safety or pharma-related legislation.

Council

At the Council level, health questions as well as health and safety at work are dealt with by the Employment, Social Policy, Health and Consumer Affairs Council (EPSCO), whereas food safety, veterinary and phytosanitary questions are being negotiated in the Agriculture and Fisheries Council. Unlike the developments in the Commission and the European Parliament, this Council setting remained largely unchanged over time.[31]

Relations with Stakeholders

In the framework of its transparency initiative since the mid-1990s, the Commission makes its stakeholder relations more transparent: before submitting legislative proposals, it consults widely so that stakeholders' views can be taken into account. Stakeholders are defined broadly and include industry, non-governmental organizations, civil society, citizens, etc. — everybody who wants to play an active role in European policy-making. They are also systematically consulted on impact assessments that the Commission produces with any given proposal. Such impact assessments evaluate the potential economic, social and environmental impact of a proposed act. In addition, the Commission uses public consultations to solicit input on its proposals.

A number of supplementary groups and structures enable citizens, interest groups and organizations to play an active part in EU activities in the field of health: the EU Health Forum is a means of informing and involving key health stakeholders in European health policy.

It disseminates information, launches ideas for debate and contributes to policy-building. It has two components: the EU Health Policy Forum,[32] which brings together 52 non-governmental umbrella organizations and advises the Commission (and EU countries, if appropriate) on health matters, and the Open Forum. The Open Forum[33] extends the work of the EU Health Policy Forum to a broader set of stakeholders in an annual flagship event. The idea is to provide a platform for networking and exchanging ideas, particularly for groups and organizations which are not normally part of the "EU circuit".

In specific health policy fields, action platforms or pacts are in operation so as to make actors work together in a multisectoral approach. Examples are the EU Platform for Action on Diet, Physical Activity and Health,[s] the EU Alcohol and Health Forum[t] and the European Pact for Mental Health and Wellbeing.[34]

In addition, a Global Health Policy Forum was set up in October 2010, right after the EU conference "Global Health — Together We Can Make It Happen" in June 2010, to solicit input from stakeholders on selected global health topics.[35] A set of five Global Health Policy Fora was set up for 2014.[36] Also, a Stakeholder Dialogue Group advises the Directorate-General for Health and Food Safety on good practice in the consultation process, not on policy content.[37]

Overall, the Commission has a well-established, clear and transparent policy on involving stakeholders in policy and legislative proposal development and listens carefully to the input given. It also has a substantial access to documents policy, which further strengthens transparency. In addition, it works in a multisectoral way with different stakeholders in platforms of action.

---

[s]The EU Platform for Action on Diet, Physical Activity and Health is a forum for European-level organizations, ranging from the food industry to consumer protection NGOs, willing to commit to tackling current trends in diet and physical activity. More information can be found at http://ec.europa.eu/health/nutrition_physical_activity/platform/index_en.htm.

[t]The EU Alcohol and Health Forum is a platform where bodies active at European level can debate, compare approaches and act to tackle alcohol-related harm. To become members, organizations must meet certain requirements and make one or more specific commitments for action. More information can be found at http://ec.europa.eu/health/alcohol/forum/index_en.htm.

External Action and International Cooperation in Health

Contrary to the gradual development of a European health policy internally for the EU, its development policy has always contained an important health component. This is all the more important as the EU and its Member States are the world's largest donor of official development assistance.

Today the EU vividly promotes health system strengthening and steps toward universal coverage and the right to health in its development policy.[38] Also, in the orientation of EU development policy that the Commission proposed in October 2011 in its "agenda for change,"[39] social protection, health and education are stressed as important areas of EU action within the area of inclusive and sustainable growth for human development. The Commission suggests continued support for social inclusion and human development through at least 20% of EU aid. The EU should support a healthy and educated population, sector reforms that increase access to quality health and education services, and develop and strengthen health systems, reduce inequalitites in health services, promote policy coherence and increase protection against global health threats so as to improve health outcomes for all. It should also support a decent work agenda and social protection schemes and floors.

For a long time, the EU's internal and external health policies were not linked with each other. It was only the EU health strategy adopted in 2007[40] and later the Communication and Council conclusions on the EU role in global health (see separate chapter) that tried to establish such a link for the first time: "In our globalized world it is hard to separate national or EU-wide actions from global policy, as global health issues have an impact on internal Community health policy and vice versa. The EC can contribute to global health by sharing its values, experience and expertise, as well as by taking concrete steps to improve health. Work can support efforts to ensure coherence between its internal and external health policies in attaining global health goals, to consider health as an important element in the fight against poverty through health-related aspects of external development cooperation with low income countries, to respond to health threats in third countries, and to encourage implementation of international health agreements such as the World Health

Organisation's (WHO) Framework Convention on Tobacco Control (FCTC) and International Health Regulations (IHR). The EU's contribution to global health requires interaction of policy areas such as health, development cooperation, external action, research and trade. Strengthened coordination on health issues with international organizations, such as WHO and other relevant United Nations agencies, World Bank, International Labour Organisation, OECD and Council of Europe, as well as other strategic partners and countries, will also enhance the EU's voice in global health and increase its influence and visibility to match its economic and political weight."[41]

The key international organization for setting standards in global health at the UN is still the World Health Organization. As early as 1972, the then European Community sought close cooperation with the WHO. This was done by exchanges of letters between the Commission and the WHO,[u] the last and most recent one being between the former Director-General of WHO, Gro Harlem Brundtland, and the then Health and Consumer Commissioner, David Byrne, dating from 2001. In 2010, a formal partnership was established between WHO EURO and the Commission to consolidate the considerable existing collaboration between the two institutions from a project-based approach to a more strategic approach, encapsulated in the jointly developed "shared vision for joint action."[42] High-level meetings and meetings of Senior Officials take place on a yearly basis.

The European Community — which was converted into the European Union by the Treaty of Lisbon — has the status of an observer, not a full member in the governing bodies of WHO, as WHO is made up of states. One notable exception is the WHO Framework Convention on Tobacco Control, to which it is a full party. It is a member of the International Health Partnership IHP+, administered by WHO and the World Bank, to

---

[u]1972: Exchange of letters between the European Commission and the Regional Committee for Europe of WHO. 1982: Exchange of letters between Commissioner Richards and WHO Director-General Mahler. 1992: Joint Statement of Intent between Mr. Prat, Director-General of DG I of the European Commission, and Mr. Adelmoumène, Deptuy Director-General of WHO. 2001: Exchange of letters between Ms. Brundtland, Director-General of WHO, and Health Commissioner Byrne, *Official Journal, Series C.* 4.1.2001, C1/7-1/11, http://eur-lex.europa.eu/LexUriServ/LexUriServ.do?uri=OJ:C:2001: 001:0007:0011:EN:PDF (last accessed 15 August 2010).

accelerate progress toward achievement of the MDGs. The EU is increasingly invited to participate in intergovernmental processes of WHO and in the work of WHO under the title of "regional economic integration organization."[v]

The EU is an important voluntary contributor to the WHO budget: in 2010/11, the European Commission alone ranked fifth on the list of the most important voluntary non-state contributors to the WHO budget. The 27 EU Member States together with the European Commission contributed, at US\$1,031,758,811, nearly 27% of the total WHO budget.[w] These contributions come from different budgets in Member States and the EU, often from development budgets.

The Commission is a full member of the FAO/WHO Codex Alimentarius, which recommends food safety standards. It speaks for the EU in the Committee on Sanitary and Phytosanitary Affairs in the World Trade Organization, which deals with food safety and animal and plant health regulations.

Just like the health strategy, the health and safety at work strategy contains a priority on promoting health and safety at international level: the EU is therefore also an observer to the International Labour Organization. There it works to promote high international labor standards on occupational health and safety.

Outside the UN, the Commission is an important funder and board member of the Global Fund to Fight Aids, Tuberculosis and Malaria and

---

[v]For a more in-depth discussion on the status of the EU in UN institutions and especially WHO, see: Eggers B, Hoffmeister F. (2006) UN–EU cooperation on publich health: the evolving participation of the European Community in the World Health Organization. In: Wouters J, *et al.* (eds.), *The United Nations and the European Union.* The Hague, pp. 155–168.

[w]Own calculations based on two WHO documents:

A65/29 Add.1, 5 April 2012, on "Voluntary contributions by fund and by donor for the financial period 2010–2011"; http://apps.who.int/gb/ebwha/pdf_files/WHA65/A65_29Add1-en.pdf.

A65/30, 5 April 2011, on "Status of collection of assessed contributions, including Member States in arrears in the payment of their contributions to an extent that would justify invoking Article 7 of the Constitution"; http://apps.who.int/gb/ebwha/pdf_files/WHA65/A65_30-en.pdf.

several other health initiatives. The Commission is a full member of the 2001 Global Health Security Initiative (GHSI) of G7 + Mexico, which is an international partnership to globally strengthen health preparedness and response to threats of biological, chemical, radio-nuclear terrorism and pandemic influenza.

As regards bilateral relations, the EU first and foremost promotes its health standards in the candidate and accession countries, as these are supposed to have the *acquis communautaire* in place once they join the EU. It also tries to promote the acquis in the countries of the European Neighborhood Policy. The EU has political cooperation agreements with many other non-EU countries. These agreements often include a clause on health, setting a mutually beneficial framework for cooperation on public health.

Some bilateral agreements are worth mentioning specifically: in 2009, specific health and food safety agreements were concluded with Russia and China. Regulatory dialogues with China, Russia and India exist on pharmaceuticals. A close collaboration with the US on different health-related matters (e.g. nanotechnology, e-health, regulatory cooperation with the US Food and Drug Administration, mutual recognition agreements on good manufacturing practices for pharmaceuticals, equivalence agreements on veterinary issues with the US, a task force on antimicrobial resistance exist as well). In 2011, an EU–US expert task force on global health was set up.[43] It will identify opportunities for joint work within the framework of the US Global Health Initiative and the EU's policy on global health, with prioritizing work on a core set of indicators to monitor greater gains in global health and strengthening health systems in partner countries in the developing world. In July 2013, the EU and the US started negotiations on a Transatlantic Trade and Investment Partnership (TTIP). This comprehensive trade agreement also contains health components, such as negotiations on SPS issues, pharmaceuticals, medical devices and cosmetics.[x] The Joint African Union–European Union Strategy and Second Action Plan 2011–2013 contains an important health and food safety component within the strategic priority of

---

[x]More on TTIP can be found at http://ec.europa.eu/trade/policy/in-focus/ttip/.

achievement of the Millennium Development Goals.[y] The European Commission also cooperates closely with the Commission of the African Union on health issues.[z] Health is an important component of EU development policy in ACP countries (Asian, Caribbean and Pacific states).

Health policy, both internal and external, should be founded on clear values. As we have seen, the Charter of Fundamental Rights gives every EU citizen the right to social security, the right of access to preventive health care and the right to benefit from medical treatment. Health care systems in the EU follow a value-based approach, with the overarching values of universality, access to good quality care, equity and solidarity. Externally, the EU promotes a human rights-based approach and the common agreed values of solidarity towards equitable and universal coverage of quality health services — and thus the strengthening of comprehensive health systems — as a basis for the EU policies in partner countries. "This support shall ensure that the main components of health systems — health workforce, access to medicines, infrastructure and logistics, financing and management — are effective enough to deliver universal coverage of basic quality care, through a holistic and rights-based approach."[aa] It is fair to say that the EU as a whole (for national

---

[y]For an overview of the EU–AU partnership: http://eeas.europa.eu/africa/continental/index_en.htm and http://www.au.int/en/partnerships/africa_eu and http://www.africa-eu-partnership.org/africa-eu-strategic-partnership.

For second action plan 2011–2013: http://www.africa-eu-partnership.org/sites/default/files/doc_jaes_action_plan_2011_13_en.pdf.

For key deliverables of second action plan 2011–2013: http://www.africa-eu-partnership.org/sites/default/files/27_07_12_key_deliverables_jaes_second_action_plan_v13_3.pdf. http://www.globalhealthguide.eu/?site=policies-and-funding&sub=development-coorperation-policies-and-health#the-africa-eu-strategic-partnership.

[z]African Union Commission / European Commission, 4th College-to-College Meeting — Joint Declaration (Addis Ababa, Ethiopia; 8 June 2010): "We will work http://europa.eu/rapid/press-release_MEMO-11-414_en.htm?locale=en together in the field of **health** on key challenges, including the access to essential medicines, sexual and reproductive health and rights, maternal and child health, social protection, and promote a comprehensive and integrated approach to all MDGs in the implementation of all requirements within the framework of the MDG Partnership." www.africa-union.org/.../EU.../College-to-...-.

[aa]Council conclusions on the EU role in global health, points 1–6.

and for EU competence) is delivering on its objectives and principles: Member States are providing healthcare and universal coverage to their citizens. Together with the European institutions, they are promoting these values and principles and the internal safety-related health-relevant legislation to the outside world.

In food safety and health and safety at work, something similar is happening: the EU tries to "export" its high standards to other countries. Better Training for Safer Food (BTSF) is an initiative to organize training in the areas of European food and feed law, plant and animal health and welfare regulations. In its development and trade policy, the EU, is committed to improving access to medicines for developing countries and has, ever since the problem was recognized, contributed to broadening access to essential medicines for developing countries and to striking a balance between the intellectual property rights of pharmaceutical companies and the need to ensure that medicines are available to poor countries based on the 2001 Doha Declaration on the WTO TRIPS agreement. In 2015, the EU even supported a permanent waiver for the least developed countries in relation to WTO rules on patents for pharmaceuticals and went further than other industrialized countries negotiators. The final outcome of the WTO negotiations was to extend the waiver for the next 17 year, thus ensuring cheaper medicines for the least developed countries.

The Lisbon Treaty has strengthened the role of the EU in external policies by setting up the new European External Action Service (EEAS) under the authority of the double-hatted High Representative for Foreign Affairs and Security Policy and Vice-President of the Commission. The High Representative has the power to coordinate the EU's external action and to represent the Union on common foreign and security policies in third countries and international organizations.[44] For the other policy areas, the Commission shall ensure the external representation of the Union.[45]

However, the full implementation of the Lisbon Treaty in external action has not yet been achieved and different interpretations of EU institutions and Member States persist. One important unresolved internal power struggle relates to the question of who is speaking for the EU — an EU actor (such as the EEAS/Commission) or the Member State holding the Presidency of the Council. Other issues address the national versus the EU competences. Such internal struggles lead to a self-induced diminishing of the influence of the EU on the world scene — independent of the question of any potential upgrading of the status of the EU in the different UN organizations.

On the latter, a first step in translating the Lisbon Treaty into direct action at UN level was resolution 65/275 of the UN General Assembly of 3 May 2011, which gives the EU the right to speak early in the debate.[46] Such a step is still missing in the health field — although it has to be noted that at the UN High Level Meeting on prevention and control of non-communicable diseases in September 2011, the EU position was expressed by the Commission. Also, the EU is increasingly speaking with a common voice in WHO.

Outlook

Overall, EU health policy has developed gradually over time. Bound by the Treaty, important health-related legislation developed on the basis of other than health articles. Internal and external policies were established rather independently from each other. Therefore, today, the EU health policy is still patchy.

Important efforts have been made in recent years to make EU health policies more consistent internally, as well as to better link the internal and external health policies. Although some policy inconsistencies were already removed — for example, the EU no longer subsidizes tobacco production while at the same time fighting tobacco consumption, which is a considerable achievement as regards policy coherence — other issues, such as health and trade or health and migration, need to be further worked on. Global health, which appeared as a concept on the EU agenda only in 2008, might contribute to achieving further policy coherence.

With increasing internal competences in health the EU was able to raise its external profile and today it speaks with a common voice on many health-related issues in WHO, in the Codex Alimentarius and in ILO. The implementation of the Lisbon Treaty is expected to strengthen this common voice.

The EU already spoke for a long time with one voice in WTO, of which the SPS Committee is the most relevant health-related component. There the EU is especially strong as it operates on the basis of extensive EU law and competence"[47] — and is the world's most important exporter and importer of foodstuffs. This strength of the EU in regulating markets already drove some researchers to see the EU as a global regulatory power.[48]

Over time, one could see that it always needed a crisis to push the EU health agenda: the BSE crisis, the dioxin crisis, the French blood scandal, 9/11, and now perhaps the financial and economic crisis. So far, the answer has always been more EU rather than less EU. If this trend continues, it will automatically strengthen the role of the EU also as a global health actor.

The EU and its Member States form the largest trading bloc in the world. Together they are also the world's largest donor of official development assistance. Therefore, their voice also matters in global health — financially, politically and economically.

References

1. European Commission. (2003) How the European Union Works. A Citizen's Guide to the EU Institutions. Office for Official Publications of the European Communities, Luxembourg, p. 5.
2. European Commission. (2008) The EU veterinarian — animal health, welfare and veterinary public health developments in Europe since 1957. Office for Official Publications of the European Communities, Luxembourg. In: Pisanello D. (2010) *EU Food Law: An introduction*. Available at http://foodlaw.ideasoneurope.eu/law-justice (accessed 15 August 2010).
3. European Union. (2007) Charter of Fundamental Rights of the European Union. *Official Journal C* 303/01, http://eur-lex.europa.eu/LexUriServ/LexUriServ.do?uri=OJ:C:2007:303:0001:0016:EN:PDF (last accessed 20 August 2010).
4. http://ec.europa.eu/europe2020/making-it-happen/index_en.htm; http://europa.eu/rapid/press-release_MEMO-11-14_en.htm.
5. http://www.consilium.europa.eu/uedocs/cms_data/docs/pressdata/en/lsa/140004.pdf.
6. European Commission. (2012) Commission Decision of 5 July 2012 on setting up a multisectoral and independent expert panel to provide advice on effective ways of investing in health. *Official Journal C* **198(06).**

7. European Commission. (2000) White Paper on Food Safety. COM (2000) 719 final. Available at http://eur-lex.europa.eu/LexUriServ/LexUriServ. do?uri=COM:1999:0719:FIN:EN:PDF (accessed 20 August 2010).
8. European Commission. (2007) White Paper Together for Health: a strategic approach for the EU 2008–2013. COM (2007) 630 final. Available at http:// eurlex.europa.eu/LexUriServ/LexUriServ.do?uri=COM:2007:0630:FIN:EN: PDF (accessed 20 August 2010).
9. European Commission. (2007) Communication from the Commission to the Council, the European Parliament, the European Economic and Social Committee and the Committee of the Regions, on a new animal health strategy for the European Union (2007–2013) where "prevention is better than cure." COM (2007) 539 final. Available at http://ec.europa. eu/food/animal/diseases/strategy/animal_health_strategy_en.pdf (accessed 20 August 2010).
10. http://europa.eu/rapid/press-release_IP-13-400_en.htm.
11. Same source as for the previous footnote.
12. European Commission. (2007) Communication from the Commission to the European Parliament, the Council, the European Economic and Social Committee and the Committee of the Regions — improving quality and productivity at work: community strategy 2007–2012 on health and safety at work.COM (2007) 62 final.
13. http://www.consilium.europa.eu/ueDocs/cms_Data/docs/pressData/en/ lsa/91929.pdf.
14. European Council. (2010) Council conclusions on the EU role in global health. 3011th Foreign Affairs Council meeting, 10 May 2010. Council of the European Union, Brussels.
15. http://www.developmentportal.eu/wcm/information/guide-on-eu-development- co-operation/eu-policies-on-international-development-assistance/policy- for-thematic-development-assistance/eus-external-policies-for-health. html.
16. http://www.developmentportal.eu/wcm/information/guide-on-eu-development- co-operation/eu-policies-on-international-development-assistance/policy- for-thematic-development-assistance/eus-external-policies-for-health. html.
17. Commission Communication and a Council Resolution on "Health and Poverty" COM (2002) 129.
18. COM (2006) 870 final.

19. http://ec.europa.eu/health-eu/doc/working_doc_strategy.pdf.
20. European Commission. (2013) A decent life for all: ending poverty and giving the world a sustainable future. COM (2013) 92 final.
21. See Communication cited under footnote 25, p. 15.
22. http://eur-lex.europa.eu/LexUriServ/LexUriServ.do?uri=OJ:L:2002:271:0001:0011:EN:PDF.
23. http://eur-lex.europa.eu/LexUriServ/LexUriServ.do?uri=OJ:L:2007:301:0003:0013:EN:PDF.
24. http://ec.europa.eu/health/programme/docs/prop_prog2014_en.pdf.
25. http://eur-lex.europa.eu/legal-content/EN/TXT/;jsessionid=5Qj3TvyCyBqb hfLZzzBttjDGh3gyXkQWYrjhrt36mChMJJlp02XX!2060916514?uri=uri serv:OJ.L_.2014.086.01.0001.01.ENG.
26. http://www.ema.europa.eu.
27. http://www.cpvo.europa.eu/documents/brochures/Brochure_EN.pdf and http://www.cpvo.europa.eu/main/en/home/about-the-cpvo/its-mission.
28. http://www.efsa.europa.eu.
29. http://ecdc.europa.eu.
30. Sources: Official homepage: http://www.europarl.europa.eu/committees/de/ENVI/home.html. Official homepage until 2007: http://www.europarl.europa.eu/comparl/envi/default_en.htm; http://de.wikipedia.org/wiki/Ausschuss_f%C3%BCr_Umweltfragen,_Volksgesundheit_und_Lebensmittelsicherheit; http://en.wikipedia.org/wiki/Committee_on_the_Environment,_Public_Health_and_Food_Safety.
31. http://www.consilium.europa.eu/policies/council-configurations/employment,-social-policy,-health-and-consumer-affairs?lang=en
32. http://ec.europa.eu/health/interest_groups/eu_health_forum/policy_forum/index_en.htm.
33. http://ec.europa.eu/health/interest_groups/eu_health_forum/open_forum/index_en.htm.
34. http://ec.europa.eu/health/mental_health/docs/mhpact_en.pdf.
35. http://ec.europa.eu/health/eu_world/events/index_en.htm#anchor0_more.
36. http://ec.europa.eu/health/eu_world/global_health/events_2014_en.htm.
37. http://ec.europa.eu/health/interest_groups/stakeholder_dialogue_group/index_en.htm.
38. For more information, see http://ec.europa.eu/europeaid/what/health/index_en.htm.

39. European Commission. (2011) Increasing the impact of EU development policy: an agenda for change. COM (2011) 637 final.
40. Cf. footnote 10 (Health Strategy).
41. http://ec.europa.eu/health-eu/doc/whitepaper_en.pdf, p. 6.
42. http://www.euro.who.int/__data/assets/pdf_file/0008/119537/RC60_edoc12. pdf, p. 29–33.
43. http://www.devex.com/en/news/us-eu-to-boost-cooperation-on-health-aid/75093?source=ArticleHomepage_Headline; http://europa.eu/rapid/press-release_MEMO-11-414_en.htm?locale=en.
44. Article 221 of the Treaty on the Functioning of the European Union. http://eur-lex.europa.eu/JOHtml.do?uri=OJ:C:2010:083:SOM:EN:HTML
45. Article 17 of the Treaty on the European Union.
46. http://daccess-dds-ny.un.org/doc/UNDOC/GEN/N10/529/10/PDF/N1052910.pdf?OpenElement; http://www.consilium.europa.eu/uedocs/cms_data/docs/pressdata/EN/foraff/124604.pdf.
47. Gree SL, Hervey TK, Mackenback JP, McKee M. (2013) Health law and policy in the European Union. *The Lancet* **381(9872):** 1135–1144.
48. Bradford A. (2003) The global rise of a regulatory superstate in Europe. *The Globalist*, 14 January 2013. Available at http://www.theglobalist.com/storyid.aspx?storyid=9871.

3

Why and How Did the EU Set a Policy in Global Health?

Canice Nolan* and Juan Garay**

The Commission adopted a Communication on the "EU Role in Global Health" on 31 March 2010. It was accompanied by three Commission staff working papers focusing on specific areas of that Communication. Shortly thereafter, the Council, in response, adopted Conclusions on Global Health. This chapter outlines the genesis of those documents, summarizes and compares their contents, and describes how the Commission and the EU more largely implements it.

The Context

Emmerling and Rys, in Chapter 2, describe how EU internal competence and action in the area of health have evolved over the last few decades. This mirrored the growing role and presence of the EU in the area of development cooperation — itself with a very important health component — and a growing recognition of the multisectoral nature of determinants of health and the need for a health-in-all-policies approach to health promotion and healthcare. Demographic and economic trends, and the

* Senior Coordinator for Global Health, DG Health and Food Safety, European Commission, Brussels, Belgium.
** Head of Cooperation Section, Delegation of the European Union in Mexico, Mexico.

acknowledgment that the increasing cost of chronic diseases to society was not a unique western problem, all contributed during the previous decade to a rethinking of the sustainability of health systems and of the role of the EU in global health. The Commission Communication of 2010 marked the end of a reflection, consultation and consolidation process and resulted in a new way of working together to address a "new" problem.

During the previous decade, SARS and H1N1, echoing previous experiences with HIV/AIDS, had sounded global alerts on global vulnerabilities. They showed how interconnected and interdependent hitherto independent countries were, with the expansion of migration and trade, *vis-à-vis* new global health risks and they showed the need for countries to accept new, globally-shared responsibilities. The contribution of the European Commission, alongside France, Germany, Italy and the United Kingdom, to the G7+ Global Health Security Initiative (see Chapter 6, by Takki) was one manifestation of the EU commitment to addressing these risks and embracing these responsibilities, but it left open questions as to how the global community — beyond the G7+ — could address them. SARS and H1N1 gave impetus to, and resulted in the 2005 revision of the International Health Regulations, which incorporated the approach of global responsibility in the prediction of, detection of and response to emergent and re-emergent health threats. It is noteworthy that even though the costs to the global economy of SARS and H1N1 were breathtaking, the driver of the response was the need to protect health rather than the economy.

Against this backdrop, the European Union itself underwent political, demographic and economic change. It expanded from 15 to 27 Member States and developed substantial geographic and thematic policies going beyond its older, trade-based origins. The adhesion of such a substantial number of Central and Eastern European countries brought to light the scale of health inequalities within and between EU Member States. With the potential addition of more candidate and potential candidate countries, tackling these became a priority and an EU policy was developed in 2009.

In parallel, the EU Health Strategy (2007–2013) identified, as one of its four objectives, the international dimension of health and the need to increase the EU role in it. Collectively, the EU and its Member States are the largest provider of development aid, but it was recognized that due to a lack of policy coordination and a clear strategy, the EU voice in global health debates was not commensurate with the level of financial and technical assistance it was contributing.

Meanwhile, EU external action in health was being challenged at global level by a development aid architecture which had focused on some specific diseases and on specific global initiatives and programs centering on them — notably those related to Millennium Development Goal (MDG) 6, on HIV/AIDS, malaria and tuberculosis. It was becoming clear that vertical programs limited in scope (focusing only on selected diseases) and in time (through a project approach) were neither contributing to the achievement of the principle of universality in the right to health, nor strengthening health systems to the point where they could deliver integrated and patient-centered healthcare. A clear sign of this effect was the fact that despite a quadrupling of health development aid in the previous decade to more than €16 billion, the progress in the "litmus test" of health systems — MDG 4 (reducing maternal mortality) — showed signs of stagnation. The aid effectiveness agenda launched in 2005 in Paris and updated during subsequent high level meetings in Accra and more recently in Busan, showed that health development aid was the most fragmented of all the aid sectors and that it required profound reform. It led to the subsequent launch of the voluntary International Health Partnership, which aimed at reviving the Sector Wide Approach of the 1990s and which worked in concert with other voluntary new powerful emergent health initiatives post-MDGs, such as the Global Fund to Fight AIDS, Tuberculosis and Malaria, the Global Alliance on Vaccines Initiative, and the growing influence of private philanthropic initiatives such as those of the Bill and Melinda Gates Foundation.

Adding to the above, there was a recognition of the need to respond to some external criticism — and irrespective of whether it was justified or not — alleging that some EU internal and external policies were having net negative effects on health outside the EU. The five main areas criticized were trade, migration, foreign policy, climate change and food security policies. The most vocal criticisms concerned the impact of the brain drain of health professionals from developing countries and the negotiation of trade agreements which, it was said, could potentially limit access to and increase the price of essential medicines in developing countries. Although the Commission disputed these, it clearly had to address the issues.

It also became increasingly clear during the decade that there was a "bias" of health research and development programs in favor of addressing the health challenges of wealthier countries. Within the envelope of a fixed global R&D budget, it was recognized that this could work to the detriment of the needs of developing countries, which bear over 80% of the global burden of disease. During the decade, one of the longest and most complicated international dialogues in health, particularly in the governing bodies of the World Health Organization (WHO), was the one addressing innovation, intellectual property rights and public health. It pitted, not always justly, the interests of the North and the South against each other. Finally, still unresolved was the issue of the timely sharing of biological information (such as an emergent H7N9 or a coronavirus with pandemic potential) from less-prepared countries most at risk of emergent diseases, with countries that have the industrial capacity to develop tools against them but also the economic capacity to prioritize their use in their own favor. In other words, how to share the benefits equitably?

With all these elements brewing, the 30th anniversary of Alma-Ata brought back, in a World Health Assembly Resolution, critical elements toward universal coverage of health services with a rights-based approach which existent non-binding or non-measurable international rights/charters/covenants had not been able to advance or hold countries accountable for lack of progress.

Against this backdrop, it gradually became more clear that the weak governance of global health — internally and externally — by WHO was hampering the development of an organized and coherent global response to the global health challenges. In the same way that low income countries saw their health systems fragmented by the effect of the balkanized global health aid architecture, the WHO budget steadily increased but gradually became dominated by earmarked projects financed by voluntary contributions to tackle specific diseases or health risks. These targeted funds came mainly from private companies and foundations or from development agencies of richer countries. Perceptions were growing that the scale of earmarked funding was distracting efforts to address the democratically agreed priorities of the World Health Assembly through its resolutions.

The Process

All those elements led to the start of a period of analysis and dialogue within the Commission in 2008. The dialogue involved many Commission services, consulting with EU Member States, international organizations, partner countries and civil society. The Commission set up a Global Health Policy Forum open to all interested stakeholders, where it discussed openly the main areas of global health challenges (it still meets today). Three Commission services shared the leadership of the process, given their direct responsibilities in issues related to global health challenges: DG Development (DG DEVCO — development policies), DG Health and Consumers (DG SANCO — EU health and consumer policies) and DG Research (DG RTD — research). The Commission services also participated in many international meetings and events, discussing with a wide range of interlocutors the potential role of the EU in the new global health challenges. With other Commission services, they prepared an issues paper in 2009 and subjected it to open consultation, including on the Internet.

The discussions were revealing. They confirmed the universality of the recognition of the need to address the global health challenges but they also revealed that individuals defined the term "global health" differently, depending on their personal experiences, the sector where they worked and the agendas of their employers. The overall vision was shared but the details of the myriad ways to achieve it were not easy to agree upon. Also, several of those countries which have developed national global health policies and strategies reported that reaching agreement and coordinating across sectors was one of the most difficult barriers to successful implementation. In the EU case, these difficulties were compounded by the challenge of creating such a framework for the EU and its then 27 Member States.

In the end it was decided that not defining global health would be the most inclusive solution. It was recognized that global health is a multisectoral area that links not only the main policy areas of development, humanitarian assistance and R&D but also, for example, trade and foreign policy. It is about worldwide improvement of health, reduction of disparities and protection against health threats. It recognized that addressing it would require coherence at *all* levels of internal and external policy whilst acting on agreed guiding principles.

It recognized that global health begins at home and that the objectives and principles applied just as much inside the EU as they did outside. In this sense the Communication foreshadowed the current UN post-2015 development process, where the eventually agreed sustainable development goals will apply to all countries.

A more immediate challenge that the Commission services faced at the time was how to capture the richness of the discussions and the scope of the actions required in a policy document with the 2400-word limit imposed on all Commission Communications (indeed, the authors faced a similar challenge in writing this chapter and for this reason did not expand on the details of the Commission staff working documents listed below).

The end result was the Commission Communication submitted to the Council, the European Parliament, the Social and Economic Committee and the Committee of the Regions in March 2010. It was accompanied by three Commission staff working documents wherein the Commission services tried to capture the detail of the above consultations and lay out in more detail how the global challenges might best be addressed with the legislative, financial and cooperation tools available to them. The three staff working papers were entitled "Contributing to Universal Coverage of Health Services Through Development Cooperation," "Global Health: Responding to the Challenges of Globalization" and "European Research and Knowledge for Global Health."

The Council discussed the Commission Communication in its working group on development, with Member States bringing elements to the discussions from their health and their research colleagues in Member State ministries back home. This all took place while the EU was transforming itself under the Lisbon Treaty and creating a unified EU External Action Service. It was during the first Council meeting on foreign policy, chaired by Baroness Ashton on 10 May 2010, that the EU adopted the conclusions on the EU role in global health, endorsing the Commission Communication and expressing the collective views of the Member States on it.

The Commission Communication

The overarching objective of the Communication was to provide a policy framework that was ambitious whilst recognizing, accommodating and redirecting, where needed, the vast amount of work already underway across the various sectors of the Commission and the Member States to promote the health of peoples around the globe. It did not, in a policy document, propose new actions but it did highlight where existing actions could be better focused or coordinated. It tried to define guiding principles for future actions and presented a number of areas where existing actions could be implemented more effectively.

A key tenet throughout the discussions was that the EU approach should also be about promoting the core values of the EU — human dignity, freedom, democracy, equality, the rule of law and respect for human rights. It should help to combat social exclusion and discrimination. It should also promote social justice and protection, as well as work for gender equality and for solidarity between people and generations. The aim of the new policy framework was to be a turning point in promoting the right to health and better addressing global health challenges.

The Communication presented four main approaches to improving global health: establish more democratic and coordinated global governance; push for a collective effort to promote universal coverage and access to health services for all; ensure better coherence between EU policies relating to health; and improve coordination of EU research on global health and boost access in developing countries to new knowledge and treatments.

(i) *Enhance global governance on health.* Several topics were dealt with under this approach. Firstly, it was felt that the EU could be more effective if it acted as one at the UN, defending where possible a single position within UN agencies. It is notable that since the Communication was issued, the number of coordinated EU statements at the WHO governing body meetings has increased. Secondly, it was considered that stronger support should be given to promotion of the leading role of WHO as the leading international voice on global health. It was recognized, however, that WHO had work to do to earn this leading role — it was not to be taken for granted. On this aspect one can only commend the courage and leadership of WHO DG Margaret Chan in launching a comprehensive reform — still ongoing — of WHO to improve its governance, management and effectiveness. Finally, the Communication advocated a more inclusive approach to global health governance. As with the previous two points, this work is underway and a key challenge on this point will be how to manage conflicts of interest.

(ii) *Progress toward universal health coverage.* The Communication stated that the EU should ensure that its development aid supports developing countries in building sustainable health systems and should promote division of labor among all actors, public and private, bringing knowledge and funding to the health sector. In relation to fostering progress toward the achievement of the health-related MDGs, the Commission expressed its intention to propose a list of priority countries, mainly the ones most off-track from the health MDGs, where the EU should concentrate its development assistance. The Commission also stated its intention to apply aid effectiveness principles agreed at Busan.

(iii) *Ensure better coherence of EU internal and external policies in relation to global health.* The Communication stipulated that all internal and external policies should be developed and implemented coherently. It stated that the EU will combine its leading roles in trade and development to create a coherent approach to global health, including also issues such as migration, security, food security, education, water and sanitation, and climate change. Some examples are given below.

(a) It promoted the implementation of a code of practice on recruitment of health workforce personnel. The Global Code of Practice, adopted by the World Health Assembly in 2011, is the key to this. Since the adoption the Commission has adopted an action plan on health workforce recruitment and is currently funding a concerted action on this topic involving at least 25 EU Member States. It is disappointing that, globally, the EU seems to be so far ahead of the rest of the world in implementing the Global Code of Practice.

(b) The Communication highlighted the need for coherent responses to situations of fragility and to addressing global health threats. In the meantime, a new legislative health threats package, Decision 1082/2013 of 22 October 2013, published in the *Official Journal* on 5 November 2013, was agreed on. It will significantly enhance the capacity of the EU to respond to health threats. In addition, the intergovernmental agreement reached at WHO on pandemic influenza preparedness should facilitate rapid exchanges of pandemic-potential viruses whilst ensuring equitable sharing of the benefits arising therefrom.

(c) On trade, the Communication stated that trade agreements should not undermine access to medicines and that development assistance should help promote countries use of the provisions and flexibilities of the TRIPS agreement in relation to access to medicines. These issues are contentious and receive a lot of policy attention, perhaps at the expense of attention that needs to be devoted to other, possibly more important causes of shortages of medicines, e.g. weak regulatory systems, market failures or fragmented markets. The EU has recently adopted legislation on falsified medicines but there is also a need at global level to fight the proliferation of falsified/substandard/spurious/counterfeit medicines. The EU is frustrated that discussions at global level have not yet been translated into actions.

(iv) *Increase global health knowledge.* The overall objective being to ensure that research and innovation produce accessible and affordable products and services and that no diseases are neglected, the Communication proposed a series of guiding principles. There should be joint priority-setting and equitable partnerships. Global (indeed any!) normative action should be evidence-based. Information and communication technologies, including e-health, should be promoted to strengthen health information systems. The EU's Seventh Research Framework Programme (FP7) includes international cooperation toward achieving health-related MDGs as well as extensive research on diseases which can devastate developing countries. For example, in the first three years of FP7 (2007–2009) alone, the EU invested over €200 million in research projects on controlling and treating HIV/AIDS, malaria and tuberculosis. Discussions are currently underway on the next R&D program — Horizon2020, which foresees 6€ billion for health research.

As stated above, the Commission Communication was accompanied by three staff working documents (which were not restricted to a 2400-word limit). These expand on the concepts, thoughts and ideas of the Communication itself and should be read in conjunction with it. This chapter will not elaborate on the details of these documents — they merit separate chapters to themselves and are adequately covered by other contributors to this book.

The Council Conclusions

One of the functions of Council Conclusions on any topic is to convert the "should" of Commission Communications to "shall" and to get endorsement of the Commission's proposals and buy-in from Member States.

The Council Conclusions framed the future EU policy on global health across EU services, institutions and EU Member States. They reaffirmed that health is a human right and confirmed that is it essential for development — foreshadowing the conclusions of the Rio+20 conference of 2012 that health is a prerequisite for the attainment of sustainable development. They uphold the EU values of solidarity toward equitable access to quality health services. They address the challenges of global health governance, global health equity and global health coherence, including global health knowledge; of reducing inequalities and protecting against global health threats. They are based on the strength of the EU as the world's largest trading and development cooperation partner, and its social model based on the responsibility of states to guarantee their citizens' rights, including social rights and the right to health, as well as a system of universal health coverage. Strengthening the leading role of WHO and its mandate to WHO requires a shift in the share of core funding versus targeted support for specific health issues. They recognize that increasing global health equity requires more equitable, aligned and effective EU health development aid, toward health systems delivering universal coverage. They acknowledge that the challengeis to enhance the EU policy coherence in five critical areas — notably trade, migration, climate change, food security and humanitarian situations — and to improve global health and especially the capacities of lower income countries to face their health needs. The research agenda also requires greater emphasis on global health priorities and greater affordability of essential health tools for those in greatest need.

It has been stated that the Council Conclusions focus too much on development aspects of global health, at the expense of traditional health concerns. It must, however, be acknowledged that they are contained in 19 paragraphs and were produced within two months whereas the Commission allowed itself 18 months and 4 documents to present its ideas. In addition, the Council is not restricted to words. The actions of the Council since 2010 across its various sectors and configurations demonstrate amply that it is cognizant of the challenges posed by global health and the need for coherence in the actions in responding to those challenges.

Conclusion

In conclusion, the EU policy in global health set a milestone and a turning point in the way to address health challenges in the EU and beyond. It provided a lens through which existing EU action could be brought into the global health focus, as well as a set of guiding principles for future action. It has improved the continued coordination of policies within the Commission and it provides a backdrop to the current discussions on EU work on health for the 2014–2020 programming period, as well as guiding discussions on the overarching post-2015 agenda.

This book is about global health but one should never forget that in reality this is all about *people*. All countries and all sectors need to join efforts to confront the fact that some 20 million people die every year from global health inequity. This means one in three deaths in the world, and the proportion has not changed in the last 20 years. The world urgently needs a profound reform to roll back this chronic tragedy, and the EU has an important role to play in this quest.

4

Trade and Health: A Healthy Relationship? The Place of Trade Policy in the EU's Global Health Agenda

Tomas Baert[*][a]

Trade policy has not escaped the greater prominence which health policy has gained in international affairs. A recent example is the interest that legislation on plain packaging of tobacco products has garnered in the context of the World Trade Organization (WTO).[b] Similarly, health policy did not stay immune to the new frontiers that trade policy acquired in the current age of globalization. Trade policies of today are said to reach "behind the border," where they touch, for example, on the intellectual property protection of pharmaceutical inventions, the procurement of medical products at large or trade in health services. So, as both trade and health policies have cast their nets wider, the interactions between them have effectively increased. This has sparked considerable debate on the mutual supportiveness and coherence of the two policy domains.

[*]Assistant to the Director-General, European Commission for Trade, Brussels, Belgium.
[a]Disclaimer: The views and opinions expressed herein are those of the author and do not necessarily reflect the views of the European Commission.
[b]On 13 March 2012, Ukraine requested consultations in the WTO regarding Australia's legislation that imposes trademark restrictions on tobacco products and packaging. The consultations have attracted the largest number of third parties in the history of WTO dispute settlement. Other WTO Members, such as the Dominican Republic, Honduras and Cuba, have equally requested consultations with Australia.

Against the background of that broader debate, this chapter considers the ways in which the EU has sought to address the health and trade nexus. Specifically, the chapter looks at whether and how the EU has oriented its trade policy to support the Union's global health agenda. An area of exclusive competence, the EU common commercial policy, as it is labeled by the Treaty on the Functioning of the European Union, is an area where the EU speaks with a single voice and leverages a vast, single market. The clear, comprehensive competence in external economic relations contrasts with the EU's role and powers in other spheres of external relations, including that of global health diplomacy. Moreover, the exercise of trade competence by the EU often results in binding and enforceable commitments under international law. Hence, if one considers the EU's performance in international affairs as a vector of the EU's legal competence, trade policy merits due consideration for its potential in advancing or at least supporting policy priorities like global health.

This chapter starts by considering the trade policy components of the EU's global health agenda as elaborated in the European Commission Communication "The EU Role in Global Health" and the May 2010 conclusions of the Council of the European Union which followed it. The first section observes how the EU's trade policy which underpins the global health agenda is essentially made up of one component of health systems, i.e. access to medicines. In this regard, intellectual property law and policy appears the main lens through which the EU has defined and viewed this challenge in the Communication. It will be explained that the EU's focus on access to medicines and on the role of intellectual property protection therein are to be seen in relation to the broader political impetus that emerged at the multilateral level on access to medicines, notably with the adoption of the Doha Declaration on the Agreement on Trade-Related Aspects of Intellectual Property Rights (TRIPS) and Public Health in the context of the World Trade Organization. The EU's bilateral trade agenda and the fear of "TRIPS-plus" provisions in free trade agreements have further added to the debate on access to medicines and the role of IPR in that context.

The second section of this chapter will elaborate on the answers the EU has provided through its trade policy to the availability and affordability of medicines. Three levels of activity are distinguished:

(1) multilateral actions, which follow commitments undertaken in the context of international regimes; (2) bilateral work in relation to specific third countries, notably in the context of free trade agreement negotiations; (3) unilateral measures which do not respond to (hard or soft) commitments made under international law.

In conclusion, this chapter will observe that while the EU has taken several initiatives in relation to access to medicines, there is more scope for plugging trade policy into the EU's global health strategy and for considering more holistically what positive contributions trade and trade policy could make to EU global health diplomacy. Indeed, the response of the EU trade policy to health has been shaped by trade politics more than by global health policies. The impact of the latter on the former is still to materialize.

The Place of Trade Policy in the EU Global Health Strategy

With a relationship that is as convoluted as it is controversial, trade and health policies offer significant scope for conflict as well as cooperation.[1] It is thus not surprising that the European Commission identified trade policy as the first of five external policies whose contribution to a global health agenda should be considered.[2] The 2010 Commission Communication on "The EU Role in Global Health" submits that, on trade:

> … the EU should work to ensure more effective use of TRIPS provisions to increase the affordability and *access to essential medicines*. The EU should support the priority actions identified in the Global Strategy and Plan of Action on Public Health, Innovation and Intellectual Property. This should address the challenges expected after 2016 when the TRIPS framework enters into force in least developed countries. The EU should continue to ensure that EU bilateral trade agreements avoid clauses which may undermine access to medicines. Generic competition and rational use of medicines are of major importance to ensure the sustainability of healthcare systems. The EU should also work at global and regional level to eliminate trade in falsified medicines e.g. through the International Medical Products

Anti-Counterfeiting Taskforce. The EU should also address further the problem of illicit drugs and its effects on health and consider the crucial role of demand reduction. The EU should also continue advocating for a better global governance of health-relevant environmental agreements.[3]

The staff working paper that accompanied the Communication added that trade policies:

... influence the economies of the EU and third countries and have a direct effect in the access to medicines, subject to global markets and patent rights, which may hinder access to affordable medicines in poor countries. TRIPS provisions theoretically enable exemptions to patent monopolies but these have not been used in an effective manner and have been further challenged by the enforcement of TRIPS in middle income countries (and major generic producers such as India) and will be further tested by the compliance of least developed countries in 2016. In addition, EU bilateral trade agreements need to ensure and facilitate the use of TRIPS provisions and assess the effects of liberalization of health services (GATS), to ensure coherence towards the principle of solidarity towards equitable and universal access to health services.[4]

Welcoming the Communication, the conclusions of the Council of the European Union of 10 May 2010 further note that:

The EU should support third countries, in particular LDCs, in the effective implementation of flexibilities for the protection of public health provided for in TRIPS agreements, in order to promote access to medicines for all, and ensure that EU bilateral trade agreements are fully supportive of this objective.[5]

Unlike the global health policy frames of third countries, which purport that an open global trading system broadly supports global health security,[6] the Commission Communication does not address the trade and health nexus in a general, horizontal manner. Rather, the Communication focuses strongly on essentially one of the components of stronger health systems, i.e. the question of access to medicines. Moreover, it does so by framing the question of the availability and affordability of essential medicines almost exclusively through the prism of intellectual property law, in particular the WTO Agreement on Trade-Related Intellectual Property Rights (TRIPS). The Communication calls both for the use of TRIPS provisions and for a response to challenges that may arise when the TRIPS minimum standard of treatment is applied to the least developed countries (LDCs). Furthermore, bilateral trade agreements, whose IP protection standards are typically based on the TRIPS Agreement, which sets a minimum standard of IP protection, are specifically identified for their possible restrictive impact on access to medicines. The Council conclusions further sharpened the focus on these specific questions.

Access to Medicines and Intellectual Property Rights

The preponderance of the references to the TRIPS Agreement and IPR law and policy in the EU's global health agenda is noteworthy. First of all, this focus implies that the breadth of the trade and health nexus is narrowed down to essentially one specific dimension, even though several trade rules are considered to relate to global health and health policies, including for example the WTO Agreements on Technical Barriers to Trade (TBT), Sanitary and Phytosanitary Measures (SPS), the General Agreement on Trade in Services (GATS) and the General Agreement on Tariffs and Trade (GATT), in addition to the TRIPS Agreement.[c] However, neither the Communication nor the staff working paper considers the health externalities of trade policy and trade liberalization in a broader, more general manner.

Second, the almost exclusive focus on the question of access to medicines is equally noteworthy, for it is a challenge that is increasingly considered by policy-makers and academics from other angles than IPR law and policy. The Communication does not, for example, touch on procurement, customs or tariff questions relating to access to medicines, which

---

[c]World Health Organization, World Trade Organization (2002), *WTO Agreements and Public Health: A Joint Study by the WHO and WTO Secretariat* (WTO, Geneva). For a study of tariffs on trade in health products, see Helbe M (2012), More trade for better health? International trade and tariffs on health products, *WTO staff working paper* (WTO, Geneva).

further highlights the centrality which the EU seemingly gives IPRs in this debate. In contrast, the US 2011 White Paper outlining the US Trade Representative's strategic initiative entitled "Trade Enhancing Access to Medicines (TEAM)" provides, for example, a broader trade policy response to the question, while also noting that trade policy alone cannot meet the challenges relating to access to medicines.[7] These notions are not explicitly part of the Commission's paper, however.

In addition, the EU's focus on IPR law and policy itself seems to be a partial one, to the extent that the Communication mostly considers the potentially restrictive impact of IPR law and policy on health policy. IPRs are intended to spur innovation, which should increase the availability of new medicines. However, the question of whether and how IPRs could reinforce or contribute to health objectives seems to receive little or no attention in the EU's policy statement. The view that IPRs can be an obstacle more than an opportunity seems to be what transpired also in the public consultation that preceded the publication of the Communication. In the context of the public consultation, the European Commission reported that "trade policies that enforce service liberalization and patent rights ... are said — among other problems — to reduce access to medicines" and "fewer voices however suggested that trade liberalization could potentially increase availability and access to medicines."[8] While the Commission detected no unanimity among stakeholders on the factors underpinning the "access gap" regarding medicines, health advocates from civil society and developing countries were said to often regard the question of IPR protection in relation to essential medicines as playing a crucial role if barriers to access are to be removed.[9]

While this is a view that the Communication has picked up, some further questions can be raised as to why access to essential medicines would be presented as essentially resulting from barriers posed by the TRIPS Agreement or from the use of flexibilities found in the Agreement. The Commission Communication refers to *essential* medicines, a term which received particular emphasis in the policy document, even though the reference to "essential" was omitted subsequently. While there is significant debate on which medicines are essential medicines, the term could be understood to refer to the World Health Organization's Model List of Essential Medicines (EML).[10] Currently in its 18th version after it was first presented in 1977, the EML contains 445 medicines and 358 molecules excluding duplicates,[11] and includes treatment options for malaria, HIV/AIDS, TB, reproductive health and non-communicable diseases (NCDs), such as cardiovascular disease, cancer, chronic respiratory disease and diabetes, based on the best available evidence.

In pioneering work published in 2004, Amir Attaran highlighted that only 17 of the 319 items on the 13th EML could theoretically be patented in developing countries, as these are the only items that have patents in developing countries that postdate 1 April 1982. Moreover, developing countries have in practice fewer essential medicines under patent or pending application than these 17, Attaran observed. Patent incidence is low and concentrated in larger markets, which Attaran saw as being linked to the fact that pharmaceutical companies decide to forgo patent protection in countries where little revenue is at stake. In this sense, patents could arguably not be a determinant of access to essential medicines when patents do not even exist 98.6% of the time. In studying the patent and exclusivity status of essential medicines for NCDs, Mackey and Lang (2012) confirmed these findings and observed that little has changed since Attaran's work was published in 2004. The authors concluded, *inter alia*, that a critical assessment is needed of non-IPR factors that may impede the affordability and accessibility of medicines.

So, while it is legitimate to consider the impact of the TRIPS Agreement on the availability and affordability of medicines at large, it is not evident to consider the agreement as the key obstacle to access to *essential* medicines. This is not to suggest that the impact of patents on essential medicines, even if only limited as a matter of principle, is not worth the EU's consideration. However, the prominence of these questions in the EU's global health agenda, at the cost of other trade rules or policies, remains striking in the face of these observations. This is perhaps even more so given that a Commission Communication from 2000 already observed that "affordability of key pharmaceuticals can only be increased and accelerated through a comprehensive synergistic approach" since "almost 90% of the products on WHO's 'essential drug list' are not patented and therefore are subject to generic competitive tendering and local production."[12]

If we are to better understand the EU trade policy tools and instruments in this area, we should consider the reasons for the prominence of an IP and access to medicines in the EU's strategy. The answer lies largely in the broader political context in which the Communication was developed, as well as in the activism of civil society and health organizations that presented patent protection as an impediment to characterize that period in particular. The above-mentioned observations that the Commission made as part of the public consultation on the EU role in global health also underscore the latter argument.

The Political Trade Policy Context for the EU Global Health Strategy

The debate about access to medicines garnered media headlines in anticipation of the expiry of the 2005 transition period for developing countries to implement the TRIPS Agreement. From 2005 onward, WTO Members (like India) which have an important pharmaceutical industry became liable for TRIPS patent protection standards, pursuant to the end of the special transition arrangements found in Article 65.4 of the Agreement. In this regard, a specific fear was that compulsory licensing could be an ineffective means of overcoming the potential barriers that may arise from patents, as Article 31(f) of the Agreement limited the use of compulsory licensing to the predominant supply of the domestic market of the Member authorizing such use. This was seen as a hindrance for developing countries to effectively use compulsory licensing when they lacked a sufficient manufacturing capacity in the pharmaceutical sector.

In response to what many feared would become a watershed in effective access to medicines by developing countries, the Doha Declaration on the TRIPS Agreement and Public Health was adopted at the WTO's Fourth Ministerial Conference in November 2001 in Doha, Qatar. The Declaration addressed the relationship between the TRIPS Agreement and public health and sought to clarify the flexibilities found in the Agreement to respond to public health objectives. The Council for TRIPS was also instructed to find an expeditious solution to the specific problem of countries with insufficient or no manufacturing capacities in the pharmaceutical sector in making a effective use of compulsory licensing under the TRIPS Agreement.[13] The solution came in the form of a WTO

General Council Decision that waived under certain circumstances (i) the obligation of exporting Members to ensure that compulsory licenses are granted only for the purpose of predominantly supplying the domestic market [Article 31(f)] and (ii) the obligation of importing Members to pay adequate remuneration to the right-holder if a compulsory license is granted [Article 31(h)].[14] A permanent amendment to the TRIPS Agreement was reached on 6 December 2005, to replace the temporary waiver of 2003.[15]

This multilateral discussion took place in a context that generally saw the focus of multilateral decision-making turn from the creation of IPRs and their enforcement to the creation and interpretation of IPR flexibilities. Some developing countries, including the so-called emerging economies, arguably regretted the inclusion of IPRs in the WTO and they began to see IPRs as an obstacle to rather than an opportunity for their economic growth and development. This trend became particularly visible as developing countries sought to recalibrate or revise IP norms through other international regimes and forums, such as the Food and Agriculture Organization, the United Nations Commission on Human Rights, or, in the case of public health, the World Health Organization.[16] Like communicating vessels, this proliferation of IP talks in non-trade forums led to a broader stagnation in the negotiating agenda of TRIPS in the WTO, as reflected for example in the inability of the TRIPS Council to agree or advance work on IPR enforcement.[17] Moreover, the multilateral deadlock in the WTO/TRIPS context made way for other avenues in which IP norm-setting and IP enforcement were considered. As such, a "forum shift" occurred also away from the WTO to plurilateral and bilateral which became alternative routes to multilateral IP norm-setting.[18]

Against this background, EU free trade negotiations became, in effect, an avenue for IPR negotiations, particularly as the EU abandoned in the fall of 2006 its *de facto* moratorium to start new free trade negotiations. The European Commission's 2006 "Global Europe" Communication projected a new generation of free trade agreements (FTAs), in which stronger rules on IP protection and enforcement, among other things, would be a key factor contributing to growth and competitiveness in Europe.[19]

As part of this agenda, which in geographical terms put the focus firmly on Asia, India became an "obvious partner" to the EU for a comprehensive bilateral trade and investment agreement.

Ever since FTA negotiations between the EU and India started in June 2007, controversy has existed about the impact of such an agreement on access to medicines. With the TRIPS Agreement setting a minimum standard of treatment for the protection of patents and other IPRs, FTAs were seen as *de facto* ratcheting up the standard of protection set by TRIPS. In any event, it would not be possible to lower the standard below the multilateral agreement and its flexibilities. In this respect, so-called "TRIPS-plus" standards were thought to impose high(er) levels of patent protection, which could have a chilling effect on the ability of Indian generic manufacturers to produce life-saving medicines. A vocal and active NGO community brought such concerns to the attention of the European Commission, which negotiates trade agreements on behalf of the EU. So, as bilateral negotiations became an alternative to multilateral norm-setting in the area of IPRs, the debate on access to medicines shifted its focus from a multilateral to a bilateral context, especially the EU–India bilateral context.

This controversy heightened as, in 2008, the Dutch customs authorities detained in a number of cases generic medicines which were in transit between India and Brazil, based on suspected patent infringements. Both India and Brazil, as well as health NGOs, saw these developments as proof of a tendency in the EU to put "patents before patients." In May 2010, India requested consultations with the EU, pursuant to the WTO Dispute Settlement Understanding. The EU undertook to review Regulation 1383/2003[20] to further clarify, in the interest of legal certainty, that the transit of medicines should not be hampered in the absence of a substantial risk of diversion of the goods to the EU market.[21]

In sum, the public and political debate on access to medicines and the role of IPRs therein have raised the profile of these matters in the EU's trade policy to a point where the EU's global health agenda has picked these up and defined them as the EU's trade policy contribution to the latter strategy. The high profile of these questions implied that other trade policy questions had received comparatively little attention in the EU's health strategy. But, before weighing the EU's trade policy contribution, let us consider what that contribution is made up of.

The EU's Trade Policy Response to Improve Access to Medicines

Three different levels could broadly be distinguished in dissecting the EU's actions on access to medicines: a multilateral, a bilateral and a unilateral level. It is worth considering these in a top-down manner, as multilateral initiatives have often shaped actions taken at the bilateral level or unilaterally. While this section briefly introduces EU trade policy actions, it is to be borne in mind, as the concluding section will further highlight, that these policies and practices were the cause much more than the consequence of the EU's global health agenda. Essentially all these initiatives pre-date the EU's global health agenda, which led further to the observation that the latter could do more to provide fresh impetus to EU trade policy actions.

EU Policy in Respect of Patent-Related TRIPS Flexibilities

While the TRIPS Agreement contains a critical minimum standard of treatment for the protection of IPRs, it also incorporates important flexibilities that can be used to deviate from that standard, including specific patent-related flexibilities. Even though they are neither defined nor enumerated by the TRIPS Agreement itself, the "TRIPS flexibilities" were increasingly identified as such in the run-up and as part of the discussions on the Doha Declaration.[22] While a study of the flexibilities and their specific implementation by the EU, whether at the EU or the EU Member State level, would fall outside the scope of this chapter,[d] it is worth con-

---

[d]An overview of the implementation of patent-related flexibilities by the EU and its Member States can be found in: World Intellectual Property Organization (2010), Committee on Development and Intellectual Property (CDIP), patent-related flexibilities in the multilateral legal framework and their legislative implementation at the national and regional levels (World Intellectual Property Organization, Geneva).

sidering the specific legislative response given by the EU to the Doha Declaration on TRIPS and public health. Not only can one find in the latter a clear expression of the EU's political commitment to access and affordability of medicines, but it is also one of the more recent EU initiatives in respect of access to medicines that is moreover enshrined in a dedicated EU regulation in the area of patent law that was otherwise not harmonized by EU law.

The Doha Declaration itself did not require any specific legal enactment by WTO members. However, its paragraph 6 invited the TRIPS Council to find an expeditious solution to the problem faced by members with insufficient or no manufacturing capacities in the pharmaceutical sector and which could therefore face problems in making effective use of compulsory licensing under the TRIPS Agreement. A response to this mandate was formulated in the form of the above-mentioned decision from the WTO General Council on the implementation of paragraph 6 of the Doha Declaration in August 2003. Following its adoption, and with a view to effectively integrating this TRIPS amendment into the EU legal order, the European Commission formulated a proposal that would extend the concept of compulsory licensing so that EU pharmaceutical companies could apply for a license to manufacture, without the authorization of the patent-holder, pharmaceutical products for export to countries in need of medicines and facing public health problems.[23] Following a rather swift co-decision procedure between the Council of the European Union and the European Parliament, Regulation 816/2006, on compulsory licensing of patents relating to the manufacture of pharmaceutical products for export to countries with public health problems, was adopted on 17 May 2006.[24]

With Regulation 816/2006, which entered into force on 29 June 2006, the EU introduced a framework for compulsory licensing that drew mostly but not exclusively on the WTO General Council decision, with procedural and administrative requirements comparable to those that can be found in voluntary licenses. Compared to the WTO General Council decision, the EU regime was broadened to cover low-income developing countries that are not or not yet a member of the WTO. It also introduced a specific price formula for the calculation of the remuneration to right holders, while maintaining the flexibilities open to countries in making use of the system.[25]

However, since its entry into force in 2006, no export licenses have been applied for, and thus no such licenses have been granted to date under the EU system. In fact, few low-income countries (other than LDCs, which are exempted from this notification requirement) have notified their general intention to use the system. The lack of interest in what is a demand-driven system is noteworthy. While it is for individual eligible importing countries to notify the specific products and quantities they seek to import, it is equally notable that exporting companies, such as generic manufacturers, have not identified this as a business opportunity and highlighted this as such to importing country governments. This begs a number of questions about the value of the instrument, especially if one considers that the EU system is not the only paragraph 6 system that lacks practical experience. Only one special export license has been granted under a paragraph 6 system today.[e]

Some of the debate on these systems has emerged in the WTO, where the effectiveness and user-friendliness of paragraph 6 systems have been discussed as part of the annual review of the decision on the implementation of paragraph 6 of the Doha Declaration.[26] While no firm conclusions have been reached, one general and plausible hypothesis in this debate that has emerged from the discussions is that alternatives to the system exist and are effectively used, including the availability of generic alternatives to patented medicines. In fact, generic alternatives were equally available from Indian manufacturers in the only paragraph 6 case to date, i.e. the supply for the triple combination ARV which Rwanda procured from a Canadian company under Canada's paragraph 6 system.

It could be observed that the paragraph 6 mechanism can generally serve a purpose even without granting a compulsory license, in so far as the utility of compulsory licensing lies in the leverage it can provide in price negotiations with pharmaceutical companies. In other words, compulsory licenses, including in the particular procurement scenario reflected by paragraph 6 of the Doha Declaration, can deliver the expected results,

---

[e]In 2007, Rwanda notified the WTO of its intention to import a triple combination antiretroviral. Following the publication of a tender won by a Canadian company, an export license was granted by Canada under Canada's Access to Medicines Regime (CAMR), which implemented paragraph 6 of the Doha Declaration.

i.e. making medicines more affordable and accessible, without such licenses being actually granted.

In its Article 19, EU Regulation 816/2006 foresees every three years a report from the European Commission on the operation of this regulation, including any appropriate plans for amendments. In the absence of any licenses being requested or granted, this review has not taken place so far. Nevertheless, there would seem to be an opportunity, for example as part of the EU's action plan on global health, to review the non-use of the system and any changes to the system that may be needed. In this respect, it would be worth further analyzing the alternatives to the system that seemingly exist and that have surfaced in the WTO debate, so as to ascertain the reasons for the limited practical use of these systems in general.

Apart from incorporating TRIPS flexibilities into its own jurisdiction, the EU has promoted the use of these flexibilities by other WTO members. In the first place, LDCs have not been required to apply TRIPS (other than Articles 3–5) pursuant to article 66 of TRIPS. This constitutes arguably the most significant flexibility from TRIPS which one could envisage. The EU has supported this transition period found in Article 66.1 and the subsequent extensions thereof by the TRIPS Council. No extension of the transition period has so far been refused, in fact. On 27 June 2002, the WTO General Council decided that LDCs will not be obliged, with respect to pharmaceutical products, to implement or apply Sections 5 and 7 of Part II of the TRIPS Agreement or to enforce rights provided under these sections until 1 January 2016.[27] While an extension by eight years of the general timeframe for implementing TRIPS was agreed on 11 June 2013, this decision was, following the request from LDCs, kept separate from the specific timeframe that was agreed for pharmaceutical products in 2002.[28]

The use and implementation of these flexibilities are also backed by technical support and cooperation with developing countries. Even though the roots of these efforts may lie outside EU trade policy, these respond to the commitments which the EU has undertaken, for example in the context of TRIPS' Article 67, on technical cooperation, and Article 66.1, on technology transfer.[f] Specific initiatives on access to medicines include

---

[f]EU technical cooperation initiatives and programs (which are not limited to access to medicines) are reported pursuant to the WTO under the respective provisions (Articles 67

the cooperation with developing countries, particularly African countries, which follow the Council Conclusions on Innovation and Solidarity in Pharmaceuticals of December 2010.[29] Another specific example is the EC/ACP/WHO Partnership on Pharmaceutical Policies, which has committed funds to support African, Caribbean and Pacific Island (ACP) countries in the development and implementation of essential medicines strategies.

Bilateral Trade Negotiations

When the EU, like other major economies, embarked on an ambitious agenda of bilateral free trade negotiations, the debate about access to medicines largely shifted from the multilateral to the bilateral level. Multilaterally, important clarifications on access to medicines had been achieved with the Doha Declaration in 2001 and the subsequent work that led to the General Council decisions in 2003 and 2005. Bilateral free trade agreements (FTAs), which the EU started negotiating again from 2006, were thought to undo these efforts by topping up multilateral commitments with bilateral TRIPS-plus commitments, at a moment when developing countries had just seen the TRIPS transition period phase-out. Both the regional focus of the 2006 "Global Europe" trade agenda on Asia (including India), and the EU's overall approach to this new generation of agreements, notably for the pursuit of state-of-the-art rules that would address behind-the-border domestic regulations in areas such as IPRs, heightened concerns from health activists and others.

As TRIPS specifies a minimum standard of treatment, WTO members can in their bilateral trade agreements not usefully maintain a standard below TRIPS, unless its falls within the TRIPS flexibilities. Hence, members invariably look over and above the TRIPS Agreement to achieve the effective protection and enforcement of IPRs, including often in areas where the Agreement is considered to have "gaps," for example compared to its own national regime. For this reason, TRIPS-plus commitments do not automatically imply that new measures or legislation is to

---

and 66.1). An overview of programs and reports can also be found in the factsheet "EU Technical Assistance Programmes in the Field of Intellectual Property," made available by the European Commission at http://trade.ec.europa.eu/doclib/docs/2013/april/tradoc_150990.pdf (accessed on 8 August 2013).

be introduced in the home jurisdiction. Often, it is about establishing a level playing field, which is pursued by introducing abroad rules similar to those that already exist at home. In doing so, some form of "hegemonic harmonization" could emerge, as partner countries may adapt or align themselves to the dominant partner in a bilateral trading relationship.[30] Hence, an important research question is whether and to what extent smaller or less-developed partners are expected to increase their regulatory standards in the context of a bilateral trade negotiation. And, if this is the case in the area of patents, what will be the effect of such higher standards on access to medicines? As we further consider the EU approach taken in respect of access to medicines in its bilateral trade negotiations, it is worth noting that the Commission Communication on "The EU Role in Global Health" did not seem to identify any specific problems in this regard, even though the tension was clearly recognized. The Communication calls on the EU to "*continue to ensure* that EU bilateral trade agreements avoid clauses which may undermine access to medicines" (emphasis added).[31]

The EU is still in the process of concluding several FTA negotiations, including with India, and hence relatively few definite data points currently exist to consider the extent to which the EU "exports" high domestic legislative standards to its trading partners and the extent to which these could affect the affordability and accessibility of medicines. In 2007, two of the newer-generation agreements were concluded, one between the EU and Cariforum and the other with Korea, which form the basis for analyzing the approach taken on access to medicines in bilateral trade relations.[32,g]

In a sole provision on patents, the EU–Cariforum Economic and Partnership agreement enumerates existing international law standards on patent protection (Article 147). However, it does so in an asymmetrical manner, since the EU undertakes more commitments than the Cariforum states, which is arguably a reflection of the development needs and priorities of the Cariforum countries, which the IP chapter has specifically

---

[g]European Union. (2011) Free trade agreement between the European Union and its Member States, of the one part, and the Republic of Korea, of the other part. *Official Journal L* **127(6):** 6–1343.

highlighted (Articles 139.2 and 139.4). In this respect, it is worth noting that the EU refrained from specifying any patent standards that may exist in the law of the EU or the Member States, which would argue against the hypothesis that the EU uses its bilateral agreements to export its own regulatory model. In addition to the reference to international standards, the EU and the Cariforum states recall and recognize the importance of the Doha Declaration (Article 147.B) and the fact that nothing in the agreement can be construed as impairing the parties' capacity to promote access to medicines (Article 139.2), which should further support the view that the agreement should not negatively affect access to medicines through the introduction of TRIPS-plus standards.

In the case of the EU–Korea FTA, a similar approach is followed as regards the confirmation of the Doha Declaration, which is explicitly said to be the basis for interpreting and implementing the rights and obligations part of the patents subsection of the agreement (Article 10.34). Unlike the agreement with Cariforum, and reflecting the more advanced stage of development of Korea, the agreement does include specific commitments on patent term extension (Article 10.35), through which compensation can be offered to patent-holders for the delays they may incur to obtain marketing approval when the patent has already been granted. Moreover, the IP chapter contains provisions on data protection and data exclusivity (Article 10.36). The inclusion of these provisions, and the absence of similar provisions in the Cariforum agreement, suggest that the EU does not introduce more advanced standards of IP protection in what could be considered an asymmetrical rather than a symmetrical relationship, contrary to what one could expect under the notion of hegemonic harmonization. In this regard, it is noteworthy that, while negotiations are still ongoing, the European Commission has publicly confirmed that an FTA with India will not introduce any kind of data exclusivity provisions and that the FTA would not require India to introduce any kind of patent term extension provision.[33]

In sum, the EU has chosen bilateral trade negotiations as an avenue to promote the full use of TRIPS flexibilities, more than as a forum for introducing TRIPS-plus standards to developing members, which could be considered as potentially affecting the affordability and accessibility of medicines.

Tiered Pricing

In parallel with the debate that took place in the context of the WTO TRIPS Agreement, the EU has pursued a system to allow pharmaceutical products (irrespective of whether they are patented) to be charged at different, discounted prices in different markets. Unlike the aforementioned actions whose roots can be traced back to WTO commitments and rules, the EU's tiered pricing system did not emanate from the latter. Not a novel concept, differentiated or "tiered" pricing was presented by the European Commission in 2000 as a means of increasing the affordability of key pharmaceuticals in a context of poverty reduction.[34] The concept was picked up in particular to accelerate action in relation to HIV/AIDS, malaria and tuberculosis in the poorest developing countries.[35]

The objective of serving specific low-income markets with low-priced pharmaceuticals was believed to be best served by a system that prevents those low-priced products from being diverted to other markets, thus avoiding the undermining of prices in high-income markets. This re-importation ban is essentially the trade policy dimension of the tiered pricing system that was introduced in EU Regulation 953/2003 (26 May 2003) to avoid trade diversion into the EU of certain key medicines.[36] To be able to use the EU tiered pricing system and avoid the re-importation into the EU of the medicines it sells outside the EU at lower prices, manufacturers are required to submit to the European Commission information about the tiered-priced products, their destination and the measures taken by the manufacturers to make the product distinguishable from identical products offered for sale inside the EU. In addition, an EU logo is to be used on the product or its packaging.

Since its introduction in 2004, the system has been used by only one manufacturer (GlaxoSmithKline), for only a handful of products, all of which were medicines for the treatment of HIV/AIDS.[37] Moreover, the volumes of registered medicines sold have significantly and steadily decreased since the introduction of the system. The Commission explains the constant drop by the fact that more patients have access to these medicines through other means or through other producers, including generic manufacturers and manufacturers that produce the medicines under voluntary licenses.[38] The Commission report omits the fact that manufacturers also find alternative ways to serve and segment markets as they adopt their own differentiated pricing regimes, without having to go through what could be considered a more bureaucratic government-driven tiered pricing mechanism. Alternative safeguards that are available to manufacturers in this respect could be the use of different trademarks or labeling for export markets, different technical regulations and product approvals or arrangements with importers or distributors of the medicines, for example.

Conclusion

While trade policy was given an important role in contributing to the EU's role in global health, this chapter observes that trade policy's answer to global health challenges (i) largely pre-dates the EU's global health agenda and (ii) is focused on only a few aspects of the global health strategy, particularly access to medicines.

The EU's trade policy actions on global health emerged in the broader political context of the last decade, when access to medicines for infectious epidemics and the trade-related intellectual property rights took center stage. The EU's actions responded essentially to multilateral commitments undertaken in the context of the World Trade Organization, much more than they have been a response to health policies, whether at the EU or the international level. The conclusion of the TRIPS Agreement and the ensuing controversy has done more for trade policy to consider public health than EU health policy has. Similarly, EU trade policy has equally far less internalized elements from the World Health Organization's global strategy and plan of action on public health, innovation and intellectual property, despite the latter's references to access to medicines and despite the specificity of some of its (non-binding) recommendations.

This implies that there is scope for plugging trade policy more and better into the EU's global health strategy. When the European Commission presented in 2012 its "trade and development" Communication entitled "Trade, Growth and Development — Tailoring Trade and Investment Policy for Those Countries Most in Need," it actually neither mentioned the contributions which trade policy could make to access to medicines in developing countries nor developed any further contribution which trade could make to the broader global health agenda. A specific action plan, currently envisaged by the Commission as a followup to the Communication on global health, would offer an opportunity for elaborating and giving effect to the contribution of trade policy to global health diplomacy. In this context, trade policy should be seen as an opportunity and not only as an obstacle to EU global health diplomacy.

The positive contributions which the EU's single trade policy could make to health policy should be considered, notably by looking specifically at how procurement, competition, customs, technical standards, trade in goods and trade in services can support health policy. Secondly, the infrequent use of the instruments put in place by the EU, such as the limited and waning use of the tiered pricing regime designed by the EU, suggests that an evaluation of existing EU policy instruments is warranted, especially at a time when the global disease burden is changing. While the limited use of these instruments could be interpreted as a welcome sign that alternatives to compulsory licensing and government-induced tiered pricing exist, a number of questions remain. Voluntary licensing, industry-led patient access programs or pricing policies may be meaningful, but are they sufficient and sustainable in the longer run? Moreover, are instruments designed specifically in response to infectious epidemics still appropriate at a time when the policy focus turns to non-communicable diseases? These and other questions deserve further consideration as trade policy's place in the EU global health agenda is further considered.

References

1. Fidler DP, Drager N, Kelley L. (2009) Managing the pursuit of health and wealth: the key challenges. *The Lancet* **373(9660):** 325–331.
2. European Commission. (2010) Communication from the Commission to the Council, the European Parliament, the European Economic and Social Committee and the Committee of the Regions: The EU Role in Global Health. COM (2010) 128. European Commission, Brussels.
3. European Commission. (2010) Communication from the Commission to the Council, the European Parliament, the European Economic and Social

Committee and the Committee of the Regions: The EU Role in Global Health. COM (2010) 128. European Commission, Brussels, p. 8.

4. European Commission. (2010) Commission Staff Working Document, Global Health — Responding to the Challenges of Globalization. SEC (2010) 380. European Commission, Brussels, p. 17.

5. Council of the European Union. (2010) Council Conclusions on the EU Role in Global Health. 3011th Foreign Affairs Council Meeting, Brussels, 10 May 2010. European Union, Brussels.

6. Labonté R, Gagnon ML. (2010) Framing health and foreign policy: lessons for global health diplomacy. *Globalization and Health* **6(14):** 19.

7. United States Trade Representative. (2011) White Paper Trade Enhancing Access to Medicines (TEAM). USTR, Washington, DC.

8. European Commission. (2010) Public Consultation on the EU Role in Global Health — Summary of Contributions. European Commission, Brussels, p. 5.

9. European Commission. (2010) Public Consultation on the EU Role in Global Health — Summary of Contributions. European Commission, Brussels, p. 38.

10. World Health Organization. (2013) WHO Model List of Essential Medicines. World Health Organization, Geneva.

11. Van den Ham R, Bero L, Laing R. (2011) The World Medicines Situation — Selection of Essential Medicines. World Health Organization, Geneva.

12. European Commission. (2000) Communication of the Commission to the Council and the European Parliament: Accelerated Action Targeted at Major Communicable Diseases Within the Context of Poverty Reduction. COM (2000) 585. European Commission, Brussels, p. 19.

13. World Trade Organization. (2001) Declaration on the TRIPS Agreement and Public Health Document. WT/MIN(01)/DEC/2. World Trade Organization, Geneva.

14. World Trade Organization. (2003) Decision of the General Council of 30 August 2003: Implementation of Paragraph 6 of the Doha Declaration on the TRIPS Agreement and Public Health. WT/L/540. World Trade Organization, Geneva.

15. World Trade Organization. (2005) Decision of the General Council of 6 December 2005 Adopting a Protocol Amending the TRIPS Agreement. WT/L/641. World Trade Organization, Geneva.

16. Helfer LR. (2004) Regime Shifting: The TRIPs Agreement and New Dynamics of International Intellectual Property Lawmaking. *Yale Journal of International Law* **29**: 1.

17. World Trade Organization. (2006) Council for Trade-Related Aspects of Intellectual Property Rights — Minutes of Meeting Held in the Centre William Rappard on 25–26 October 2006. IP/C/M/52. World Trade Organization, Geneva.

18. Mercurio B. (2012) Beyond the text: the significance of the Anti-Counterfeiting Trade Agreement. *Journal of International Economic Law* **15(2)**: 361–390.

19. European Commission. (2006) Global Europe: Competing in the World — A Contribution to the EU's Growth and Jobs Strategy. COM (2006) 567. European Commission, Brussels.

20. Council Regulation (EC) No. 1383/2003 of 22 July 2003 concerning customs action against goods suspected of infringing certain intellectual property rights and the measures to be taken against goods found to have infringed such rights. (2003) *Official Journal L* **196**: 7–14.

21. European Commission. (2012) Guidelines of the European Commission Concerning the Enforcement by EU Customs Authorities of Intellectual Property Rights with Regard to Goods, in Particular Medicines, in Transit Through the EU. European Commission, Brussels.

22. World Intellectual Property Organization. (2010) Committee on Development and Intellectual Property (CDIP), Patent-related Flexibilities in the Multilateral Legal Framework and Their Legislative Implementation at the National and Regional Levels. World Intellectual Property Organization, Geneva, p. 11.

23. European Commission. (2004) Proposal for a Regulation of the European Parliament and of the Council on Compulsory Licensing of Patents Relating to the Manufacture of Pharmaceutical Products for Export to Countries with Public Health Problems. COM (2004) 737. European Commission, Brussels.

24. Cornides J. (2007) European Union adopts regulation on compulsory licensing of pharmaceutical products for export. *The Journal of World Intellectual Property* **10(1)**: 70–77.

25. European Parliament. (2007) Access to Essential Medicines: Lessons Learned Since the Doha Declaration on the TRIPS Agreement and Public

Health, and Policy Options for the European Union. European Parliament, Brussels, p. 3.

26. World Trade Organization. (2010) Annual Review of the Decision on the Implementation of Paragraph 6 of the Doha Declaration of the TRIPS Agreement and Public Health. World Trade Organization, Geneva.

27. World Trade Organization. (2002) Decision of the Council for TRIPS of 27 June 2002 — Extension of the Transition Period Under Article 66.1 of the TRIPS Agreement for Least Developed Country Members for Certain Obligations with Respect to Pharmaceutical Products. IP/C/25. World Trade Organization, Geneva.

28. World Trade Organization. (2013) Decision of the Council for TRIPS of 11 June 2013 — Extension of the Transition Period Under Article 66.1 for Least Developed Country Members. World Trade Organization, Geneva.

29. Council of the European Union. (2010) Council Conclusions on Innovation and Solidarity in Pharmaceuticals. 3053rd Employment, Social Policy, Health and Consumer Affairs Council Meeting. Brussels, 6 December 2010. European Union, Brussels.

30. Sampson GP, Woolcock S (eds.). (2003) *Regionalism, Multilateralism, and Economic Integration: The Recent Experience.* United Nations University Press, Tokyo.

31. European Commission. (2010) Communication from the Commission to the Council, the European Parliament, the European Economic and Social Committee and the Committee of the Regions: The EU Role in Global Health. COM (2010) 128. European Commission, Brussels.

32. European Union. (2008) Economic Partnership Agreement between the CARIFORUM States, of the one part, and the European Community and its Member States, of the other part. *Official Journal L* **289:** 3–1955.

33. European Commission. (2013) Access to Medicines: The EU–India Free Trade Agreement Negotiations, 17 May 2013. Available at http://trade.ec.europa.eu/doclib/docs/2013/april/tradoc_150989.pdf (accessed on 8 August 2013).

34. European Commission. (2000) Communication of the Commission to the Council and the European Parliament: Accelerated Action Targeted at Major Communicable Diseases Within the Context of Poverty Reduction. COM (2000) 585. European Commission, Brussels.

35. European Commission. (2001) Communication from the Commission to the Council and the European Parliament: Programme for Action: Accelerated

Action on HIV/AIDS, Malaria and Tuberculosis in the Context of Poverty Reduction. COM (2001) 96. European Commission, Brussels.
36. European Union. (2003) Council Regulation (EC) No. 953/2003 of 26 May 2003 to avoid trade diversion into the European Union of certain key medicines. *Official Journal L* **135**: 5–11.
37. European Commission. (2012) Annual Report 2010–2011 on the Application of Council Regulation (EC) No. 953/2003 of 26 May 2003 to Avoid Trade Diversion into the European Union of Certain Key Medicines. COM (2012) 775. European Commission, Brussels.
38. *Ibid.*

General References

Attaran A. (2004) How do patents and economic policies affect access to essential medicines in developing countries? *Health Affairs* **23(3)**: 155–166.
European Commission. (2008) Commission Communication "Safe, Innovative and Accessible Medicines: A Renewed Vision for the Pharmaceutical Sector." Brussels, 10 December 2008. COM (2008) 666 final.
European Commission. (2009) Executive Summary of the Pharmaceutical Sector Inquiry Report. Brussels, 8 July 2009. COM (2009) 351 final.
Mackey TK, Liang BA. (2012) Patent and exclusivity status of essential medicines for noncommunicable disease. *PLoS ONE* **7(11)**.

5

EU Global Health Priorities: Migration and Mobility

Davide Mosca* and Caroline Schultz†

Introduction

In line with the principles of solidarity, fundamental rights and social inclusion delineated in the Lisbon Treaty and reiterated in the Europe 2020 Strategy, the Council Conclusions on the EU Role in Global Health (2010)[1] highlight the need to take action on three aspects: improve health, reduce inequalities, and increase protection against global health threats. All three of these aspects are linked to the topic of migration and mobility.

There are approximatelymarg 232 million international migrants today. If current rates of international migration continue, the number could reach 405 million by 2050.[a] Adding the estimated 740 million internal migrants to the picture, there are about one billion migrants today, a seventh of the currently seven billion people on the planet.[b] Facilitated by faster and more

*Director, Migration Health Department, International Organization for Migration, Geneva, Switzerland.

†Migration Health Programme Coordinator, International Organization for Migration, Migration Health Division, Geneva, Switzerland.

[a]United Nations Department of Economic and Social Affairs (UNDESA), 2013.

[b]The United Nations' definition of a migrant is used here: an individual who has resided in a foreign country for more than one year irrespective of the causes, voluntary or involuntary, and the means, regular or irregular, used to migrate [IOM (2011): Glossary on Migration].

affordable transport and communication technologies as well as transnational migrant networks, modern migration is increasingly global, multidirectional and dynamic, often involving temporary or circular movements. Most migrants move because they expect to improve their livelihoods and well-being elsewhere. Differentials in wages and in workforce supply and demand across and within countries (often linked to demographic changes), lack of opportunities or unstable conditions due to natural or man-made disasters, the existence of positive migration examples within the community, and individual factors such as transnational family ties, all influence individuals' decision to migrate. Some of the people on the move are skilled migrants, such as health professionals; others are lower- or semi-skilled migrants who work in the construction, hospitality and agricultural sectors, or as domestic and home care workers.

In 2011, 33.3 million non-nationals were living on the territory of an EU Member State, accounting for 6.6% of the EU-27 population. More than one third of these people (12.8 million) were nationals of another EU Member State (i.e. intra-EU migrants), and the rest (20.5 million) were nationals of a country outside the EU (usually referred to as third country nationals).[2] It is estimated that about 1.9–3.8 million irregular migrants reside in EU Member States.[3]

The EU has recognized the need to address migration in a coherent way: the European Commission's reform proposal for the Global Approach to Migration and Mobility (GAMM), published in November 2011, builds on the Global Approach to Migration first adopted in 2005 and stresses the interdependence between migration and foreign policy and development. It delineates the thematic and geographical priorities of the EU's external migration policy and the instruments to achieve them, and also makes reference to health.

Migration and mobility to and within the EU has implications for health outcomes inside and outside the EU and for the European Community's role in global health. The European Commission recognized this and identified two main aspects of migration as part of the EU's role in global health: (1) effectively managing the migration of health professionals to ensure adequate distribution and provision of health professionals inside and outside the EU; (2) ensuring the health of migrants, both inside and outside the EU. In its communication to the Council, the Commission[4] stated, "EU Member States should ensure that their migration policies do not undermine the availability of health professionals in third countries whilst respecting the individual freedom of movement and personal and professional aspirations. ... EU Member States should step up their efforts to ensure that everyone — including migrants — in the EU has access to quality health services without discrimination."

If both these health-related aspects of current migration dynamics are consistently addressed, health and socio-economic inequalities in health will be reduced and subsequent social cohesion and protection against global health will be enhanced. However, as stated in the Commission Communication, this requires coherence of all internal and external policies and actions.

The EU's Role in Global Health: Migrants' Health

The Commission Communication on the EU Role in Global Health[4] mentioned the health of migrants in one sentence: "EU Member States should step up their efforts to ensure that everyone — including migrants — in the EU has access to quality health services without discrimination". However, this sentence was removed in the subsequent Council Conclusions on the EU Role in Global Health,[1] which seems indicative of the current political climate regarding migration in the EU. As Cecilia Malmström, European Commissioner for Home Affairs, noted in her speech in April 2012, in the wake of the economic crisis, the political climate "has turned sour, some would even say toxic. ... We have not seen as many populist and xenophobic parties in European national parliaments since before the Second World War."

There are two main reasons for the EU to step up action on migrants' health and to make it a central theme with regard to their role in global health:

(1) *Coherence of internal and external EU policies is crucial for the EU to remain a credible global actor.* The EU has an interest in leading the global health debate — toward universal coverage and ensuring the human right to health.[c] If seeking to engage in the global health debate as

---

[c]See for instance the European Commission's 2007 White Paper "Together for Health: A Strategic Approach for the EU 2008–2013," which proposed "strengthening the EU's

a powerful actor, the EU needs to align external and internal policies on health. The importance of this is recognized in the Commission Communication, which acknowledges that "increased coherence between relevant internal and external policies will reinforce the EU as a global actor".[4] The Communication argues that "[the] EU should ensure that *all relevant internal or external policies* contribute to promoting equitable and universal coverage of quality health services."[4] The Council reiterates this in its Conclusions (2010),[1] calling on the EU and its Member States "to act together in all relevant internal and external policies and actions by prioritizing their support on strengthening comprehensive health systems in partner countries, which are central to all global health challenges."

As the EU is promoting equitable and universal coverage of quality health services as part of its strategy on global health, it should start at home, by ensuring the realization of migrants' right to health within the EU, regardless of their legal status. This should include, among other things, social protection in health, such as access to healthcare services and health insurance, and access to safe living and working conditions. Given the principles of solidarity and human rights that the EU was built on,[5] ensuring that migrants can realize their right to health is an ethical imperative, beyond its strategic benefits.

(2) *From a public health, economic and social perspective, protecting migrants' health is in the EU's best interest.* Europe 2020, the EU's growth strategy, mentions that "[a] major effort will be needed to combat poverty and social exclusion and reduce health inequalities to ensure that everybody can benefit from growth."[6] The increasing diversity of populations in Europe creates new challenges for health systems, which have to adapt in order to remain responsive.[7] A major global health goal that has direct relevance to the health of migrants is reduction in disparities. These disparities create and sustain adverse health outcomes and are

---

voice in Global Health" as one of its principles and maintained that "the EC and its Member States can create better health outcomes for EU citizens and for others through sustained collective leadership in global health" (EC, 2007).

often exacerbated for migrants by conditions surrounding the migration process.

Guaranteeing migrants' equitable access to healthcare and health promotion makes practical sense — it is cost-effective and improves public health outcomes, as well as necessary for integration and productivity, and thus for regional and global development, which is captured by the slogan "Health is wealth."[d] Promoting migrants' use of primary healthcare and early treatment and including them into disease-control programmes will reduce the need for costly emergency care and related high costs for the health system.

Communicable diseases of public health interest such as HIV and Tuberculosis, as well as non-communicable diseases (NCDs), are more prevalent among the foreign-born population in Europe. For instance, research has shown that migrants from South Asia residing in Europe face higher risks of acquiring NCDs than the population in both their countries of origin and the European host country; and[8] have identified migration as a social determinant of health as the predominant reason for this discrepancy. Mitigation and management of the global spread of diseases is thus a second global health goal that has direct relevance to migration health.

EU Regulatory Framework, Strategies, and Action on Migrants' Health

The right to health of every human being, including migrants, is officially enshrined in many EU (and international) legally binding human rights treaties.[9] The Treaty of the EU (the Lisbon Treaty) states in Article 168, "A high level of human health protection shall be ensured in the definition and implementation of all Union policies and activities."[e] Regarding

---

[d]See the European Commission DG Sanco website, http://ec.europa.eu/health/health_policies/health_in_eu_initiatives/index_en.htm.
[e]See also the European Social Charter (1961) and Revised Charter of 1996, Article 11; the Council of Europe Convention on Human Rights and Biomedicine of 1997, Article 3; and the Charter of Fundamental Rights of the EU (2000), Article 35.

developments and actions by EU Member States, the past decade has witnessed important progress on migrant health within the EU.[f]

In 2006, "Health in All Policies"[g] was the main health theme of the Finnish EU Presidency, which supports a horizontal, intersectoral approach to health. This paved the way for putting the issue of migration and health on the European agenda during the Portuguese EU Presidency in 2007. The conference "Health and Migration in the EU: Better Health for All in an Inclusive Society"[10] led to the adoption of the Council Conclusions on Health and Migration in the EU (December 2007),[11] which highlighted the link between the health of migrants and that of all EU citizens.

These Council Conclusions (2007a)[12] invited Member States to integrate migrant health into national policies and to facilitate access to healthcare for migrants. They also called on the European Centre for Disease Prevention and Control (ECDC) to produce a comprehensive report on migration and infectious diseases in the EU, focusing on tuberculosis, HIV and vaccine preventable diseases, to inform policy and public health responses. In response to the call, ECDC has published a number of reports since 2008.[h] The EU Directorate General for Health and Consumers (DG Sanco), the DG Research and the EU Agency for

---

[f]This also applies to the wider European Region: in November 2011, the Committee of Experts of the Council of Europe (CoE) adopted the Recommendation CM/Rec (2011) 13, on mobility, migration and access to healthcare. This Recommendation supports the CoE, its Member States, and its partners in collective efforts to acknowledge and adequately address issues around mobility, migration and health, and ultimately protect migrants' health in the European Region.

[g]"Health in All Policies addresses the effects on health across all policies such as agriculture, education, the environment, fiscal policies, housing, and transport. It seeks to improve health and at the same time contribute to the well-being and the wealth of the nations through structures, mechanisms and actions planned and managed mainly by sectors other than health" (Stahl *et al.*, 2006: xviii).

[h]These include: ECDC (2009): *TECHNICAL REPORT, Migrant Health: Access to HIV Prevention, Treatment and Care for Migrant Populations in EU/EEA Countries*; ECDC (2011): *TECHNICAL REPORT, Improving HIV Data Comparability in Migrant Populations and Ethnic Minorities in EU/EEA/EFTA Countries: Findings from a Literature Review and Expert Panel.*

Fundamental Rights (FRA) have supported a number of large projects in the EU dealing with migration and health in the last few years.[i] Recently, IOM was awarded a direct grant within the 2012 EC Public Health Programme to work on fostering health provision for migrants, the Roma and other vulnerable groups.

The process initiated and led by European countries largely influenced the agenda of the 61st World Health Assembly (WHA) in 2008,[13] which adopted Resolution 61.17, Health of Migrants. In the followup, the Ministry of Health and Social Policy of Spain co-hosted the "Global Consultation on Health of Migrants" with WHO and IOM during the Spanish Presidency of the Council of the EU (2010).[1] This consultation took stock of progress made on the implementation of the WHA Resolution and produced an operational framework based on the four pillars of the Resolution: (1) legal and policy frameworks on migrant health; (2) migrant-friendly health systems/services; (3) networks, partnerships and multi-country collaboration on migrant health; and (4) monitoring migrant health (WHO/IOM/Government of Spain, 2010).[14]

In March 2011, the European Parliament (EP) adopted a Resolution called "Reducing Health Inequalities in the EU," which calls on Member States to tackle health inequalities in access to healthcare for undocumented migrants. Although non-binding, this is a significant step forward in ensuring equitable access to healthcare for all, with no discrimination linked to administrative status or financial resources.

Despite the leadership role of the EU in bringing migrant health to the European and global health agenda, the last few years have seen setbacks rather than progress in migrants' access to health in Europe, fueled principally by anti-migrant sentiments and austerity measures as a result of the economic crisis. Generally, undocumented migrants still face major barriers to health in Europe. As the EU Agency for Fundamental Rights (FRA)

---

[i]These include: "Health Care in NowHereLand — Improving Services for Undocumented Migrants in the EU" (led by the University of Vienna), "Assisting Migrants and Communities: Analysis of Social Determinants of Health and Health Inequalities" (AMAC, led by IOM, Brussels), and "Development of Recommendations for Integrating Socio-cultural Standards in Health Promoting Offers and Services" (led by the Austrian Red Cross).

(2011)[15] says, "[Most] European countries entitle irregular migrants to emergency care only and this is not always granted cost-free." There is still considerable need for implementation and harmonization of policies and practices across different government sectors and EU Member States to ensure both internal and external coherence of migrant-inclusive policy approaches.

The EU should therefore seize the opportunity of addressing migrant health in a coherent way, for at least three reasons. First, migrants are entitled to the human right to health, and realizing this right is necessary for EU Member States to comply with the foundations of human rights and solidarity that the EU is built on. Not only is this an ethical imperative, but also, persistent non-compliance with these self-set principles will greatly diminish the EU's credibility, not only in the Global Health Debate. Second, including migrants — regardless of legal status – in the public health systems, and offering them access to migrant-sensitive health services,[j] is cost-effective and conducive to public health. Third, health is a migrant's main asset and a prerequisite for being able to contribute to the development of both origin and destination countries. Thus, ensuring that migrants can build on this asset is in line with the European Consensus on Development, which was adopted by the three EU institutions in December 2005.[16]

Moreover, the EU could set a powerful example on the inclusion of migrants' right to health to other countries and regions in the world. This would include advocating the implementation of WHA Resolution 61.17 on the Health of Migrants, and putting the issue on the agenda of global forums on both health and migration, for instance in the context of the debate on the post-2015 development framework and the one on "Global Health and Foreign Policy" spearheaded by the Oslo Declaration (2007).[17]

---

[j]Migrant-sensitive health systems, also referred to as migrant-friendly health systems, consciously and systematically incorporate the needs of migrants into health financing, policy, planning, implementation and evaluation, including such considerations as the epidemiological profiles of migrant populations, relevant cultural, language and socio-economic factors, and the impact of the migration process on health (Fortier, 2010).

The EU's Role in Global Health: Migration of Human Resources for Health

The migration and mobility of health professionals, especially from developing countries (the so-called brain drain), has been a global development concern for decades. The 2006 WHO World Health Report estimated a global shortfall of almost 4.3 million health personnel, with 57 countries (most in Africa and Asia) facing severe shortages. Migration of health professionals occurs for a set of reasons, including relatively low wages, poor working conditions and lack of further professional development opportunities in the countries of origin, and growing demand for health professionals in developed countries, as a result of accelerating demographic changes in combination with inadequate domestic health workforce planning (WHO/IOM/CDC, 2005).[18] While this is a serious development concern for many countries, one should also note that health professionals with a migration background can act both as agents of development for their home countries and as mediators for migrant-friendly health services in countries of destination.[19]

Many EU countries are relying highly on foreign-trained health workers, although "mobility flows are difficult to quantify with accuracy."[20] In the face of an ageing population,[k] with severe consequences for public welfare and social security systems across Europe, the current forecasted shortage of health personnel compels EU Member States to act. Within the EU, the situation is especially alarming in certain health professions, such as nursing and medical specializations.[l] In total, the Commission estimates a potential gap of one million healthcare workers by 2020.[m,6]

---

[k]"Between 2008 and 2060 the population of the EU-27 aged 65 and over is projected to increase by 66.9 million" (EC, 2008:3).

[l]For instance, Slovakia faces shortages of nurses, midwives, physiotherapists, radiological assistants and paramedics, while in Italy numbers of newly trained nurses are unable to replace those due to retire. Germany has serious difficulties in training enough graduates, and Romania, France, Hungary and Austria report unfilled specialist training places (EC, 2012a).

[m]Labor shortages are generally not inevitable, but can be addressed by sound public policies. Shortages in specific sectors are often used to recruit migrants as "cheap labor," who then face working and living conditions which are often unacceptable for a large part of

The EU has good reasons to be concerned about health worker mobility. Firstly, intra-EU health worker mobility means that less developed regions within the EU are faced with severe shortages in the health sector. Secondly, in light of a shortage of health workers especially in developing countries, the EU must ensure that their Member States' health workforce training and recruitment policies do not counteract EU development goals by depriving already struggling third countries of much-needed health personnel.

The lack of comparable data is a major constraint on addressing issues about the mobility of health workers. Although there have been numerous studies on health worker mobility, there is a significant "lack of up-to-date, comparable data and information in the EU, for example on numbers of health workers, [both] in training and in employment, their specializations, their geographical [distribution], age, gender and country of provenance."[21,20,22] Therefore, this chapter largely quotes anecdotal evidence from country reports.[n]

Mobility of Human Resources for Health Within the EU — Issues, Strategies and Policy Responses

The Commission Communication and the Council Conclusions on the EU Role in Global Health[4,1] refer only to the movement of health professionals *to* and *outside* the EU, not *within* — however, to discuss the EU's role in global health, it is necessary to look at intra-EU health worker mobility as well.

Recent studies funded by the EC Directorate General Research[o] found "an undersupply of health professionals [particularly in] rural and sparsely

---

the "domestic" workforce in industrialized countries (Ruhs and Anderson, 2011; MoHProf, 2012a: 133).

[n]Efforts to collect comparable data have been initiated. For instance, the OECD, WHO and Eurostat agreed on the need for a common strategy for the joint collection of health statistics in 2004 and have developed a framework for joint data collection including a questionnaire on human resources for health, using "new sets of indicators, harmonized and agreed definitions" (WHO RO for Europe, 2012).

[o]These studies include (1) Health Professional Mobility and Health Systems (PROMeTHEUS) in 17 European countries (http://www.euro.who.int/__data/assets/pdf_file/0017/152324/e95812.pdf); (2) Mobility of Health Professionals to, within and from

populated areas, for example in Denmark, Finland, France, Germany, Romania, and an oversupply of doctors in some urban areas, particularly in Germany."[4] In general, and EU-wide, the lack of health professionals in rural areas is of concern.[p] Further findings include a distinct east–west asymmetry for doctors, nurses and dentists, meaning that shortages are most severe in eastern EU Member States.

After the EU enlargement in 2004 and 2007, the internal market was gradually opened to workers from new Member States. This led to out-flows from the 12 new members, especially to the UK, Germany, Ireland, Italy, Spain and Austria. A substantial share of those working in Italy and Austria are employed in the home care system.[23] Flows of registered health workers from the EU10[q] were smaller than expected, yet flows from Bulgaria and Romania were significant. These two countries,which joined the EU in 2007, experience critical shortages in certain health professions.[r]

Several European Community Directives directly or indirectly regulate the mobility of health professionals within the EU. The *Working Time Directive* 2003/88/EC, issued in 2004, limits weekly work to 48 hours. As this also affected salaried doctors who had often been working longer hours, many Member States would have needed to recruit large numbers of additional staff in a very short time to comply with the Directive, which is why a transitional period was introduced.[21] It is unclear how successful this Directive has been, though, as it "seems to have led to creativity in

---

the EU (MoHPROF) in 25 countries in Europe, North America, Asia and Africa (http://www.mohprof.eu/LIVE/); and (3) Registered Nurse Forecasting (RN4CAST) study (http://www.rn4cast.eu/en/index.php).

[p]In Germany, for instance, "rural areas, particularly in East Germany, show a considerable lack of general practitioners" (MoHProf, 2012b). In Sweden, many physicians and dentists leave rural areas once they have finished their specialist education (MoHProf, 2012b).

[q]The 10 countries that joined the EU in 2004: Cyprus, the Czech Republic, Estonia, Hungary, Latvia, Lithuania, Malta, Poland, Slovakia and Slovenia.

[r]Bulgaria has one of the lowest numbers of nurses per capita in the European region, and one of the lowest densities of pharmacists in the EU (MoHProf, 2012b). In Romania, the number of health professionals has increased in recent years, but is still low in comparison to European countries. In 2009, the president of the Romanian College of Physicians announced that in the last two years 5000 Romanian physicians had left the country (MoHProf, 2012b).

attempts by both health systems and health professionals to avoid its implications."[23] The Directive 2005/36/EC, *on the recognition of professional qualifications*, harmonizes qualifications to enable free movement of EU-trained health workers within the EU by a system of "automatic recognition" which *de facto* restricts access to the EU labor market of health workers from outside the European Economic Area (EEA).[s] In recent years, intra-EU migration of health professionals appears to have increased relative to migration from outside the EU — at least in some EU countries: in 2009, "Austria, Belgium, France, Germany and Italy receive[d] their foreign health professionals predominantly from the European free-movement area,"[22] while the UK and Spain still received foreign health personnel predominantly from third countries.

Mobility of Human Resources for Health to and from the EU — Issues and Policy Responses

Health is a prerequisite for sustainable development. Some sub-Saharan countries, for instance, experience emigration rates of health personnel to OECD countries above 50%, causing considerable staff shortages in the health sector.[24,t] The 2005 EU Strategy for Action on the Crisis in Human Resources for Health in Developing Countries, which both the Commission[4] and the Council Conclusions on the EU Role[1] reference and support, acknowledges that "[there] is a global market for health workers, but it is a distorted market, shaped by global inequity in health care provision and the capacity to pay workers, rather than by health needs

---

[s]The Directive has been amended several times since it came into force. In 2011, a public consultation was held; a summary of the 370 contributions can be found at http://ec.europa.eu/internal_market/qualifications/docs/news/20110706-summary-replies-public-consultation-pdq_en.pdf.

[t]For instance, the expatriation rate for doctors in Mozambique is 64.5%, in Sierra Leone 58.4%, in Liberia 54.2%, and in Angola 63.2%, according to the OECD (2007; figures for 2000). Taking into account data on health worker migration from 2000 to 2008, a joint OECD/WHO Policy Brief (2010) summarizes that "[despite] recent trends showing signs of stabilization or decline in a few countries, overall migration of health personnel to OECD countries is still on the rise."

and the burden of disease,"[25] and encourages Member States to address the issue in partnerships with sending countries.

Country reports from the Mobility of Health Professionals (MoHProf) project give insights into the general trends of health worker mobility from developing countries to the EU.[26] Along with the US, Canada and Australia, the EU is one of the top destinations for health professionals from developing countries.[u] All in all, health worker migration from outside the EU is currently decreasing rapidly, due to stricter implementation of EU legislation as well as the economic crisis in the EU.

All 27 EU Member States experience emigration of health professionals, mainly to the US, Canada and Australia. Australia receives EU health workers mainly from the UK, and to a lesser extent from Italy. Canada experiences "high inflows from EU countries, especially from France and the UK," and "[in] 2007 ... 3% of its foreign registered nurses were Polish by background."[23] Since the onset of the economic crisis, especially medical graduates from Ireland and the UK have increasingly been seeking entry to the US.[23]

At the global level, the *WHO Code of Practice on the International Recruitment of Health Personnel* was adopted at the 63rd World Health Assembly, in 2010. It aims to "establish and promote voluntary principles and practices for the ethical international recruitment of health personnel" (Article 1.1) and "discourages the active recruitment of health personnel from developing countries facing critical shortages of health workers" (Article 5.1). It emphasizes the importance of equal treatment for migrant health workers and the domestically trained health workforce

---

[u]For instance, Ghana has lost about 50% of its professional nurses to the UK, the US and Canada in the last decade. In 2005, Indian medical graduates constituted 10.9% of the UK physician workforce, and Ireland was the second most favorite EU country for health worker migration from India. In Morocco it has been reported that in 2008 five private Spanish and Italian investors built nursing and paramedic schools in northern Morocco to train local students for European markets. The Philippines has long been known for training health workers for "export"; however, stays in the EU are mostly regarded as transitory, and the final destinations are the US and Gulf states. The same applies to Egypt, where informants and stakeholders often refer to EU Member States as temporary destinations for skills accumulation through education, training or work.

(Articles 4.4 and 4.5), and honors the right of any individual, including health personnel, to leave any country and to migrate to any other country that wishes to admit and employ them (Article 3.4). Although the Code is not legally binding, Member States should periodically report to the WHO Secretariat on progress in the implementation of the Code. The WHO Director General will report on progress for the first time during the WHA in May 2013.

The commitment of the EU and some of its Member States on ethical recruitment started before the adoption of the WHO Code, and goes beyond it as well, with legally binding rules (such as those contained in EU directives) on health worker recruitment. For example, the EU Blue Card Directive (2009/50/EC) states, "Member States should refrain from pursuing active recruitment in developing countries in sectors suffering from a lack of personnel. Ethical recruitment policies ... should be developed in key sectors, for example the health sector" (Article 22).

Already in 2007, the Council Conclusions welcomed the European Programme for Action to Tackle the Critical Shortage of Health Workers in Developing Countries (2007–2013),[27] which had been developed by the European Commission in 2006.[16] In it the Council "recognizes that adequate financial resources are needed to ensure sustainable solutions to the human resource crisis in the wider context of health sector financing in developing countries."

An Action Plan for the EU Health Workforce, published by the EC in 2012, makes the link between intra-EU health worker mobility and migration of third country health personnel, mentioning that health worker migration within the EU and to non-EU countries has "increased the reliance on the recruitment of healthcare professionals from outside the EU."[v,4]

---

[v]This Staff Working Document identifies four areas of action "to promote a sustainable workforce for health": (1) forecasting workforce needs and improving workforce planning methodologies; (2) anticipating future skills needs in the health professions; (3) sharing good practice on effective recruitment and retention strategies for health professionals; (4) addressing the ethical recruitment of health professionals.

Progress Toward Better Management of Health Worker Mobility: Country Examples from the EU/EEA

Regarding implementation of the WHO Code, as of 30 August 2012, 18 of the 27 EU Member States had submitted a national progress report to WHO.[w] Four others have designated a national authority, but not submitted a report yet.[x] Five countries did not have designated national authorities.[y] Most of the countries reporting action focused on translating the Code into the national language and raising awareness across stakeholders as first steps.[20]

Many EU Member States have started developing guidelines and implementing actions to better plan their health workforce and manage health worker mobility.

For instance, the UK Department of Health adopted a Code of Practice in 1999, but this applies only to the National Health Service (NHS), not to private employers.[23] According to the NGO Action for Global Health,[1] the UK Code was "only partially successful given the expansion in the number of private recruitment agencies that enable migrants to enter the NHS 'via the back door'."[z]

In order to mitigate health worker shortages in rural South Africa, the UK and South Africa, in the context of their bilateral agreement, have started to deploy trainee doctors from the UK to rural and underresourced hospitals in South Africa with the Out of Programme Experience (OOPE) project.[aa,23] EU Member States have also been funding projects

---

[w]These countries were: Austria, Belgium, Cyprus, the Czech Republic, Denmark, Estonia, Finland, Germany, Hungary, Ireland, Italy, Latvia, the Netherlands, Poland, Slovenia, Spain, Sweden and the UK.

[x]Portugal, Romania, Lithuania and Slovakia.

[y]Greece, Malta, Luxembourg and Bulgaria and France.

[z]Similarly, Norway and the Netherlands have both issued workforce strategies that set limits for active state recruitment or by promoting recruitment via bilateral agreements. Another step in the right direction could be the Commission-funded EU Joint Action on Health Workforce Planning and Forecasting, which is to be launched in December 2012 (Jorens, 2012).

[aa]Ireland's Health Service Executive (HSE) is also exploring bilateral agreements with a number of countries, to address issues related to the recruitment of health personnel,

in the context of IOM's Migration for Development in Africa (MIDA) Programme, which helps to mobilize competencies acquired by African nationals abroad for the benefit of Africa's development. For instance, the program facilitated Ghanaian health professionals' living in the Netherlands, the UK and Germany to strengthen the health systems and human resources for health capacity in Ghana, and qualified Somali health professionals from Finland to contribute to the rehabilitation and development of regional health sectors in northern Somalia.[bb] A similar program has been implemented by the Centre for International Migration and Development (CIM) on behalf of the German Federal Ministry for Economic Cooperation and Development (BMZ).[cc]

Conclusion

This chapter has described some of the most relevant EU actions and strategies related to migration and global health. With regard to health worker migration, the Commission and the individual EU Member States have often been at the forefront of global action and seem well on their way to complying with self-set rules and the WHO Code of Practice. However, a lot of gaps still need to be addressed, to ensure a good distribution of quality health personnel within Europe as well as globally.

Moreover, the chapter has argued that not only the mobility of health workers is an issue of concern for the EU's role in global health, but also migrants' health. If the Commission and the Council do not take action to ensure that EU Member States comply with Community and international law on migrants' right to health, including social protection in health, the EU's credibility as a powerful normative actor in global health will be adversely affected.

---

circular migration, training and capacity building in source countries (Dussault *et al.*, 2012).

[bb] See the IOM website, https://www.iom.int/cms/mida (accessed 4 December 2012).

[cc] This *Returning Experts Programme* "supports the professional integration of university graduates and experienced experts from developing, emerging and transition countries, who have completed their training in Germany and are interested in returning to their countries of origin" (CIM 2012).

To ensure policy coherence, the EU needs to step up action to remove barriers to migrants' health, both in its Member States and by supporting, or even initiating, global action on this issue. For instance, migrant health should be made an integral part of important international discussions on migration and development, as well as high level meetings and commitments on global health issues, such as the thematic discussion on health within the post-2015 development framework, which is currently being discussed. The EU could be a model for how societies should incorporate migrant health as an important part in ensuring sustainable health systems.

Commitments made at EU and global level on both sets of issues, such as the WHO Code, national initiatives on ethical recruitment of health professionals or the WHA Resolution on the Health of Migrants, need to be carefully implemented, and implementation needs to be monitored. Therefore, it is indispensable to step up actions on collecting comparable data of both health worker mobility and migrant health, on the basis of commonly agreed upon definitions of terms and indicators. Moreover, coherence between policies and strategies drafted by the different Directorate Generals of the European Commission is of the utmost importance.

If both these health aspects of migration are managed well, with coherent internal and external policies and actions that are in line with the principles of solidarity and human rights that the EU is built on, overall health will be improved, health and socio-economic inequalities reduced, and protection against global health threats enhanced.

References

1. Action for Global Health. (2011) Addressing the Global Health Workforce Crisis: Challenges for France, Germany, Italy, Spain and the UK. Available at http://ec.europa.eu/health/eu_world/docs/ev_ 20110915_rd02_en.pdf.
2. Eurostat. (2012) Migration and Migrant Population Statistics. Data from October 2011. Available at http://epp.eurostat.ec.europa.eu/statistics_explained/index.php/Migration_and_migrant_population_statistics.
3. Karl-Trummer U, Novak-Zezula S, Metzler B. (2010) Access to health care for undocumented migrants in the EU: a first landscape of NowHereLand. *Eurohealth* **16(1)**.

4. European Commission. (2010a) Communication: The EU Role in Global Health. COM (2010) 128 final. Available at http://ec.europa.eu/development/icenter/repository/COMM_PDF_COM_2010_0128_EN.PDF.

5. European Union. (2007) Treaty of Lisbon Amending the Treaty on European Union and the Treaty Establishing the European Community. *Official Journal C* **306(01)**.

6. European Commission. (2010b) Communication: Europe 2020 — A Strategy for Smart, Sustainable and Inclusive Growth. COM (2010) 2020 Final. Available at http://eur-lex.europa.eu/LexUriServ/LexUriServ.do?uri=COM:2010:2020:FIN:EN:PDF.

7. Rechel B, Mladovsky P, Devillé W, *et al.* (eds.). (2011) *Migration and Health in the European Union*. Open University Press, Maidenhead, UK.

8. Davies AA, Blake C, Dhavan P. (2011) Social determinants and risk factors for non-communicable diseases (NCDs) in South Asian migrant populations in Europe. *Asia Europe Journal* **8(4):** 461–473.

9. Pace P. (2007) Migration and the Right to Health — A Review of International Law. International Migration Law No. 19. IOM, Geneva. Available at http://publications.iom.int/bookstore/free/IML_19.pdf.

10. Eurohealth: Migration and health in the European Union, Volume 16, Number 1, 2010.

11. Migrant health policy: The Portuguese and Spanish EU Presidencies by Maria-José Peiro and Roumyana Benedict (see attached) an

12. European Council. (2007a) Draft Council Conclusions: Health and Migration in the EU. Available at http://register.consilium.europa.eu/pdf/en/07/st15/st15609.en07.pdf.

13. World Health Assembly. (2008) Health of Migrants. WHA Resolution 61.17. Available at http://apps.who.int/gb/ebwha/pdf_files/WHA61-REC1/A61_REC1-en.pdf.

14. International Organization for Migration. (2010) The World Migration Report 2010: The Future of Migration: Building Capacities for Change. IOM, Geneva.

15. European Union Agency for Fundamental Rights (FRA) "Access to healthcare in 10 European Union Member States" (p. 3).

16. European Commission. (2006) A European Programme for Action to Tackle the Critical Shortage of Health Workers in Developing Countries (2007–2013). COM (2006) 870 final. Available at http://eurlex.europa.eu/LexUriServ/LexUriServ.do?uri=COM:2006:0870:FIN:EN:PDF.

17. Ministers of Foreign Affairs of Brazil, France, Indonesia, Norway, Senegal, South Africa and Thailand. (2007) Oslo Ministerial Declaration — global health: a pressing foreign policy issue of our time. *Lancet* **369:** 1373–1378. "Oslo Ministerial Declaration — global health: a pressing foreign policy issue of our time." *The Lancet* Volume 369, No. 9570, pp. 1373–1378, 21 April 2007, Celso Araorim (Brazil); Philippe Douste-Blazy (France); Hasan Wirayuda (Indonesia); Jonas Gahr Store (Norway); Cheikh Tidiane Gadio (Senegal); Nkosazana Dlamini-Zuma (South Africa); Nitya Pibulsonggram (Thailand). http://www.thelancet.com/journals/lancet/article/PIIS0140-6736(07)60498-X/abstract.

18. WHO, IOM, Centers for Disease Control and Prevention. (2005) Health & Migration: Bridging the Gap. International Dialogue on Migration No. 6. Available at http://www.iom.int/jahia/webdav/site/myjahiasite/shared/shared/mainsite/published_docs/serial_ publications/RedBook6_eng.pdf.

19. Davies AA, Mosca D, Frattini C. (2010) Migration and Health Service Delivery. *World Hospital and Health Services — The Official Journal of the International Hospital Federation* **46(3)**.

20. Dussault G, Perfilieva G, Pethick J. (2012) Implementing the WHO Global Code of Practice on International Recruitment of Health Personnel in the European Region, Draft Policy Brief for Discussion at the RC 62 Technical Briefing 2, Malta, 11 September 2012. Available at http://www.euro.who.int/data/assets/pdf_file/0020/173054/Policy-Brief_HRH_draft-for-RC62-discussion.pdf.

21. European Commission. (2008) Green Paper on the European Workforce for Health. COM (2008) 725 final. Available at http://ec.europa.eu/health/ph_systems/docs/workforce_gp_en.pdf.

22. Wismar M, Maier CB, Glinos IA, *et al.* (eds.). (2011) Health Professional Mobility and Health Systems: Evidence from 17 European Countries. World Health Organization 2011, on behalf of the European Observatory on Health Systems and Policies. Available at http://www.euro.who.int/__data/assets/pdf_file/0017/152324/e95812.pdf.

23. Mobility of Health Professionals. (2012a) Mobility of Health Professionals — Health Systems, Work Conditions, Patterns of Health Workers' Mobility and Implications for Policy Makers. Bonn, Germany, March 2012. Available at http://www.mohprof.eu/LIVE/DATA/National_reports/national_report_Summary.pdf.

24. OECD. (2007) Part III: Immigrant health workers in OECD countries in the broader context of highly skilled migration. In *International Migration Outlook*, Sopemi 2007 edition. OECD, Paris.
25. European Commission. (2005) EU Strategy for Action on the Crisis in Human Resources for Health in Developing Countries. COM (2005) 642 final. Available at http://eurlex.europa.eu/LexUriServ/site/en/com/2005/com2005_0642en01.pdf.
26. Mobility of Health Professionals. (2012b) National Profiles. Available at http://www.mohprof.eu/LIVE/national_profiles.html.
27. European Council. (2007b) Conclusions of the Council and the Representatives of the Governments of the Member States Meeting Within the Council on a European Programme for Action to Tackle the Critical Shortage of Health Workers in Developing Countries (2007–2013). Council of the European Union, Brussels.

6

EU Global Health Priorities: Climate Change

Annika Herbel* and Arne Niemann†

Introduction

Over the last two decades, the European Union (EU) has emerged as a leading actor — or even as the "undisputed leader"[1] — in regional and international environmental politics.[2-6] In this context, "climate change" has successfully entered the European agenda and has become a "high politics" issue at the international level.[5] For example, in the context of the Kyoto Protocol, after the withdrawal of the United States in mid-2001, the EU has successfully supported and promoted its ratification.[4,6] The meteorological and also economic impacts of climate change have been widely recognized and explored.[7] Although the interaction between climate change and health has been highlighted by health and climate scientists for decades, the health sector is almost not at all represented in UNFCCC negotiations.[8]

Climate change, or global warming, poses serious threats to global health, especially affecting the poorest countries that are already suffering the worst health and other climate change effects, such as food and water shortages.[9] Several aspects of global health will be affected by the effects of climate change. First, disease vectors and carriers (mosquitoes, ticks, rodents) will have more fertile conditions and be able to alter geographical

*University of Heidelberg, Germany.
†University of Mainz, Germany.

ranges, which will bring them into closer contact with the human population. Second, higher temperatures due to climate change will impact on air
quality, particularly in urban environments, which may increase the
concentration of allergenic aero-pollens and the risks of respiratory and
cardiovascular diseases, too. Third, and maybe most importantly, global
warming has an effect on the scarcity of clean water. It will get more
and more difficult to have access to clean water, which will add to diarrhea illnesses. Moreover, the scarcity of clean water and other ecosys-
tem changes may increase food shortages. In particular, poor countries
in southern regions will suffer these effects.[10]

This chapter will address the following questions: What is the legal basis
for EU climate change policy or external climate action? How does the EU
address the health effects of climate change? And what is the EU's international role in combating climate change (in regard to health effects)?

Climate Change as a Threat to Global Health

The EU (especially in the form of the Commission) recognized climate
change as a threat to human health in its White Papers on the EU Health
Strategy 2008–2013 and on climate change.[11] The EU Health Strategy
states that action is needed on "emerging health threats such as those
linked to climate change, to address its potential impact on public health
and health care systems."[12] It foresees, in particular, action on adaptation
to climate change. In the White Paper on climate change, this aspect is
taken up and complemented by surveillance and control measures to be
explored by the WHO and EU agencies, such as epidemiological surveillance, the control of communicable diseases and the effects of
extreme events.[11] In 2010, the Commission published a communication
on "The EU Role in Global Health," where it is again highlighted that
climate change is a main factor in global health and that the EU would
"take global health objectives into account in implementing the collective
commitment by developed countries, in December 2009, for new and
additional resources at the 15th Conference of Parties."[13] The Commission
staff working document accompanying the Communication further states
that the EU already plays a leading role in committing to CO_2 emission
reduction targets and in the development of renewable energies. This

should be complemented by the promotion of new, healthier lifestyles to encourage more responsible and sustainable use of natural resources. In terms of global funding mechanisms, climate change conventions are seen as a source that should contribute to mitigation and adaptation measures of health services worldwide.[14] In the Council Conclusions following the Communication, climate change is identified as one of five priorities influencing global health. The EU should therefore "include consideration of health issues in the adaptation and mitigation strategies in developing countries in environmental and climate change policies and actions."[15] Yet, references to explicit challenges related to climate change cannot be found. The Council Conclusions rest rather general in relation to what the EU can do to fight global health challenges; for example, the Council "calls on the EU and its Member States to act together in all relevant internal and external policies and actions by prioritizing their support on strengthening comprehensive health systems in partner countries, which are central to all global health challenges," but does not prescribe how this should be achieved (*ibid*.: 2).

In reaction, the EU established several actions and projects to implement in particular the monitoring and control measures that were called for in the EU Health Strategy. They encompass, for instance, EUROHEIS (European Health and Environment Information System for Risk Assessment and Disease Mapping), which improves analysis, reporting and dissemination of environmental health information; EUROSUN, to monitor ultraviolet exposure in the EU and its effect on the incidence of skin cancers and cataracts; or HIALINE, which looks at the effects of climate change on airborne allergens.[a]

The EU at UNFCCC Climate Change Negotiations: Legal Basis

Mitigation and adaptation to climate change are considered two important components in the fight against health effects of climate change. They are central topics in the United Nations Framework Convention on Climate

---

[a]Available at http://ec.europa.eu/clima/sites/change/what_is_eu_doing/health_en.htm (accessed on 2 July 2012).

Change (UNFCCC) negotiations, and therefore the EU's role in the UNFCCC context will be analyzed in more detail. Within the context of the UNFCCC, the EU is recognized as a Regional Economic Integration Organisation (REIO) alongside its member states and participates as such at the Conference of the Parties (COP) meetings. The reason for this is that climate change falls within the sphere of shared competence between the EU and its Member States.[3,5] All UNFCCC matters, as well as the Kyoto Protocol, fall under shared competence (Article 4.2 TFEU). This split in competences leads to so-called mixed agreements, where neither the EU nor the Member States have the exclusive power to execute those.[4,16] They both decide "on their respective responsibilities for the performance of their obligations under the Convention" and do not exercise their rights concurrently.[17] According to Article 18 of the Convention, if an issue falls under exclusive EU competence, the EU has the right to vote with the number of votes equal to the number of Member States that are Parties to the Convention. A regional economic integration organization shall not exercise its right to vote if any of its Member States exercises its right, and vice versa. Usually, it is the Council Presidency held by an EU Member State and the Commission speaking on behalf of the Union during the COP meetings.[4] Moreover, in 2010, the Commission created two new Directorates-General, one for Energy and one for Climate Action, in order to develop and implement international and domestic climate action policies and strategies, and to lead international climate negotiations.[18]

In 2004, a system of "lead negotiators" and "issue leaders" was introduced to enhance the efficient use of expertise within the EU and to show greater coherence and continuity during the negotiations. This system entails lead negotiators over a longer period of time from various Member States, other than the current Council Presidency, and from the Commission. In cooperation with the issue leaders, the lead negotiators develop the common EU position for the negotiations.[5] Recently, since the negotiations on a post-2012 agreement have become much more political, additional issue leaders and lead negotiators have been introduced for the Ad Hoc Working Group on Further Commitments for Annex I Parties under the Kyoto Protocol (AWG-KP) and the Ad Hoc Working Group on Long-Term Cooperative Action under the Convention (AWG-LCA).[19] At the COP16 meeting in Cancun in 2010, for example, the team of negotiators for the AWG-LCA entailed the UK (lead), Poland, France and Germany.[20] The Commission provided the lead negotiator for the AWG-KP.[21]

Global Health at UNFCCC COP Negotiations

Although the EU takes part in the UNFCCC process and has recognized the importance of climate change as a threat to global health, the topic is neither explicitly mentioned in the Council Conclusions for COP15 (Copenhagen, 2009) nor in those for COP16 (Cancun, 2010) or COP17 (Durban, 2011). At the Copenhagen summit itself, where a post-Kyoto agreement should have been negotiated, the parties only adopted the so-called Copenhagen Accord, which was a general political statement without any binding framework for future climate cooperation.[22] The parties only agreed to "take note" of it and decided on the last day to extend the mandates of the AWG-LCA and the AWG-KP, which should present their results at the COP16 meeting in Cancun in December 2010.[27] The actual outcome of the negotiations was "little more than the lowest common denominator."[24] This was a major setback for the EU, as it had had contrary objectives and had been "sidelined" during the final hours of the negotiations.[25] Its degree of actorness — in terms of its capacity to behave actively and deliberately in relation to other actors — was only moderate.[26] In addition, the Union's effectiveness, in terms of goal attainment, was low, as it could not attain its two main objectives: playing a leadership role at the conference and the establishment of a legally binding agreement.[26] The EU was internally divided on issues such as emission reduction targets, climate finance or land use, land use change and forestry (LULUCF), and could not advance a common position here. Moreover, its objectives seem to have been too ambitious in comparison with other major negotiating parties, such as the US, China or Brazil. The constellation of these actors was very unsuitable for the EU (*ibid.*).

The EU's Role at the COP16 Negotiations

The main focus of the COP16 meeting in Cancun was on the two-track negotiating process to enhance long-term cooperation under the

Convention and the Protocol. Originally, this should have been already completed at the COP15 meeting in Copenhagen, but as many issues remained unresolved, the mandates of the two working groups had been expanded until Cancun. The expectations for Cancun were rather modest and several issues were identified beforehand where a balanced package of outcomes might be possible. During the two weeks, the parties were negotiating these issues in plenary sessions, contact groups, informal consultations and bilateral meetings. During the second week, the negotiations were taken up at the ministerial level.[27] The outcome of the COP16 meeting was the Cancun Agreements, one 30-page decision under the Convention and one 2-page decision under the Kyoto Protocol. Together, they are to be seen as a "Copenhagen Accord plus," since they further elaborate and complement the Copenhagen Accord.[28]

The EU's overarching objective for the negotiations in Cancun was to make stepwise progress toward establishing a post-2012 climate change regime building on the Kyoto Protocol and in this context to integrate the political guidance given in the Copenhagen Accord into a balanced set of decisions so as to pave the way for a global and comprehensive legally binding framework in the future. The EU would be willing to consider a second commitment period under the Kyoto Protocol if this was part of a wider outcome including the perspective of a global and comprehensive framework.[29] A legally binding text was not envisaged as an explicit short-term outcome of Cancun.[30] In direct comparison with 2009, the EU attained most of the objectives it was heading for during the negotiations. Most importantly, the negotiations proved that the multilateral climate process was still alive. This EU goal was fully achieved.[19,31,32] Also, the trust in the UN negotiating process was restored and Connie Hedegaard was happy that the UN process had been saved (The Guardian, 16 December 2010).[33]

In sum, the conference succeeded in "keeping the UN climate process alive" and "averting serious damage to multilateralism more broadly."[28] Besides saving the process, the participating parties agreed on the so-called Cancun Agreements. Here, important progress on substance was made in several areas, such as anchoring the mitigation pledges of developing and developed countries in the UN process, or the establishment of a Green Climate Fund, which was also one of the EU's main goals before the negotiations. Yet, it has to be acknowledged that the goals of the EU were less ambitious and much more modest at Cancun than at Copenhagen. At Copenhagen, the Union was striving for the "big bang," a new international agreement combating climate change, whereas at Cancun the EU downsized its aims and set more moderate (or more realistic) objectives that were easier to achieve and more reconcilable with those of other major negotiating parties.

The actor constellation and the interplay between other key negotiating parties and the EU seem to have been different. The US and China, the world's two largest emitters, pursued a more constructive approach in public, as far as it concerned the negotiating process, and showed more willingness to find an agreement. Before the start of the negotiations, the US and China approached each other and tried to overcome their differences of opinion. US negotiator Jonathan Pershing seemed to be optimistic. Still, he did not name any concrete points where the two countries made progress.[33] When it comes to the goals and objectives of the other key negotiating parties, the EU's main aims of securing the multilateral UN climate negotiating process and the translation of the Copenhagen Accord into a balanced package of decisions were highly compatible with other parties' preferences. The EU pursued rather modest and more realistic objectives that were closer to the positions of the US and the BASIC countries. Almost every participant of the summit shared the wish to secure the UN process after Copenhagen and to avoid another failure in order to prevent countries from diverging from the UNFCCC process and thus deterring international climate change cooperation. In this sense, Cancun was widely perceived as a "stepping stone" toward a future agreement.[27] The disaster of Copenhagen played an essential role in the course of the Cancun negotiations. It reconciled the negotiating parties in the wish to avoid another failure and to show that the climate change negotiating process was still alive.

Moreover, over the year 2010, the EU shifted its negotiating strategy and its approach to the international climate change process in reaction to Copenhagen. The EU realized that it was completely unrealistic to achieve a comprehensive and global agreement in one or two years. It then decided to do it "step by step" — what was then called the "stepwise" or "incremental" approach.[19] The new EU strategy constituted a shift of focus/attention to build alliances with new partners. Connie Hedegaard shifted the EU focus away from China and the US. She was looking for coalitions with countries willing to move forward. The EU, for example, actively participated in the Cartagena Dialogue for Progressive Action. It was able to impact on several points of the COP16 agenda together with those progressive countries, such as the acknowledgment that existing pledges needed to be strengthened, a process for clarifying these pledges as well as an ambitious work program for the future elaboration of frameworks for reporting.[28] In the context of the Global Climate Change Alliance, launched by the Commission in 2007 to deepen dialogue and cooperation on climate change between the EU and developing countries, EU representatives met with representatives of Asian developing countries in May 2010 in Dhaka, Bangladesh, and agreed to work closer together in order to mobilize international support for the fight against climate change. Besides the policy dialogue, the EU provided technical and financial support.[35] Alliance building has in the meantime become significant, because it has the capacity to prevent a complete deadlock in the UN climate negotiating process. It can additionally be used as a means of exerting pressure on parties that are not participating in those alliances which might then enhance the chance of a compromise in the framework of formal negotiations.[36]

The formation of alliances with new partners was accompanied by the abolition of the strategy to "lead by example" and to show goodwill in order to encourage others to move forward, too. Before the COP16 conference, Commissioner Hedegaard announced that the Union would not lead the way unconditionally anymore; instead, it would enter into a commitment only if others did so, too. Hence, the EU would not automatically sign a new international agreement, and in particular the US would have to commit to binding greenhouse gas emissions reduction targets.[34] At the same time, the EU was willing to consider a potential second commitment period under the Kyoto Protocol only under certain conditions: as part of a wider outcome and including the perspective of the global and comprehensive framework in which all major economies are engaged and committed to binding reduction targets.[29]

The EU's Role at the COP17 Negotiations

At the COP17 meeting in Durban in December 2011, the Parties to the Convention reached a compromise "to launch a process to develop a protocol, another legal instrument or a legal outcome under the Convention applicable to all Parties, through a subsidiary body under the Convention hereby established and to be known as the Ad Hoc Working Group on the Durban Platform for Enhanced Action."[37] This AWG should develop an agreement until no later than 2015 and the agreement should come into effect and be implemented until 2020. In addition, countries agreed on a second commitment period under the Kyoto Protocol. The second commitment period is to begin on 1 January 2013 and to end on either 31 December 2017 or 31 December 2020.[38]

The EU position for the COP17 summit is outlined in the Council Conclusions. The EU still preferred a "single global and comprehensive legally-binding agreement," but was at the same time open to a second commitment period under the Kyoto Protocol as part of a transition toward a legally binding framework.[39,40] In contrast to the Cancun climate change conference, the conditions for a further commitment under the Kyoto Protocol were delineated in the Council Conclusions, too: the roadmap and deadline for a comprehensive and legally binding global framework should enter into force until 2020, the essential elements of the Kyoto Protocol should be preserved, its environmental integrity guaranteed and its architecture further enhanced.[39,40] So, at the core of the Durban negotiating agenda was operationalizing the Cancun agreements, achieving a balanced package that would extend the Kyoto Protocol, and paving the way for the process to find a followup agreement.[38]

At the Durban conference, health was — for the first time since 1992 — taken note of within the UNFCCC framework as a key goal of climate policies and as a priority in climate mitigation and adaptation actions.[41] The UK-based Climate and Health Council, the NGO Health Care Without Harm and the Nelson R. Mandela School of Medicine at the University of KwaZulu Natal, in partnership with the World Health Organization, the World Medical Association and the International Council of Nurses, organized on 4 December 2011 the first Climate and Health Summit as a side event parallel to the COP17 summit. The event hosted over 200 participants from more than 30 countries, who adopted the Durban Declaration[b] and the Health Sector Call to Action.[c,42] The signers of the Durban Declaration call on the COP17 negotiators to recognize the health benefits of climate mitigation and to take "bold and substantive action" to reduce global greenhouse gas emissions, to ensure greater health sector representation on national delegations and within the bodies of the UNFCCC, to adopt a strong second commitment period of the Kyoto Protocol and to negotiate a "fair, ambitious and binding agreement," consistent with the Prescription for a Healthy Planet, endorsed by more than 130 health organizations in Copenhagen in 2009, by 2015 (Durban Declaration on Climate and Health).[43] The signers comprise mainly NGOs — neither states nor the EU.

The EU continued with the negotiating strategy that it had developed for the COP16 summit. First, it stayed with its stepwise approach instead of aiming at the adoption of a new legally binding agreement.[39] Second, it kept on building alliances with African and smaller states. The Alliance of Small Island States (AOSIS) decided to form an alliance with the EU as well as with the least developed countries (LDCs), as they feared that there would be no second commitment period under the Kyoto Protocol.[44] They altogether tried to push for an ambitious outcome and they were in this context ready to take up concrete obligations.[45] Hence, for the first time, the states of the Cartagena Dialogue and other LDCs openly supported the EU position and joined its demand for a new climate agreement.[46,47] At the same time, the group G77 did not act homogenously in public anymore. Many developing countries were no longer willing to tolerate China's and India's refusals to undertake climate action, and to release them from their responsibility. They were concerned that both countries did not advocate the developing countries' interests.[44,46] The alliance between the EU, the AOSIS and the LDCs brought "a sense of direction and pace into the negotiations as the countdown to the end of the

---

[b]Available at http://www.climateandhealthcare.org/wp-content/uploads/2011/12/Durban-Declaration-on-Climate-and-Health-Final.pdf (accessed on 12 Febuary 2013).
[c]Available at http://www.climateandhealthcare.org/wp-content/uploads/2011/12/Durban-Global-Climate-and-Health-Call-to-Action-Final.pdf (accessed on 12 February 2013).

Conference began".[38] Third, the EU took a "hardline stance" and, again, would not lead by example anymore, as already at the COP16 conference.[48] Overall, the EU was able to give impetus to the negotiations and the text which was finally followed most of the EU roadmap: "The EU drafted the script for the central plot in Durban by setting out their stall early in the process and offering to do the heavy lifting to save the Kyoto Protocol within the context of a roadmap that put up a challenge to other parties — developing and developed".[38] It also seems that Connie Hedegaard had quite a lot of influence on the negotiating process as she drafted the EU strategy to build alliances with developed and developing countries and forced China to acknowledge to take on commitments, too. In turn, she offered the extension of the Kyoto Protocol, and thus she managed to take the US in, too.[43] Generally speaking, the EU took up a leadership role again at the Durban conference and was quite successful in achieving its own goals as well as an outcome with substance.

The EU's Role at Rio+20

The United Nations Conference on Development, Rio+20, on 20–22 June 2012, was dominated by the concept of a green economy, which was also advanced by the EU as a means of achieving sustainable development globally.[49] In the Union's view, a economy is essential to promote "human health and well-being and hence eradicate poverty" (*ibid.*). It aimed at the adoption of a green economy roadmap with timetables for specific goals, objectives and actions. Furthermore, the EU saw the work on sustainable development goals (SDGs) as an important element of progress, also with regard to the review process of the Millennium Development Goals (MDGs). The outcome of the Rio+20 conference was the resolution "The Future We Want,"[50] which contained several important health references in the end. However, it had taken common efforts from health ministries all over the world to get such health related language into the resolution.

Conclusion and Outlook

The EU — in particular the European Commission — recognized the importance of the relationship between climate change and global health in its White Papers on the EU Health Strategy 2008–2013 and on climate change.[11] Yet, it did not focus on this issue in the actual climate change negotiating process, nor does it seem that the EU pulled its weight to put health on the negotiating agenda. Other controversial topics were in the foreground, such as the second commitment period under the Kyoto Protocol, the process to find a successor agreement, or climate finance. The EU's role in climate change negotiations changed over the years, from a leader during the last two decades to a sidelined or marginalized actor at Copenhagen. Copenhagen constitutes a break in the history of climate change. Afterward, the EU "learned from its mistakes" and adopted a new negotiating strategy that encompassed, *inter alia,* a "stepwise approach" to adopting new climate legislation, the building of alliances with AOSIS and LDCs which are willing to move forward, too, and the end of the so-called "leading by example." For example, it imposed conditions for the continuation of the Kyoto Protocol, which it did not do before Copenhagen. As a result, it apparently regained some of the leadership it had lost at the Copenhagen conference.[51] However, at the most recent summit in Doha in 2012, EU internal conflicts over reduction targets came up again and weakened the EU's negotiating position. It became clear that the EU would reach the 20% reduction target earlier, by 2015, and other states pressured the EU to adopt a more ambitious target which was openly blocked by Poland during the final plenary session.[52,53] So, it seems that the EU's role in climate change negotiations has not yet been consolidated and is still very much subject to the negotiating context and EU internal divisions or disputes. As regards health aspects in climate change policies, the EU seems to be a follower of developments rather than a leader.

References

1. Kelemen RD. (2010) Globalizing European Union environmental policy. *Journal of European Public Policy* **17(3):** 335–349.
2. Bretherton C, Vogler J. (2006) *The European Union as a Global Actor.* Routledge, London.
3. Groenleer M, van Schaik L. (2007) United we stand? The European Union's international actorness in the cases of the International Criminal Court and the Kyoto Protocol. *Journal of Common Market Studies* **45(5):** 969–998.

4. Lacasta NS. *et al.* (2002) Consensus among many voices: articulating the European Union's position on climate change. *Golden Gate University Law Review* **32(4):** 352–353.

5. Oberthür S, Roche Kelly C. (2008) EU leadership in international climate policy: achievements and challenges. *The International Spectator* **43(3):** 35–50.

6. Vogler J. (2009) Climate change and EU foreign policy: the negotiation of burden sharing. *International Politics* **46(4):** 469–490.

7. McMichael AJ, Woodruff ER, Hales S. (2006) Climate change and human health: present and future risks. *The Lancet* **367(9513):** 859–869.

8. Wiley LF. (2010) Mitigation/adaptation and health: health policymaking in the global response to climate change and implications for other upstream determinants. *The Journal of Law, Medicine & Ethics* **38(3):** 629–639.

9. St Louis ME, Hess JJ. (2008) Climate change: impacts on and implications for global health. *American Journal of Preventive Medicine* **35(5):** 527–538.

10. Wiley LF, Gostin LO. (2009) The international response to climate change: an agenda for global health. *The Journal of the American Medical Association* **302(11):** 1218–1220.

11. European Commission. (2009) White Paper Adapting to Climate Change: Towards a European Framework for Action. Brussels, 1 April 2009. COM (2009) 147/4.

12. European Commission. (2007) White Paper Together for Health: A Strategic Approach for the EU 2008–2013. Brussels, 23 October 2007. COM (2007) 630.

13. European Commission. (2010a) Communication from the Commission to the Council, the European Parliament, the European Economic and Social Committee and the Committee of the Regions: The EU Role in Global Health. Brussels, 31 March 2010. COM (2010) 128.
Guigner, S. 2009. The EU and the health dimension of globalization: Playing the World Health Organization Card. In The European Union and the social dimension of globalization: How the EU influences the world, eds. J. Orbie and L. Tortell, 131–147. Routledge Abingdon.

14. European Commission. (2010b) Commission Staff Working Document Global Health — Responding to the Challenges of Globalisation. Brussels, 31 March 2010. SEC (2010) **380:** 18.

15. Council of the European Union. (2010a) Council Conclusions on the EU Role in Global Health. 3011th Foreign Affairs Council Meeting, Brussels, 10 May 2010, p. 4.
16. Lenschow A. (2010) Environmental policy: contending dynamics of policy change. In: Wallace H, Pollack MA, Young AR (eds.), *Policy-Making in the European Union*. Oxford University Press, Oxford, pp. 307–330.
17. UNFCCC. (1992) Text of the Convention. Available at http://unfccc.int/essential_background/convention/background/items/2853.php (accessed on 14 December 2011).
18. European Commission. (2010c) Commission Creates Two New Directorates-General for Energy and Climate Action. Brussels, 17 February 2010. IP/10/164.
19. Interview with EU Council Secretariat representative by telephone. 19 January 2012.
20 Emerson E, *et al.* (2011), *Upgrading the EU's Role as Global Actor — Institutions, Law and the Restructuring of European Diplomacy*. Brussels: Centre for European Policy Studies.
21. Interview with European Commission delegate by telephone. 10 January 2012.
22. Hunter D. (2010) Implications of the Copenhagen Accord for Global Climate Governance. *Sustainable Development Law & Policy* **10(2):** 4–15, 56–57.
24. Falkner R, Stephan H, Vogler J. (2010) International climate policy after Copenhagen: towards a "building blocks" approach. *Global Policy* **1(3):** 252–262.
25. Kilian B, Elgström O. (2010) Still a green leader? The European Union's role in international climate negotiations. *Cooperation and Conflict* **45(3):** 255–273.
26. Groen L, Niemann A. (2013) 'The European Union at the Copenhagen Climate Negotiations: A Case of Contested EU Actorness and Effectiveness'. *International Relations* **27(3):** 308–324.
27. IISD. (2010) *Earth Negotiations Bulletin* **12(498)**. COP16 Final, 13 December 2010. Available at http://www.iisd.ca/climate/cop16/ (accessed on 14 December 2011).
28. Oberthür S. (2011) Global climate governance after Cancun: options for EU leadership. *The International Spectator* **46(1):** 5–13.
29. Council of the European Union. (2010b) Environment Council of Ministers Conclusions. Brussels, 14 October 2010. 14957/10.

30. Hedegaard C. (2010a) Speech at the plenary debate on preparations for the Cancún Climate Conference (29 November–10 December). European Parliament plenary debate, Strasbourg, 24 November 2010. SPEECH/ 10/687.

31. Hedegaard C. (2010b) Speech at the European Parliament plenary debate on the outcome of the Cancún Climate Conference. Strasbourg, 14 December 2010. SPEECH/10//55.

32. Interview with German delegate by telephone. 21 February 2012.
    Bialek D. (2010) How trust was restored at Cancún. The Guardian, 16 December 2010. Available at http://www.guardian.co.uk/environment/ 2010/dec/16/cancun-climate-change-conference-2010-climate-change (accessed on 13 February 2012).

33. *Spiegel Online*. (2010) USA verkünden Annäherung mit China. 30 November 2010. Available at http://www.spiegel.de/wissenschaft/natur/0,1518,731894, 00.html (accessed on 13 February 2012).

34. *Spiegel Online*. (2010) EU will nicht mehr Vorreiter spielen. 14 September 2010. Available at http://www.spiegel.de/wissenschaft/natur/0,1518,717450, 00.html (accessed on 13 February 2012).

35. European Commission. (2010d) Global Climate Change Alliance Regional Conference for Asia. Brussels, 31 May 2010. IP/10/642.
    Seidler C. (2010) Klimapolitiker feiern Cancún-Kompromiss. *Spiegel Online*, 11 December 2010. Available at http://www.spiegel.de/wissenschaft/ natur/0,1518,734136,00.html (accessed on 25 February 2012).

36. Fischer S, Leinen J. (2010) Kurskorrekturen auf dem Weg nach Cancún: Die Europäische Union in der internationalen Klimapolitik. *Friedrich-Ebert-Stiftung Internationale Politikanalyse*. Available at http://library.fes.de/ pdf-files/id/ipa/07635.pdf (accessed on 14 September 2011).

37. UNFCCC. (2011) Report of the Conference of the Parties on its seventeenth session, held in Durban from 28 November to 11 December 2011. Available at http://unfccc.int/resource/docs/2011/cop17/eng/09a01.pdf (accessed on 19 November 2011).

38. IISD. (2011a) *Earth Negotiations Bulletin* **12(534)**. COP17 Final, 13 December 2011. Available at http://www.iisd.ca/download/pdf/enb12534e .pdf (accessed on 19 November 2011).

39. Council of the European Union. (2011) Environment Council of Ministers Conclusions. Brussels, 10 October 2011. 15353/11.

40. European Commission. (2011) Durban must deliver a roadmap for climate action by all major economies. European Commission Press Release. IP/11/1436.

41. World Health Organization. (2011) Health issues gain traction at UN climate conference. Available at http://www.who.int/globalchange/mediacentre/events/2011/durban_conference_update/en/index.html (accessed on 20 November 2012).

42. IISD. (2011b) First Global Climate and Health Summit Adopts Durban Declaration. 4 December 2011. Available at http://climate-l.iisd.org/news/first-global-climate-and-health-summit-adopts-durban-declaration (accessed on 20 November 2012).

43. The Guardian (2011). Durban talks: how Connie Hedegaard got countries to agree a climate deal. 11 December 2011. Available at http://www.guardian.co.uk/environment/2011/dec/11/connie-hedegaard-duban-climate-talks (accessed on 15 January 2013).
    World Health Organization. (2011) Health issues gain traction at UN Climate Conference. Available at http://www.who.int/globalchange/mediacentre/events/2011/durban_conference_update/en/index.html (accessed on 20 November 2012).

44. Banerjee SB. (2012) A climate for change? Critical reflections on the Durban United Nations Climate Change Conference. *Organization Studies* **33(12):** 1761–1786.

45. South African Government News Agency. (2011) EU teams up with smaller states at COP17. Available at http://www.sanews.gov.za/south-africa/eu-teams-smaller-states-cop17 (accessed on 20 November 2012).

46. Dröge S. (2012) Die Klimaverhandlungen in Durban, *Stiftung Wissenschaft und Politik Aktuell*. Available at http://www.swp-berlin.org/de/publikationen/swp-aktuell-de/swp-aktuell-detail/article/klimaverhandlungen_in_durban.html (accessed on 15 January 2013).

47. The Guardian (2011). African nations move closer to EU position at Durban climate change talks. 8 December 2011. Available at http://www.theguardian.com/environment/2011/dec/08/african-eu-durban-climate-change (accessed on 15 January 2013).

48. The Guardian (2011). EU takes hardline stance at UN climate talks. 30 November 2011. Available at http://www.guardian.co.uk/environment/2011/nov/30/europe-hardline-un-climate-talks (accessed on 19 November 2012).

Vidal J, Harvey F. (2011) African nations move closer to EU position at Durban climate change talks. *The Guardian*, 8 December 2011. Available at http://www.guardian.co.uk/environment/2011/dec/08/african-eu-durban-climate-change (accessed on 15 January 2013).

49. Council of the European Union. (2012) Rio+20: Pathway to a Sustainable Future — Council Conclusions Brussels, 9 March 2012.

50. United Nations. (2012) The Future We Want: Resolution Adopted by the General Assembly, 11 September 2012. A/RES/66/288.

51. Groen L, Niemann A, Oberthür, S. (2012) 'The EU as a global leader? The Copenhagen and Cancún UN climate change negotiations'. *Journal of Contemporary European Research* **8(2):** 173–191.

52. The Guardian (2012). Doha climate talks: EU weakened over new emission targets. 23 November 2012. Available at http://www.guardian.co.uk/environment/2012/nov/23/doha-climate-talks-eu-weakened-emissions (accessed on 15 January 2013).

53. Seidler C. (2012) Brechstangen-Taktik bringt Klima-Kompromiss. *Spiegel Online*, 8 December 2012. Available at http://www.spiegel.de/wissenschaft/mensch/klimagipfel-in-doha-al-attija-haemmert-entscheidungen-durch-a-871774.html (accessed on 15 January 2013).

7

Research, Development and Innovation for Global Health

*Stephen A. Matlin** and Samantha Battams*†

There is no single Commission or Council document that defines the EU's principles, policies and strategies on research, development and innovation (RDI) for global health. Some elements are stated in a range of documents or in lower level Commission staff working papers such as the Commission Staff Working Document "European Research and Knowledge for Global Health" [SWC (2010) 381 final] of 31 March 2010, which accompanied the Commission's Communication on the EU role in global health; some may be deduced from diverse EU policies and strategies. This chapter attempts to draw these together, examine them for coherence and consistency, and point out gaps and future needs.

We first consider the concept of global health, as set out in official EU documents, along with the scope of RDI. Second, we consider the EU's policy goals in RDI and how it is meeting them. Third, we explore key challenges for current EU policy on RDI. Fourth, we reflect upon the key messages and conclusions on the EU's role in global health RDI.

*Senior Fellow, Global Health Programme, Graduate Institute of International and Development Studies, Geneva; Adjunct Professor, Institute of Global Health Innovation, Imperial College London; and Head of Strategic Development in the International Organization for Chemical Sciences in Development.

†Associate Professor and Public Health Programme Director, Torrens Universit, Australia and Senior Lecturer, Southgate Institute of Health, Society & Equity, Flinders University, South Australia.

Introduction: Scope of the Field

Global Health

To date, there is no widely agreed definition of "global health" and it is often used interchangeably with other terms, such as "public health" and "international health." The absence of consensus on the scope of the field[1-7] creates potential for confusion about the scope and purpose of relevant research.

The EU sets out its role in the Council Conclusions on the EU's Role in Global Health[8] and in the related EC Communication.[9] The latter, while acknowledging the lack of a broadly agreed definition of "global health," considers that it is

> . . . about worldwide improvement of health, reduction of disparities, and protection against global health threats. Addressing global health requires coherence of all internal and external policies and actions based on agreed principles.

The Commission Staff Working Document[10] amplifies why collective action at global level is needed for R&D for global public goods lacking in fields that would benefit health in low and middle income countries (LMICs).

In 2008 the EU had articulated a new health strategy, including global health, in a White Paper.[11,12] This notes that:

> The EC can contribute to global health by sharing its values, experience and expertise, as well as by taking concrete steps to improve health. Work can support efforts to ensure coherence between its internal and external health policies in attaining global health goals, to consider health as an important element in the fight against poverty through health-related aspects of external development cooperation with low income countries, to respond to health threats in third countries, and to encourage implementation of international health agreements such as the World Health Organization's (WHO) Framework Convention on Tobacco Control (FCTC) and International Health Regulations (IHR).

The strategy defines four fundamental principles for EU action on health: a strategy based on shared health values; "health is the greatest wealth"; health in all policies; and strengthening the EU's voice in global health.

The approach that the strategy proposes for the EU includes:

- The EU Member States and the Commission can create better health outcomes for EU citizens and for others through sustained collective leadership in global health.
- In a globalized world it is hard to separate national or EU-wide actions from global policy, as global health issues have an impact on internal Community health policy and vice versa. The EU can contribute to global health by sharing its values, experience and expertise, as well as by taking concrete steps to improve health.
- The EU's contribution to global health requires interaction across policy areas such as health, development cooperation, external action, research and trade. Strengthened coordination on health issues with international organizations, e.g. the WHO and other relevant UN agencies (such as the International Labour Organization), the World Bank, the OECD and the Council of Europe, as well as other strategic partners and countries, will also enhance the EU's voice in global health and increase its influence and visibility to match its economic and political weight.

Research, Development and Innovation (RDI)

Both research and development (R&D) take place within innovation environments that are regulated to different extents at national, regional and global levels, and enable the processes and products they generate to be brought into practical use. In the health field, RDI has yielded a large number of products and healthcare technologies[13] that have not only improved health but also contributed substantially to wealth on a global scale. The global health research and innovation system addresses innovation failures in science, the market or public health, which has been crucial to reducing health inequities.[14]

The social determinants of health approach, reflected in "health in all policies" embraced by the EU,[15] has been mirrored by a broadening of the fields seen as relevant to RDI for global health, in particular:

- *Research for health*[16] is research in any discipline(s) undertaken to understand the impact on health of policies, programs, processes, actions or events originating in any sector and encompassing biological, economic, environmental, political, social and other determinants of health.
- *Innovation for health and health equity* is an initiative in any sector(s) that takes up novel ideas, inventions or processes and applies them to achieving improved health and greater health equity.[17] The Europe 2020 agenda stresses that a combination of social innovation (involving new ways to manage people, processes and information) and technological innovation is essential.[18,19]

Intersectoral and interdisciplinary[20] action is fundamental to both practice and research in global health. As noted by MacLachlan,[21] the concept of research for health[22] is broad and, as endorsed in the Bamako Call for Action on Research for Health,[23] requires that we "rethink our approach to research in global and public health and to complement narrow research specializations with a new cadre of researchers who have expertise concerning the context and process of research, as well as its content, and the interplay of these knowledge domains." MacLachlan considers that the new approach could greatly facilitate better research utilization, helping policy-makers and practitioners work through more evidence-based practice and across traditional research boundaries.

Elements of the EU's Role in RDI for Global Health

In this section we consider the EU's policy goals in relation to RDI for global health and examine how the EU is meeting these goals, including through its stance on UN health debates and initiatives.

Policy Goals

The Council Conclusions (Paragraph 18)[8] call on the EU and its Member States "to promote effective and fair financing of research that benefits the health of all," with the EU ensuring that "innovations and interventions produce products and services that are accessible and affordable." This should be achieved by:

- "Working towards a global framework for research and development that addresses the priority health needs of developing countries and prioritises pertinent research actions to tackle global health challenges in accordance with the WHO Global Research Strategy."
- Building research capacity in public health and health systems.
- Exploring models that disassociate the cost of R&D and the prices of medicines in relation to the WHO Global Strategy and Plan of Action on Public Health, Innovation and Intellectual Property.
- Ensuring that EU public investments in health research secure access to the knowledge and tools generated as a global public good.
- Strengthening and balancing the complete health research process of innovation, implementation, access, monitoring, and evaluation, and promoting international cooperation in research.
- Improving health information systems of partner countries and the collection of quality and comparable data and statistics to enable benchmarking and inform on the impacts of global and national policies on social determinants in health, including the adoption of equity indicators.
- Taking into account evidence when setting normative action regarding products and technology, while taking into account the precautionary principle.

With these recommendations, the Council drew heavily from the Commission's Communication on the EU Role in Global Health[9] (Paragraphs. 3.4 and 4.4), thus largely following the Commission's suggestions on research and health R&D.

Against this background of goals and aspirations that the EU has set out, how has the EU actually performed? We examine this question from three broad perspectives:

- Engagement in global policies and partnership initiatives.
- Funding for global health R&D.
- Capacity-strengthening for R&D in LMICs.

EU Engagement in Global Health R&D Policies and Partnership Initiatives

UN debates and initiatives

HIV/AIDS. Global health has gained increasing political importance in international affairs[24,25] and has been addressed by the UN General Assembly (GA) on several occasions, the first being a Special Session (UNGASS) on HIV/AIDS in 2001, at which a statement[26] made by the Head of the EC Delegation, on behalf of the European Community, included three key paragraphs on R&D aspects:

14. The EC also underlines the importance of global rules on intellectual property rights in promoting investments in new medicines, and especially vaccines....

15. The EC recalls the right of the members of the World Trade Organisation (WTO) to invoke the relevant provisions of the Agreement on Trade-Related Intellectual Property Rights (TRIPS) to address national health policy concerns... by, *inter alia*, using discretion to grant compulsory licenses in certain exceptional circumstances provided the conditions of Article 31 of the TRIPS Agreement are fulfilled....

16. It is also our intention to increase significantly the financial support for R&D.

Up to today, the Commission has also been one of the major funders of the Global Fund on AIDS, TB and malaria.

Non-communicable diseases (NCDs). A UN high level meeting[27] on NCD prevention and control in 2011 generated a GA political resolution.[28]

This recognized that NCDs are a worldwide problem and the largest single cause of mortality globally (with 80% of deaths occurring in LMICs), which can be largely prevented or reduced with an approach that incorporates evidence-based, affordable, cost-effective, population-wide and multisectoral interventions. As regards research, the meeting called for an approach that:

- Encourages alliances and networks, bringing together national, regional and global actors for the development of new medicines, vaccines, diagnostics and technologies.
- Strengthens international cooperation, *inter alia*, by promoting the development and dissemination of appropriate, affordable and sustainable transfer of technology on mutually agreed terms and the production of affordable, safe, effective and quality medicines and vaccines.
- Promotes actively national and international investments and strengthens national capacity for quality research and development, while continuing to incentivize innovation.
- Supports and facilitates NCD-related research, and its translation, to enhance the knowledge base for ongoing national, regional and global action.

Delivering the EU's statement at the UN meeting, the then-Commissioner for Health and Consumer Policy, John Dalli,[29] noted that "NCDs' heavy impact on people's health, as well on economic development, requires efficient coordinated action at global level," and that "the EU is determined to take forward the declaration in partnership with the global community."

The need for new technologies for NCDs, including R&D on pharmaceuticals and diagnostics, especially to meet the conditions experienced in LMICs, has also been highlighted in the literature.[30] Although most health R&D globally is invested in NCDs, the specific focus of attention on health technologies suited to the prevention and treatment of NCDs in LMICs remains a neglected field. The importance of this is illustrated by examples such as the problematic access to drugs for breast cancer[31] and for hepatitis C.[32,33]

The Commission has instituted an "action" on chronic NCD research activities, which will identify and analyze current EU-funded, as well as national and regional, research programs and initiatives on chronic NCDs. This will map the scale, scope and fields of NCD research activities, with a view to identifying potential overlaps, synergies, gaps and opportunities for collaboration, which should contribute to developing evidence-based policies supporting coordinated approaches in chronic NCD research.[34]

Health and foreign policy. The UN Secretary General's report[35] for a 2010 GA debate on health and foreign policy identified the health-related challenges that must be addressed by foreign policy-makers and the key foreign policy issues that have a significant impact on health, including the need for:

- Ensuring access to/or affordability of medicines, including through fostering innovation; implementing the Global Strategy and Plan of Action on Public Health, Innovation and Intellectual Property.
- Implementing the right to use, to the full, the provisions contained in the TRIPS Agreement.
- Overcoming disagreements on the sharing of the benefits (vaccines, drugs, diagnostics) that might arise from conducting research on samples of biological materials obtained in surveillance and response for pandemics such as avian influenza A (H5N1).

The report concludes, "The level of foreign policy involvement and interest in global health has grown dramatically, making the relationship between global health and foreign policy an increasingly important issue for the UN, WHO, many intergovernmental organizations and processes and national Governments... [reinforcing] the importance of concerted and sustained international cooperation...."

EU responses to this growing connection between foreign policy and global health have included the creation in 2005 of the European Centre for Disease Prevention and Control (ECDC) as an EU agency charged with strengthening Europe's defences against infectious diseases[36] and the inclusion of health activities within the EU–Africa strategic partnership established in 2007.[37] The combined work of the EU and other regional organizations such as the Association of Southeast Asian Nations (ASEAN), the African Union (AU) and the Pan American Health Organization

(PAHO) is considered to have contributed to strengthening health systems, increasing accessibility to health coverage and facilitating dialogue among member states, international institutions, and non-state actors.[38]

Intellectual property (IP). The EU's stance on matters relating to IP and TRIPS has not consistently matched the ideal of the EC's statement to the 2001 UNGASS (see above). For example:

- The EU's initial position in bilateral trade negotiations with LMICs has sometimes proposed removing TRIPS flexibilities and instead required new obligations not only exceeding TRIPS requirements, but also surpassing the EU's own legal regime, such as in negotiations with some Latin American countries.[39]
- A number of European-based NGOs such as Wemos have expressed concern that recent trade negotiations such as the Trans-Atlantic Trade and Investment Partnership threaten to undermine public health, with fears of more data protection for certain treatments (e.g. diagnostics) and poorer access to such treatments and generic medications.[40]
- In 2010, Brazil and India requested consultations pursuant to the WTO Dispute Settlement Understanding against the EU over the seizure of generic drugs in transit through the Netherlands, complaining that EU and Dutch regulations apparently allowed customs officials to detain goods in transit to Latin America and Africa through European ports and airports on grounds of infringing IP rights. Although no IP rights were infringed by either the manufacturer or the recipient (the drugs not being under patent in either country), Dutch patents on the medicines blocked release of the goods in transit under the EU's application of patent rights. Brazil and India claimed in two rounds of consultations that this violated WTO rules and required Members to provide freedom of transit through their territories. They also invoked a breach of the Doha Declaration on TRIPS and Public Health, which confirmed that the agreement "can and should be interpreted and implemented in a manner supportive of WTO Members' right to protect public health and, in particular, to promote access to medicines for all."[41] Responding to this, the Commission published guidance and also, in the review of Regulation 1383/2003,[42] clarified, in the interest

of legal certainty, that the transit of medicines should not be hampered in the absence of a substantial risk of diversion of the goods onto the EU market.[43]

Globally coordinated action on health R&D

One concern of global health is R&D for the creation of global public goods,[44,45] including diagnostics, prevention and treatment for diseases predominantly found in poor countries and for which market mechanisms have hitherto failed to provide solutions. The last decade has seen a succession of global efforts to address this issue,[46] leading to agreement on a WHO Global Strategy and Plan of Action on Public Health, Innovation and Intellectual Property (GSPOA). The EU (Member States and EC) as well as strong advocacy from civil society, played a significant role in the inter-governmental negotiations leading to its formulation and subsequent adoption.[9,47] At the 68th WHA, the extension of the Global Strategy and Plan of Action on Public Health, Innovation and Intellectual Property was supported after initial delay, largely due to leadership towards compromise by South Africa. As we saw in the previous part, the EU Council Conclusions on the EU Role in Global Health call on the EU and its Member States to ensure that innovations and interventions produce products and services that are accessible and affordable, to be achieved through, among other actions, exploring models that disassociate the cost of R&D and the prices of medicines in relation to the GSPOA, including the opportunities for EU technology transfer to developing countries. The EC Staff Working Document on the European research and knowledge for global health[10] observes that new approaches to incentives, financial mechanisms and coordination of stakeholders are necessary to address the very different issues when either no product exists to address specific health needs of the poor or existing medical products are not accessible and affordable for poor communities.

The Commission has been a major supporter of the WHO's implementation of the GSPOA, including through provision by EuropeAid of (1) financing for work by the Special Programme for Research & Training in Tropical Diseases (TDR) to develop a platform for research needs on infectious diseases of poverty as well as a comprehensive overview of global research investments in this area (€2 million); in partnership with TDR, financing of establishment of sustainable innovation networks at regional level in order to build capacity, manage, facilitate coordination and provide funds for health product R&D innovation in Africa, Asia and Latin America, and enhance South–South collaboration (€5 million); and (3) in a joint initiative with WHO and others, financing to identify the main challenges and obstacles to local production of pharmaceuticals, vaccines and diagnostics relevant to public health needs of developing countries, as well as related transfer of technology, and to provide evidence-based recommendations on their feasibility and sustainability (€2.184 million).[48]

Global Health R&D Convention. Following agreement on the GSPOA, a followup process was set in place by the WHO to operationalize some of its key areas, including the financing and coordination of R&D for health products especially needed by LMICs. An Expert Working Group examined this area, but its 2010 report[49] was not broadly accepted. Subsequently a Consultative Expert Working Group (CEWG) on R&D: Financing and Coordination was established and the key recommendation of its 2012 report was for a binding international R&D convention,[50,51] which would address the dearth of drugs for diseases predominantly or exclusively affecting poor countries, by delinking the costs of R&D from the prices of medicines, generating public funds to finance R&D and a coordinated priority-setting mechanism to allocate the resources. The proposals were discussed by the World Health Assemble in 2012; subsequently in November 2012 at an a Open Ended Meeting of Member States which WHO was asked to organize to consider the matter further; and then by Executive Boards and World Health Assembliles in 2013–15.[52,53,54,55] In following up the CEWG Report, there was little appetite by countries for engaging in negotiations for a Global Health R&D Convention. However, other elements in the proposals did receive support — for the establishment of a Global Health R&D Observatory; for the organization and conduct of a set of Demonstration Projects; and for the creation of a pooled fund for voluntary contributions towards R&D for diseases of relevance to LMICs. Each of these is valuable in its own right as a step to strengthen global capacities in health R&D; but in addition they support one another and could help to pave the way for a Global Health R&D Convention at some later time.

The 2010 Council Conclusions on global health recognized the need for a global R&D framework and supported the GSPOA. Support for the follow-up process to the GSPOA and CEWG afforded an important opportunity for the EU to demonstrate its practical commitment to its global health principles. However, there has been no concrete EU support for the follow-up to the CEWG proposals. In the early stages the EU supported delaying debates, probably reflecting the ambiguous and still evolving positions of its own Member States on this controversial[56,57] issue. At the 65th WHA, the EC expressed the view that more clarity and discussion were required before entering into a legally binding global R&D agreement[58] and supported a draft resolution which just "noted" the CEWG report and called for informal in-depth discussions on the CEWG which were not limited to the recommendations of the CEWG.[59] At the following 62nd Session of the WHO Regional Committee for Europe, the EU statement[60] emphasized that *"the solutions should be found through strengthening coordination"* and *"it did not support legal reform."* The emphasis on "coordination" reflects an aspect of the position in the EC Communication, which also stresses the importance of joint priority setting in research processes; safeguarding access to knowledge; research capacity building in LMICs; translating research and knowledge generated into policy and practice; and the need to link with others for the development of health information systems. Significant advances[61] were made in the follow-on to the CEWG report at the 66th WHA in May 2013, which approved the draft resolution from the November 2012 Open Ended Meeting of Member States and also the "decision point" proposed[62] by the USA. The CEWG resolution contains three areas of action: establishing a global health R&D observatory; setting up demonstration projects; and developing norms and standards to better collect data on health R&D. The establishment of a global health R&D observatory, based in the Special Programme in Tropical Diseases at WHO, has made considerable progress and the observatory is due to launch in 2016.[63] A process for establishing demonstration projects has also been agreed and a number were selected by open completion and funded through voluntary contributions.[64] The EC has not, to date, made any contributions to either the global observatory of demonstration projects.[65]

EU Funding for Global Health R&D

Framework programs for research and technological development (FPs)

The EU budget, including funds for research, is proposed by the European Commission and forwarded to the budgetary authority — the European Parliament and the Council, which discuss, agree on and adopt the budget. If there is disagreement between Parliament and Council, they engage in a process of conciliation. The final decision rests with the Parliament.[66]

The EU's main instrument for supporting research and building the European Research Area (ERA)[67] involves successive multi-year FPs, the first (FP1: €3.75 billion), from 1984 to 1988, up to the seventh (FP7: €55 billion), from 2007 to 2013. The Research Framework Programme for 2014–2020, Horizon 2020, has a financial envelope of €79.4 billion.[68] Most FP funds go to research actors in Europe and beyond, co-financing research, technological development and demonstration projects. The highly competitive grants are determined on the basis of calls for proposals and a peer review process.[69]

A number of important health research initiatives were supported by earlier FPs, including health systems research (HSR). A report[70] by an independent expert panel in 2004 on 20 years of experience of support for HSR in the EC INCO-DEV program for S&T cooperation in research for development concluded that it had made a significant contribution to funding HSR and building the capacity of institutions and individuals in both Europe and developing countries and contributed to the creation of solid partnerships. The areas highlighted for further attention included encouraging more HSR learning and capacity development and transfer of existing knowledge through equitable North–South, South–South and South–North partnerships; greater investment in further strengthening capacities both for research and for using research findings, particularly in developing countries; the need for clear prioritization mechanisms; and greater support for the development and maintenance of Regional Health System Observatories to collect and disseminate regionally based evidence.

EU research framework programme 7

The seventh Research Framework Programme was structured into four types of activities: transnational cooperation on policy-defined themes (Cooperation), investigator-driven research based on the initiative of the research community (Ideas), support for training and career development of researchers (People), and support for research capacities (Capacities).

Within the "Cooperation" program (overall budget €32.413 billion for 2007–2013), Health was one of ten thematic areas and, with a budget of €6.1 billion, the biggest research area. The ICT (eHealth) Theme contained an additional €450 million. The objective was the following:

> Improving the health of European citizens and increasing the competitiveness and boosting the innovative capacity of European health-related industries and businesses, while addressing global health issues including emerging epidemics. Emphasis will be put on translational research (translation of basic discoveries in clinical applications, including scientific validation of experimental results), the development and validation of new therapies, methods for health promotion and prevention including promotion of child health, healthy ageing, diagnostic tools and medical technologies, as well as sustainable and efficient healthcare systems.

The areas of translational research highlighted included major infectious diseases that are major threats to public health, and chronic diseases.[71,72]

International cooperation is an integral part of the Theme and is of particular importance for areas addressing global health problems, such as antimicrobial resistance, HIV/AIDS, malaria, tuberculosis, neglected diseases and emerging pandemics. Specific cooperation actions, implemented through bi-regional dialogues as well as within the context of the MDGs and adapted to local needs and through partnerships, may include: health policy research, health systems and healthcare service research, maternal and child health, reproductive health, control and surveillance of neglected communicable diseases. International cooperation includes actions designed to enhance the participation of researchers and research institutions from third countries in the thematic areas; specific cooperation actions where there is mutual interest in cooperating on particular topics selected on the basis of the scientific and technological level and the needs of the countries concerned; cooperative activities targeted at developing and emerging countries, focusing on their particular needs in fields such as health, including research into neglected diseases.

The aim is that international cooperation supports and promotes "European competitiveness" through strategic research partnerships with third countries, including highly industrialized and emerging economies in science and technology. This will be done by engaging the best third country scientists to work in and with Europe; developing cooperation to generate, share and use knowledge through equitable research partnerships (taking into account the international, country, regional and socio-economic contexts); and enhancing EU competitiveness and global sustainable development. These actions will be the subject of targeted calls, and particular attention is to be paid to facilitating the access of the relevant third countries, notably developing countries, to the actions.

Support for unforeseen policy needs may address, for example, living and work conditions, health impact assessment, risk assessment, statistical indicators, management and communication in the public health domain, as well as obligations under international health treaties, including the Framework Convention on Tobacco Control and the International Health Regulations.

An Interim Evaluation[73] found that FP7 was on course overall and making a significant contribution to EU science and the development of the ERA, but also identified weaknesses.

Several of these weaknesses have significant consequences for RDI for global health, especially in the area of the creation of global public goods such as drugs, vaccines and diagnostics for neglected diseases. For example, among the recommendations of the Interim Evaluation for reform was that research effort should increasingly be focused on "grand challenges" — including some significant for global health generally, like climate change and aging.

Following the Interim Evaluation, an EC Communication presented a strategic approach to enhancing and focusing EU international cooperation in research and innovation.[74] This noted that the EU (the Member States and the EC) is a world leader in research and innovation, responsible for 24% of world expenditure on research, 32% of high impact publications and 32% of patent applications, while representing only 7% of the population. Nevertheless, the Communication acknowledged that critical mass was lacking in many cases and the strategy driving the development of the actions was not always clear. It proposed a strategic approach to enhancing and focusing the Union's international cooperation activities in research and innovation, in particular with a view to preparing for the implementation of Horizon 2020, which would be the main instrument for implementing the EC's international research between 2014 and 2020.

Global challenges are seen as important drivers of research and innovation; and Horizon 2020 will be fully open to participation from all over the world, with country groupings highlighted to include both:

- *Industrialized countries and emerging economies*, where the main objective will be to increase the EU's competitiveness, to jointly tackle global challenges through common innovative solutions, and to develop enabling technologies by accessing new sources of knowledge.
- *LMICs*, where the emphasis will be on complementing the EU's external policies and instruments by building partnerships — in particular, bi-regional partnerships — to contribute to the sustainable development of these regions and address challenges such as the green economy, climate action, improved agriculture, food security and health. This includes supporting the MDGs and their possible successors, strengthening demand-led research and innovation for development, and delivery of the outcome of the Rio+20 conference, such as through the transfer of climate technologies. The strategy stated that the EU's external policies will aid in building up research capacity, including in developing countries.

Support for R&D relevant to health in LMICs

Collectively (EU Member States and the Commission), the EU is the world's largest development assistance donor, providing more than half of total aid flows to LMICs. The Commission alone accounts for 13% of total aid flows — €12.3 billion in 2009 — through programs which promote the MDGs as well as sectors crucial for sustainable development, such as infrastructure, climate and energy. In the health field, EU contributions have included support for policies and services as well as for vertical programs to reduce maternal and child mortality and combat infectious diseases,[75] although overall EC aid for health has not kept pace[76] with the last decade's global increase in development assistance for health.[77]

With respect to EU support for R&D related to health in LMICs, five areas are examined below.

1. *Millennium Development Goals (MDGs)*. The importance of research to underpin the MDGs has been emphasized.[78–81] Key EU policy and program documents[82–84] on the MDGs rarely mention the need for research to support their achievement, and neither research nor research capacity strengthening in LMICs appears to feature in the Commission's Technical Assistance Programmes for HIV/AIDS, Tuberculosis and Malaria.[85] However, the Commission makes use of research to examine progress toward the MDGs[86] and the FP7 Health Theme included a mandate on research to serve the MDGs under "international cooperation." To date, including the special Call on Africa (see "Focus on Africa," point 5 below), some 35 research projects are currently supported or under negotiation in this area through "specific international cooperation actions" corresponding to approximately €97 million.[87,88] The objective is to make Europe's contribution more effective so as to better accompany LMICs in getting back on track toward achieving health-related MDGs. The research support aims to provide a scientific base for International Cooperation Partner Countries to improve their health service delivery, including aspects of accessibility, effectiveness, efficiency and quality of care and user-friendliness. The mandate also covers public health concepts and interventions beyond health services through cross-sectoral and multidisciplinary research approaches. These actions on particular priorities, such as health systems, health policy, maternal and child care, reproductive health and neglected communicable diseases, aim to reinforce the research and cooperative capacities of candidate, neighborhood, developing and emerging countries. Particular attention is paid to facilitating access to these actions for these countries, particularly LMICs.

Research on neglected infectious diseases is performed under the FP Activity "Translational Research in Major Infectious Diseases: To Confront Major Threats to Public Health." In particular, the Framework Programmes provide funding for research on HIV/AIDS, malaria and TB.[89] Funding by both the EC (FP6) and other states or global bodies peaked in the middle of the last decade and subsequently declined.[90–92] Notwithstanding the 2001 UNGASS commitment, the EC's funding for research on HIV/AIDS vaccines and microbicides has remained below about 3% of the global total (EC investment in 2006 was about US$23 million, or 2.9% of the global total, around the peak year for the global total), and in 2011 the EC funding declined steeply from the previous year. In 2010, the EC invested US$20 million in HIV vaccine R&D, but in 2011 this decreased by about 50% to US$10 million. Similarly, the EC funded US$7.1 million (<3% of the global total) for R&D on microbicides in 2009, falling to US$6.7 million in 2010.[93–95] TB funding in FP6 and FP7 projects has focused on vaccine research (42% of the total EU funding), followed by basic research (17%), drugs (16%), clinical research and epidemiology (13%), and diagnostics (12%).[96] Overall, the Commission contributes about a quarter of the total EU funding for R&D on poverty-related neglected diseases, the rest coming directly from individual Member States, with these combined efforts not only benefitting LMICs but also contributing to EU jobs, investment, integration and the protection of European citizens.[97] In comparative terms, the Commission has been a modest but significant contributor to funding for neglected disease R&D: Throughout the five-year period 2007–2011, the top three public funders were the US, the UK and the Commission, with the last contributing US$113.5 million (5.8%) of the total.[98]

2. *Innovative Medicines Initiative (IMI).* Recognizing the challenge of declining[99] innovation in the pharmaceutical industry — globally and in the EU in particular — IMI has been established as a joint undertaking between the EU and the European Federation of Pharmaceutical Industries and Associations, as the largest initiative to boost pharmaceutical innovation in Europe and speed up development of better and safer medicines for patients. FP7 contributed €1 billion to the IMI research programme and Horizon 2020 will contribute €1.638 billion during its lifetime.[99] Out of more than five dozen projects under way, only a handful are of relevance to LMICs, addressing diseases such as Ebola and TB.[100]

3. *Capacity strengthening for R&D in LMICs.* The FPs have provided opportunities for institutions in Africa, Asia and South America to participate actively in EC projects on poverty-related diseases.[101] In addition, a major EU initiative has been the establishment of the European and Developing Countries Clinical Trials Partnership (EDCTP), based in The Hague and with an Africa hub in Cape Town.[102] The EDCTP aims to accelerate the development of new vaccines and drugs for HIV/AIDS, malaria, TB and other diseases relevant to LMICs by supporting clinical trials in Africa in partnership with African countries. Since its inception in 2003, EDCTP has developed a large portfolio of work in conducting clinical trials, supporting training, capacity building and networking. Clinical research capacities in the sub-Saharan Africa have been developed and strengthened under EDCTP with the number of participating sub-Saharan African countries rising since 2006, with more than 230 projects listed in the EDCTP's cumulative project compendium in June 2014.[103]

The EDCTP has supported 75 ethics and regulatory building capacity activities, notably in countries with almost non-existent capacity. It has fostered the establishment of four regional clinical research networks of excellence (in East, West, Central and Southern Africa) and provided over 300 research and training awards to African researchers, including 45 senior fellowships. Over 50% of clinical trials and over 70% of other projects funded by the EDCTP have been led by African researchers, and

African co-leadership and co-ownership have also been provided via African representation in the governance structure and advisory bodies of the EDCTP.

EDCTP was subject to independent external reviews, in 2007[104] and 2009,[105] which concluded that it has been particularly successful in working with researchers and clinicians in Africa and in providing a unique platform for a genuine dialogue between African and European researchers. The reviews recommended the continuation of EU support for a second 10-year programme (EDCTP2) during which shortcomings in the first programme could be addressed.

A further independent external evaluation was conducted in 2014,[106] while EDCTP2 was approved by the European Parliament on 15 April 2014 and the European Council on 6 May 2014. The overall strategy of EDCTP2 was not revised: it will continue to support clinical development of new or improved diagnostics, drugs, vaccines and microbicides against HIV/AIDS, tuberculosis and malaria. However, in addition, EDCTP2 will also support studies on neglected infectious diseases and will support all clinical trial phases (I to IV). The geographical focus of EDCTP2 will remain on sub-Saharan Africa, although collaborative research with other LMICs outside sub-Saharan Africa could be envisioned when possible and desirable. The European Union will provide a contribution of up to €683 million for the 10-year programme (2014–2024), provided this is matched by contributions from the European Participating States.[107]

4. *Research to enhance equity.* As highlighted in an independent Expert Report,[108] action by the EU to improve health in third countries and address social determinants of health through policy coherence is underpinned by Article 168 of the Treaty on the Functioning of the EU. This specifies that:

> ...the Union and the Member States shall foster cooperation with third countries and the competent international organizations in the sphere of public health, and that a high level of human health protection shall be ensured in the definition and implementation of all Union policies and activities.

The Communications on "The EU Role in Global Health" and "Solidarity in Health: Reducing Health Inequalities in the EU" reinforce the EU's commitment to reduce health inequalities, including through its role in global health. The Expert Report observes that global health (and health equity) could be incorporated to a greater extent in the implementation of the European Consensus on Development. It recommends that the EU consider adopting health (and health equity) as a cross-cutting issue. This would follow up the Council Conclusions on Health in All Policies from 2006 and the Oslo Ministerial Declaration, which calls for making "impact on health" a point of departure and a defining lens to examine key elements of foreign policy and development strategies. The Report notes that policy areas including research are important for confronting global health inequalities, and makes repeated references to the importance of influencing research priorities to improve the monitoring of health inequalities and of adopting a social-determinants-of-health approach.

The opportunity for more effective cooperation between the EU and the US to address global health inequities has been stressed by Garay.[109] In a personal capacity, he has also made the case[110] for a new global health framework based on global shared values of present and future equity and recognizing the right to health in an operational and accountable (and demandable) way, ensuring coherence with other key policies such as trade, migration, food security and the environment.

Beyond the support for R&D on drugs for poverty-related diseases already discussed, there are few examples so far where the EC has implemented any of the above approaches in the field of research to underpin reductions in inequities in global health.

5. *Focus on Africa.* The Joint Africa–EU Strategy under the Africa–EU Strategic Partnership launched by the EU and the African Union in 2007 included EU commitments to strengthen cooperation in science, technology and scientific research for development; to promote further research, particularly on vaccines and new medicines for both major and neglected diseases, and on issues relating to waterborne diseases, as well as on the clinical effectiveness of traditional medicine; and to strengthen cooperation to build scientific and technological capacities and the development of science and technology and innovation systems in Africa as a contribution to achieving the MDGs; with implementation of the Joint Strategy being effected through successive Action Plans.[111] Action under the EU Framework Programme FP7 included an "Africa Call" in 2010, implemented jointly by: Theme 1 — "Health"; Theme 2 — "Food, Agriculture and Fisheries, and Biotechnology"; and Theme 6 — "Environment (including climate change)." The aim of this call was to address some of the Science & Technology objectives of the Africa–EU Strategic Partnership, putting emphasis on "Water and Food Security" and "Better Health for Africa." This call had a multidisciplinary approach involving various scientific and technological research fields, such as food, agriculture, health, land and water resources, including their inter-action with climate change. It aimed principally to strengthen local capacities in the relevant science and technology fields and their appli-cations, also through appropriate training activities and exchange of staff. The indicative total call budget was €63 million, of which €39 million was for Theme 1 — "Health."[112]

Horizon 2020 (FP8) and Europe 2020

Horizon 2020, the successor to FP7 for 2014–2020, was designed to be closely aligned to Europe 2020[113] which places a strong emphasis on R&D for the progress of Europe: at its heart *"is the conviction that we need R&D and innovation to create smart, sustainable growth and get Europe out of the current economic crisis."*

Horizon 2020 aims to be a centre-piece of the EU's drive to create new growth and jobs in Europe; to provide a boost to top-level research in Europe, including the European Research Council; to strengthen industrial leadership in innovation, including through investment in key technologies, greater access to capital and support for SMEs; and to help address major societal challenges like climate change, developing sustainable transport and mobility, making renewable energy more affordable, ensuring food safety and security, or coping with the chal-lenge of an aging population. It also aims to help bridge the gap between research and the market. International cooperation will be an important priority, with the Marie Sklodowska-Curie Actions receiving an increase to €6.1 billion in 2014–2020, allowing the EU to support more than 65,000 researchers. The European Institute of Innovation and Technology will receive €2.7 billion in 2014–2020 to enhance links between higher education, research and business, and to support entrepreneurial start-ups and specialized postgraduate training.

The initial budget set for Horizon 2020 was close to €80 billion,[114] but this has already been reduced by skimming of several billion to pay for other activities.[115] Within the overall budget[116] for 2014–2020, the area of "Excellence in Science" was allocated 31.7% (over €24 billion) and the area of "Health, Demographic Change and Wellbeing" was allocated 9.70%.

During the formative stages of Horizon 2020, hopes and concerns were expressed about the extent to which it will be structured and organized to deal with a range of global health R&D problems, including support for trans-disciplinary innovation along the spectrum from basis sciences to health product development and clinical delilvery.[117,118] It has been felt in many quarters that Europe's health research is not reaching its potential: promising discoveries do not get to patients as rapidly as anticipated with excellent breakthroughs in basic science not being pursued. Europe's innovators are relocating outside Europe and national healthcare systems are trying to cope with increasing costs in a time of economic and demographic change. Moreover, despite similar infrastructures and technologies and well as common challenges facing health disciplines in Europe, there is significant fragmentation in research programmes and insufficient cross-talk between diseases and disciplines.[119] While strengthening support for EDCTP and the Innovative Medicines Initiative (see above), Horizon 2020 appears to do little to address to wider issues in global health or the structural factors that would facilitate R&D for global health.

RDI for global health in EU development policy

The "Mobilising European Research for Development Policies" initiative, supported by the EC and several Member States, seeks to enhance the European perspective of some of the most pressing contemporary development issues of our time through knowledge, innovation and building common ground between the European research community and policy-makers. The main outcome of this initiative is the publication of yearly reports in the series European Report on Development.[120] The themes covered to date in the series include "Overcoming Fragility in Africa,"[121] "Social Protection for Inclusive Development,"[122] Confronting Scarcity: Managing Water, Energy and Land for Inclusive and Sustainable Growth"[123] and "Global Action for an Inclusive and Sustainable Future";[124] and "Financing and other means of implementation in the post-2015 context.[125]

Ethics, Regulatory and Legal Roles and RDI for Global Health

The EU's European Medicines Agency (EMA, formerly EMEA)[126] is responsible for the scientific evaluation of medicines developed for use in the EU. The EMA is involved in a number of areas of policy and practice that have important consequences for health in LMICs, including:

Clinical trials

Standards

Since 2005, the EMA has implemented revisions to the pharmaceutical legislation, to place increased emphasis on the ethical standards required of clinical trials conducted in third countries and included in Marketing Authorisation Applications submitted in the European Economic Area (EEA). A system of routine Good Clinical Practice (GCP) inspection has been in place since 2006. Two key factors in selecting sites and studies for routine inspection are the presence of vulnerable populations (including children) and of investigator sites in LMICs. Both the review process and the inspection program have been expanded.[127] The EMA has engaged in wide consultations on its approach and the promotion of high ethical and clinical standards globally.[128,129]

However, research indicates that the EMA and equivalent national bodies have not always carried out the ethical checks required by Directive 2003/63/EC.2,3. For example, studies on approved drugs in the EU revealed cases in which the EMA and national authorities devoted little to no attention to the ethical aspects of the clinical trials submitted and they accepted unethical trials as well as trials of poor quality.[130]

An EC–EMA conference[131] on the operation of the Clinical Trials Directive highlighted issues of importance regarding non-commercial sponsors of clinical trials (who could include not-for-profit organizations such as Product Development Partnerships for neglected diseases) and the tensions between ensuring compliance with all necessary standards such as GCP and the need to minimize over-burdensome costs and procedures damaging to noncommercial research and to investment in it. The idea of a differential application of the legislation, using a risk-based approach, was proposed.

The EMA's "Road Map to 2015" recognizes the need to address the impact of globalization in the pharmaceuticals sector:[132]

> ... characterised by: the increasingly global nature of research, develop-
> ment, manufacturing and clinical-trial activities; challenges relating to the
> movement of clinical research to developing countries, to ethical standards
> and to regulatory and supervision arrangements in non-EU countries; the
> attendant need for closer and more intense cooperation between interna-
> tional partners.

The strategic areas on which the Road Map focuses include stimulation of medicines development in areas of unmet medical needs, neglected diseases and rare diseases. The Road Map also promises to facilitate access to medicines, with a focus on activities designed to reduce the productivity gap that currently exists in the development of medicines. It notes that EMA collaboration with the Commission's Directorate-General Research has so far been rather fragmented and aims to create a platform for dialogue to improve input into the EU research agenda for medicines.

Capacity strengthening

A major element of the EU's work in capacity strengthening for clinical trials has been the combined support of the Commission and some

Member States for the EDCTP (see above). In addition, the Commission has supported the Paediatric European Network for Treatment of AIDS (PENTA),[133] which, among other activities, has helped strengthen capacity for conducting high quality, ethical clinical trials in a number of LMICs. The EMA has been a collaborator with PENTA.[134]

Registration of drugs predominantly for use in LMICs

There are major weaknesses in regulatory authority capacity in Africa to handle the pipeline of new products being developed specifically for diseases prevalent mainly in LMICs. In the past, most new drugs for neglected diseases (NDs) have been first registered with a well-established Western medicines regulatory authority (MRA) such as the US FDA or EMA, but this can delay access for African patients since African regulatory authorities often wait for the Western MRA decision before commencing action; and it puts the ND product decisions in the hands of regulators that have less experience in tropical disease products, presentations and epidemiology, and that are not accountable for the needs and safety of target African patients.

To overcome these shortcomings, policy-makers have developed regulatory pathways tailored for ND products. The EMA's Article 58, established by the EU in 2004, aims to facilitate and assist LMIC registration of medicines by providing the same scientific assessment ("opinion") on products used outside the EU as for those inside the EU. Article 58 combines stringent review standards, efficiency (the average review time is 2.5 months), and structured input from WHO disease experts from disease-endemic countries. However, it has been little utilized, as it has lacked incentives for product developers.

A study by Moran *et al.*[135] has made six recommendations to create an efficient integrated system of national, regional, and international approvals to achieve an optimal drug registration approach for Africa that can reliably evaluate safety, efficacy, and quality of drugs for African use.

Key Challenges for Current European and Global R&D Policy

A forum on R&D for global health, which included discussion of the CEWG report,[136] articulated that furthering the global research and innovation agenda will require that:

- *Research policies are informed by evidence of health need*, oriented to achieving health equity and strongly guided by principles of affordable access to knowledge and products generated.
- The results of global health research be made readily available to policy-makers and the public through more extensive and *effective knowledge translation*.
- A *comprehensive research agenda* be developed for global health, for use by policy-makers, funders and researchers.
- The *process of priority-setting* for global R&D be done with wide *stakeholder participation*, including engagement between researchers, funders and policy-makers and with the involvement of LMICs.
- The *capacities of LMICs be strengthened* and utilized to engage in research, development and innovation for health and in policy development and priority-setting regarding research, development and innovation, at both the national and the global level.
- *Consortia conducting research and innovation for global health be expanded* and engage diverse players, including the public and private sectors, ensuring that the health needs and priorities of poorer as well as richer populations are met.
- To underpin all of the above, *comprehensive global metrics* be developed and used regarding resourcing of research and innovation for global health, as proposed by the Consultative Expert Working Group on Research and Development: Financing and Coordination (CEWG) in the creation of a global observatory function.[50]

In the following, we discuss three different types of challenges for European and global health research: (1) content/issue challenges, (2) governance challenges and (3) political/implementation challenges.

Content/Issue Challenges

Balancing the need for economic growth with equity concerns

Potential tension between objectives of economic growth, sustainable development and global health should be examined in the research context. Pratt and Loff have suggested that international research is too often focused on new medical interventions and the "economic competitiveness" of countries, rather than collaborative health systems research informing policy which is important for the development of successful health interventions in developing countries.[137] Pratt and Loff particularly highlight the need for resources focused on research into health policy and systems in order to achieve the current MDGs — a priority also established by the WHO Task Force on Health Systems Research and the Mexico Statement on Health Research. They argue that the dearth of health policy and systems research is the result of "the laws and policies governing research in high-income countries," especially those which emphasize the economic function and "economic competitiveness" of research, including technology transfer, laws and infrastructure aiming at the development of disease-focused, licensed marketable products. Pratt and Loff argue that such research policies have diverted attention away from research into health policy and systems and global health equity. Ostlin *et al.*[138] suggest that a paradigm shift is required in order for health research to address health equity concerns, and based on stakeholder consultations, they propose four areas for the development of research on health equity:

(1)   global factors and processes that affect health equity
(2)   structures and processes that differentially affect people's changes to be healthy within a given society
(3)   health system factors that affect health equity, and
(4)   policies and interventions to reduce health inequity.

Capacity building in LMICs; promoting health equity and sustainable development

The value-driven approach to global health that the EU espouses demands working toward equity in health between and within countries. The EU's adoption of the Paris Principles require that it engage LMICs at all stages in the design, ethical review, management, execution and follow-up of RDI processes that concern them; and that it contribute to capacity building so that LMICs can derive the maximum benefit from current activities and be the creators and owners of their own health RDI in the future. Capacity building will be particularly important for the development of health metrics systems and ethical review processes.

In addition, any knowledge translation involving LMICs must take into account local contexts. Frenk and Chen[139] highlight the need to put evidence into practice, taking into account the particular context of countries, and state:

> ...all nations must participate in the advancement and sharing of research-generated knowledge, along with developing the capacity to not just adopt the evidence, but to adapt it to local circumstances. We are now ideally situated to expand global networks of collaboration and develop consortia of national and regional centers of excellence.

Innovation policy and global public goods

The need for collective global action to create global public goods for health has been highlighted by the recent call for a Framework Convention for Global Health. The pressure to create global public goods through RDI has also been highlighted through the report of the CEWG, as discussed above.

Governance Challenges

Meeting the challenge of the multisectoral and multidisciplinary nature of global health

Important corollaries of the EU's conceptualization of global health are the need for related RDI to be designed, structured, conducted and translated in ways that recognize the transnational character of global health; that involve many disciplines within and beyond the health sciences (in alignment with a social determinants approach) and promote transdisciplinary approaches and interdisciplinary collaborations; that synthesize population-based prevention with individual-level clinical care; and are inherently equity-oriented. This will necessitate multisectoral and multidisciplinary governance of global health research and a "health in all policies" framework, which may highlight areas of policy incoherence.

Stakeholder participation, transparency and accountability

It is desirable that global health research be accountable and responsive to communities and different types of needs (felt need, expressed need, normative or evidence-based need, comparative need), which may entail a range of stakeholders being part of all stages of research, including governance processes. As Frenk and Chen[140] point out, there is currently a "democratic deficit" in global health governance, where international organizations are accountable to Member States rather than their communities. Whilst transparency is important for proper governance, ethical review and translation of research, in some instances the ideal of transparency may need to be balanced with concerns related to health security (i.e. brought about by gain-of-function research; see below).

New ethical challenges and gain-of-function research

A number of ethical challenges have arisen from international health research conducted within LMICs by organizations based in high-income countries (such as the Kano trovafloxacin trial conducted by Pfizer). They have highlighted the continued need for capacity building when it comes to research involving LMICs, particularly for ethical review processes.

There are also many new ethical issues that have arisen from health research in our globalized world which require proper ethical review. We are currently seeing the sharing of viruses for research purposes, and experiments designed to increase the transmissibility of viruses (e.g. H5N1), referred to as "gain of function" research. This has resulted in scientists associated with the Foundation for Vaccine Research declaring such research to be "morally and ethically wrong" and calling for an ethical review and high-level investigation into such research.[141,142] There was a self-imposed temporary moratorium on gain-of-function research amidst ethical debates, but this subsequently ceased.[143] Such review of ethical challenges for global health research should be considered at the global level.

Political/Implementation Challenges

As governments face internal challenges such as those brought about by the global economic crisis, political and implementation challenges arise for taking action on global health research policies. In addition, policy incoherence between areas such as trade and global health (e.g. in relation to access to medicines[144]) may bring about political challenges for furthering global health research and the development of global public goods. The resolve of the EU and its member countries to meet commitments made to global health is being tested and can only be judged by the practical outcomes that emerge in the years ahead, including the extent to which Horizon 2020 is adapted to accommodate the trans-disciplinary field of global health R&D.

Conclusion

The EU has articulated a definition of global health and has developed and agreed on principles on the role that it should play in this field. Through interventions and positions taken by EU representatives in a range of discussions in the UN and other global fora and through the programs and actions funded by the EU Budget — notably including the Framework Programs for research and innovation; support for the EDCTP; and capacity building through actions such as the Call for Africa — the EU has demonstrated practical support for global health and for the necessary research, development and innovation to underpin it.

The field of global health is rapidly evolving, driven by major global forces including globalization, the imperative of reforming global governance structures and mechanisms, the struggle to complete the Doha Round, and the momentum building toward the post-2015 development goals and toward new mechanisms of international cooperation on R&D for neglected diseases. The EU faces significant challenges in sustaining its support for global health, including in the area of research, development and innovation, as it strives to accommodate to these changes and to contemporary internal pressures such as financial stringency and the need to enhance policy coherence within and across sectors.

References

1. Koplan JP, Bond TC, Merson MH, *et al.* (2009) Towards a common definition of global health. The *Lancet* **373:** 1993–1995. Available at www.globalbrigades.org/media/Global_Health_Towards_a_Common_Definitition.pdf.
2. Kickbusch I, Lister G (eds.). (2006) European Perspectives on Global Health — A Policy Glossary. European Foundation Centre, Brussels. Available at www.ilonakickbusch.com/kickbusch-wAssets/docs/EFC_EPGH.pdf.
3. Kickbush I. (2006) The need for a European strategy on global health. *Scandinavian Journal of Public Health* **34:** 561–565. Available at http://sjp.sagepub.com/content/34/6/561.long.
4. Kickbusch I. (2002) Global Health — A Definition. Yale University. Available at www.ilonakickbusch.com/kickbusch-wAssets/docs/global-health.pdf.
5. Fried LP, Bentley ME, Buekens P, *et al.* (2010) Global health is public health. The *Lancet* **375:** 535–537. Available at www.thelancet.com/journals/lancet/article/PIIS0140-6736%2810%2960203-6/fulltext#article_upsell.
6. Beaglehole R, Bonita R. (2012) What is global health? *Global Health Action* **3:** 5142. Available at http://globalhealthcenter.umn.edu/documents/whatisglobalhealth.pdf.
7. Rowson M, Willott C, Hughes R, *et al.* (2012) Conceptualising global health: theoretical issues and their relevance for teaching. *Globalization and Health* **8:** 36. Available at www.globalizationandhealth.com/content/pdf/1744-8603-8-36.pdf.
8. EU Council Conclusions on the EU Role in Global Health. (2010) Council of the European Union 3011th Foreign Affairs Council Meeting, 10 May 2010. European Union, Brussels. Available at http://www.eu-un.europa.eu/articles/en/article_9727_en.htm.
9. Communication from the Commission to the Council, the European Parliament, the European Economic and Social Committee and the Committee of the Regions. (2010) The EU Role in Global Health. COM (2010) 128 final. European Commission, Brussels. Available at http://

ec.europa.eu/development/icenter/repository/COMM_PDF_COM_2010_0128_EN.PDF.

10. European Commission. (2010) Commission Staff Working Document: European Research and Knowledge for Global Health: Accompanying Document to the Communication to the Council, the European Parliament, the European Economic and Social Committee and the Committee of the Regions. SEC (2010) 381. European Commission, Brussels. Available at http://ec.europa.eu/development/icenter/repository/SEC2010_381_EN.pdf.

11. European Commission. (2007) White Paper — Together for Health: A Strategic Approach for the EU 2008–2013. COM (2007) 630 final. SEC (2007) 1374; 1375; 1376. European Commission, Brussels. Available at http://ec.europa.eu/health-eu/doc/whitepaper_en.pdf.

12. Together for Health: A Strategic Approach for the EU 2008–2013.(2010) European Parliament Resolution of 9 October 2008 (2008/2115(INI)). *Official Journal C* **9E:** 56–64. Available at http://eur-lex.europa.eu/LexUriServ/Lex UriServ.do?uri=OJ:C:2010:009E:0056:0064:EN:PDF.

13. Howitt P, *et al.* (2012) Technologies for global health. *The Lancet* **380:** 507–535. Available at www.thelancet.com/journals/lancet/article/PIIS0140-6736%2812%2961127-1/fulltext#article_upsell.

14. Matlin SA, Samuels GMR. (2009) The Global Health Research and Innovation System. *The Lancet* **374(9702):** 1662–1663. Available at www.thelancet.com/journals/lancet/article/PIIS0140-6736%2809%2961912-7/fulltext.

15. Ståhl T, Wismar M,Ollila E, *et al.* (2006) Health in All Policies: Prospects and Potentials. Finnish Ministry of Social Affairs and Health. Available at www.euro.who.int/__data/assets/pdf_file/0003/109146/E89260.pdf.

16. Matlin SA, Evans T, Hasler J, *et al.* (2008). Signposts to research for health, *The Lancet* **372(9649):** 1521–1822. Available atwww.thelancet.com/journals/lancet/article/PIIS0140-6736(08)61630-X/fulltext.

17. Matlin SA. (2008) The scope and potential of innovation for health and health equity. In: Gehner M, Jupp S, Matlin SA (eds.), *Global Forum Update on Research for Health, Volume 5: Fostering Innovation for Global Health*. Pro-Brook, London, pp.13–20. Available at www.isn.ethz.ch/isn/Digital-Library/Publications/Detail/?id=93556&lng=en.

18. European Commission. (2010) Europe 2020 Flagship Initiative: Innovation Union. Communication from the Commission to the European Parliament, the

Council, the European Economic and Social Committee and the Committee of the Regions. Brussels, 6 October 2010. COM (2010) 546 final. Document SEC (2010) 1161, p. 8. Available at http://ec.europa.eu/research/innovation-union/pdf/innovation-union-communication_en.pdf#view=fit&pagemode=none.

19. European Commission. (2012) State of the Innovation Union 2011: Report from the Commission to the European Parliament, the Council, the European Economic and Social Committee and the Committee of the Regions. Brussels, 2 December 2011. COM (2011) 849 final. EC Directorate-General for Research and Innovation, p. 11. Available at http://ec.europa.eu/research/innovation-union/pdf/state-of-the-union/2011/state_of_the_innovation_union_2011_brochure_en.pdf#view=fit&pagemode=none.

20. A definition of "interdisciplinary research" is that it has "as its starting point an integrated research question to which different disciplines contribute by bringing their own perspective, and ideally thinking through the research issue from more angles. Thus an interdisciplinary research project will from the very outset produce a research question that more accurately approximates the complexity of the real world in which policy and practice decisions must be made."
MacLachlan M, Carr SC, McWha I (eds.). (2008) *Interdisciplinary Research for Development: A Workbook on Content and Process Challenges.* Global Development Network, New Delhi, p. 16.

21. MacLachlan M. (2009) Rethinking global health research: towards integrative expertise. *Globalization and Health* **5:** 6. Available at www.biomedcentral.com/content/pdf/1744-8603-5-6.pdf.

22. IJsselmuiden C, Matlin SA. (2006) Why Health Research? Research for Health Policy Briefings. Council on Heath Research for Development & Global Forum for Health Research, Geneva. Available at http://announcementsfiles.cohred.org/gfhr_pub/assoc/s14844e/s14844e.pdf.

23. Editorial. (2008) The Bamako call to action: research for health. *The Lancet* **372(1855).** Available at www.who.int/entity/rpc/news/Bamako%20call%20to%20action%20%20thelancet%20281108.pdf.

24. Kickbusch I. (2011) Advancing the Global Health Agenda. UN Chronicle. Available at www.un.org/wcm/content/site/chronicle/home/archive/issues 2011/7billionpeople1unitednations/advancingtheglobal-healthagenda.

25. Ministers of Foreign Affairs of Brazil, France, Indonesia, Norway, Senegal, South Africa and Thailand. (2007) Oslo Ministerial Declaration — global health: a pressing foreign policy issue of our time. *The Lancet* **369(9580)**: 1373–1378.

26. Statement by John B. Richardson, Head of the Delegation of the European Commission, on behalf of the European Community on the occasion of the 26th Special Session of the General Assembly of the UN on HIV/AIDS. (2001) United Nations, 27 June 2001, New York. Available at www.un.org/ga/aids/statements/docs/ecE.html.

27. United Nations high-level meeting on noncommunicable disease prevention and control. (2012) World Health Organization, Geneva. Available at www.who.int/nmh/events/un_ncd_summit2011/en.

28. United Nations. (2012) Political Declaration of the High-Level Meeting of the General Assembly on the Prevention and Control of Non-communicable Diseases. Resolution adopted by the General Assembly 66/2, 24 January 2012. United Nations, New York. Available at www.who.int/nmh/events/un_ncd_summit2011/political_declaration_en.pdf.

29. Commissioner Dalli delivers first EU statement at UN General Assembly. (2011) *Health & Consumer Voice*, October 2011 edition. Available at http://ec.europa.eu/dgs/health_consumer/dyna/consumervoice/create_cv.cfm?cv_id=762.

30. Nundy S, Han E. (2012) New Technology Needs for Noncommunicable Diseases in Developing Countries: A Landscaping Study. Results for Development Institute, Washington, DC. Available at http://healthresearchpolicy.org/assessments/new-technology-needs-noncommunicable-diseases-landscaping-study.

31. Unger-Saldana K. (20 14) Challenges to the early diagnosis and treatment of breast cancer in developing countries. World J Clin Oncol. 5(3), 465–477. Available at www.ncbi.nlm.nih.gov/pmc/articles/PMC4127616/.

32. Ford N., *et al*. (2012) Chronic hepatitis C treatment outcomes in low- and middle-income countries: a systematic review and meta-analysis. Bull. World Health Organization, 2012; 90: 540–550. doi: 10.2471/BLT.11.097147. Available at http://www.who.int/bulletin/volumes/90/711-097147/en/.

33. TAG. (2015) Gilead: Stop Blocking Access to Hepattis C Treatment. Treatment Action Group, Press Release 5 May 2015. Available at http://www.treatmentactiongroup.org/hcv/2015/gilead-stop-blocking-HCV-access.

34. FP7 Action Programme. (2012) HEALTH.2013.4.1-6: Mapping Chronic Non-communicable Diseases Research Activities. Available at www.2020-horizon.com/Mapping-chronic-non-communicable-diseases-research-activities-i1203.html.

35. Note by the UN Secretary-General. (2009) Global Health and Foreign Policy: Strategic Opportunities and Challenges. UN General Assembly Debate on Health and Foreign Policy, 64th Session, 2009. Agenda item 123, paper A/64/365. Available at www.who.int/entity/trade/foreignpolicy/FPGH.pdf.

36. European Centre for Disease Prevention and Control (ECDC). Available at www.ecdc.europa.eu/en/Pages/home.aspx. Available at www.ictsd.org/downloads/bridges/bridges14-3.pdf.

37. Fidler D, Drager N. (2009) Global Health and Foreign Policy: Strategic Opportunities and Challenges. Background Paper for the Secretary-General's Report on Global Health and Foreign Policy. World Health Organization, Geneva. Available at www.who.int/trade/events/UNGA_Background_Rep3_2.pdf. Available at http://ictsd.org/downloads/bridges/bridges14-3.pdf.

38. The Global Health Regime: Issue Brief. (2012) Council on Foreign Relations, Washington, DC. Available at www.cfr.org/health-science-and-technology/global-health-regime/p22763. Available at http://eur-lex.europa.eu/LexUriServ/LexUriServ.do?uri=OJ:L:2003:196:0007:0014:EN:PDF.

39. Seuba X, García JF. (2010) Intellectual property and public health in the EU–CAN FTA. *Bridges* **14(3):** 15–16. Available at http://ec.europa.eu/taxation_customs/resources/documents/customs/customs_controls/counterfeit_piracy/legislation/guidelines_on_tranist_en.pdf.

40. Wemos. (2015) Dutch Parliament visiting Brussels 20 April 2015: TTIP and Health Risks. Amsterdam: Wemos. Available at www.wemos.nl/files/Documenten%20Informatief/Bestanden%20voor%20Governance/20150415%20TTIP%20and%20Health%20def.pdf.

41. EU challenged on generics seizures. (2010) *Bridges* **14(3):** 9.

42. European Council. (2003) Council Regulation (EC) No. 1383/2003 of 22 July 2003 concerning customs action against goods suspected of infringing certain intellectual property rights and the measures to be taken against goods found to have infringed such rights. (2003) *Official Journal L* **196:** 7–14. Available at www.who.int/intellectualproperty/report/en/.

43. European Commission. (2012) Guidelines of the European Commission concerning the enforcement by EU customs authorities of intellectual property rights with regard to goods, in particular medicines, in transit through the EU. European Commission, Brussels. Available at: http://apps.who.int/gb/ebwha/pdf_files/ A61/ A61_R21-en.pdf.

44. Kaul I, Grunberg I, Stern MA (eds.). (1999) *Global Public Goods: International Cooperation in the 21st Century.* Oxford University Press, New York. Available at http://ec.europa.eu/health/eu_world/docs/ev_20100610_rd05_en.pdf.

45. Stiglitz JE. (2012) A Breakthrough Opportunity for Global Health. Project Syndicate. Available at www.project-syndicate.org/commentary/a-breakthrough-opportunity-for-global-health. Available at www. who.int/phi/documents/RDFinancingwithiSBN.pdf.

46. Public Health, Innovation and Intellectual Property Rights. (2006) Report of the Commission on Intellectual Property Rights, Innovation and Public Health. World Health Organization, Geneva. Available at www.who.int/phi/CEWG_Report_5_April_2012.pdf.

47. Global strategy and plan of action on public health, innovation and intellectual property. 61st World Health Assembly Paper WHA61.21, 24 May 2008. Geneva: WHO 2008, 48pp. Available at http://apps.who.int/gb/CEWG/pdf/A65_24-en.pdf.

48. European Commission. (2010) Improving Access to Medicines and Effective Health Services Through Innovation and Technology Transfer — The EU Contribution to the Global Strategy and Plan of Action on Public Health, Innovation and Intellectual Property. EuropeAid. European Commission, Brussels. Available at http://apps.who.int/gb/CEWG/pdf/A65_24-en.pdf.

49. Research and Development Coordination and Financing. (2010) Report of the WHO Expert Working Group. World Health Organization, Geneva. Available at http://apps.who.int/gb/ebwha/pdf_files/WHA65/A65_R22-en.pdf.

50. Work Health Organization. (2012) Consultative Expert Working Group on Research and Development: Financing and Coordination. Research and Development to Meet Health Needs in Developing Countries: Strengthening Global Financing and Coordination. World Health Organization, Geneva. Available at www. who.int/phi/1-cewg_secretariat_paper-en.pdf.

51. Rottingen JA, Chamas C. (2012) A new deal for global health R&D? The recommendations of the Consultative Expert Working Group on Research and Development (CEWG). *PLoS Med* **9:** e1001219. Available at http://journals.plos.org/plosmedicine/article?id=10.1371/journal.pmed.1001219.

52. CEWG. (2012) Consultative Expert Working Group on Research and Development: Financing and Coordination. Geneva, WHO, 198pp. Available at http://apps.who.int/gb/CEWG/pdf/A65_24-en.pdf.

53. WHO. (20 L 2) Follow up of the report of the Consultative Expert Working Group on Research and Development: Financing and Coordination. World Health Assembly Paper WHA65.22, Agenda item 13.14, 26 May 2012. Geneva, WHO. Available at http://apps.who.int/gb/ebwha/pdf_files/WHA65/A65_R22-cn.pdf.

54. WHO. (2012) Open-ended meeting of Member States on the follow-up of the report of the Consultative Expert Working Group on Research and Development: Financing and Coordination. Report by the Secretariat. Geneva: WHO, Paper A/CEWG/3, 2 November 2012. Available at www.who.int/phi/1-cewg_secretariat_paper-en.pdf.

55. WHO. (2015) Follow-up of the report of the Consultative Expert Working Group on Research and Development: Financing and Coordination. Report by the Director-General to the 68th World Health Assembly. Geneva: WHO, Paper WHA68.34, Agenda item 17.4, 10 April 2015. Available at http://apps.who.int/gb/ebwha/pdf_files/WHA68/A68_34-en.pdf.

56. IP-Watch. (2013) Debate Erupts At WHO Over "Consensus" On Financing R&D For The Poor. Ip-Watch, 28 January 2013. Available at www.ip-watch.org/2013/01/28/debate-erupts-at-who-over-consensus-on-financing-rd-for-the-poor/.

57. KEI. (2013) WHO Director-General Chan throws down the gauntlet on the CEWG process: "Let's fight this out at the Assembly!" Knowledge Ecology International, 26 January 2013. Available at http://keionline.org/node/1643.

58. European Union. (2012) WHO 65th World Health Assembly (Geneva, 21–26th May 2012) EU Statement, Consultative Expert Working Group on Research and Development: Financing and Coordination, Agenda item 13.14. Available at http://keionline.org/node/1419.

59. de Tarso Lugon Arantes P. (2012) Intense R&D negotiations during the 65th World Health Assembly, Health Diplomacy Monitor, Volume 3(4) 21–3. Available at www.ghd-net.org/sites/default/files/Health%20Diplomacy%20Monitor%20Volume%203%20Issuc%204.Pdf.

60. EU. (2012) 62nd Session of the WHO Regional Committee for Europe, Malta 10–13 September 2012, EU Statement 'Consultative Expert Working Group on Research and Development: Financing and Coordination (CEWG)' (item 3). Available at www.eeas.europa.eu/delegations/un_genevaldocuments/eu_statements/who/2012–0910_whorc62_cewg.pdf.

61. RH Hermann. (2013) World Health Assembly: As Members Approve Health R&D Decisions, US Says Time To "Put Our Money Where Our Mouth Is". Intellectual Property Watch, 27 May 2013. www.ip-watch.org/2013/05/27/world-health-assembly-as-members-approve-health-r-us-says-time-to-put-our-money-where-our-mouth-is/.

62. WHO. (2013) Follow-up of the report of the Consultative Expert Working Group on Research and Development: Financing and Coordination. Outcome of the informal drafting group on the draft decision proposed by the delegation of the USA. Agenda Item 17.2, paper A66/B/Cnf./2, 27 May 2013. Available at www.ip-watch.org/weblog/wp-conten/uploads/2013/05/CEWG-decision-point-May-2013.pdf.

63. IP Watch. (2015) WHO Advances R&D Financing Effort; Global R&D Observatory To Launch In January. Intellectual Property Watch, 24 May 2015. Available at www.ip-watch.org/2015/05/24/who-advanccs-r-global-rd-observatory-to-launch-in-january/.

64. WHO. (2015) CEWG Demonstration Projects: Background and Process. Geneva: WHO. Available at www.who.int/phi/implimentation/cewg_background_process/en/.

65. KEI. (2014) TDR and the Pooled Fund for R&D: WHO demonstration projects and CEWG follow-up. Washington DC: Knowledge Ecology International. Available at http://keionline.org/node/2076.

66. European Commission. (2012) Financial Programming and Budget: How is the Budget Decided? European Commission, Brussels. Available at http://ec.europa.eu/budget/explained/management/deciding/decide_en.cfm.

67. European Research Area: A Unified Research Area in Which Researchers, Scientific Knowledge and Technology Circulate Freely. Available at http://ec.europa.eu/research/era/index_en.htm.

68. EC. (2014) EC Budget: Multiannual Financial Framework. Brussels: European Commission. Available at http://ec.europa.eu/budget/mff/programmes/index_en.cfm#horizon2020.

69. European Commission. (2007) FP7 in Brief. Available at http://announcementsfiles.cohred.org/gfhr_pub/assoc/s14809e/s14809e.pdf.

70. Van Damme W, *et al.* (2004) North–South Partnerships for Health Systems Research: 20 Years of Experience of EC Support. European Commission Dictorate-General for Research, Brussels. Available at http://announcementsfiles.cohred.org/gfhr_pub/assoc/s14835e/s14835e.pdf.

71. Council of the European Union. (2006) Decision No. 1982/2006/ec of the European Parliament and of the Council of 18 December 2006 concerning the Seventh Framework Programme of the European Community for research, technological development and demonstration activities (2007–2013). *Official Journal L* **412:** 1–41.

72. Council of the European Union. (2007) Council decision of 19 December 2006 concerning the specific programme "Cooperation" implementing the Seventh Framework Programme of the European Community for research, technological development and demonstration activities (2007 to 2013) (2006/971/EC). *Official Journal L* **54:** 30–80.

73. Interim Evaluation of the Seventh Framework Programme. (2010) Report of the Expert Group. Final Report, 12 November 2010.

74. Communication from the Commission to the European Parliament, the Council, the European Economic and Social Committee and the Committee of the Regions. (2012) Enhancing and Focusing EU International Cooperation in Research and Innovation: A Strategic Approach. Brussels; 8 September 2012. COM (2012) 497 final. European Commission, Brussels. Available at www.consilium.europa.eu/uedocs/cms_Data/docs/pressdata/EN/genaff/115157.pdf.

75. European Commission. (2010) EU Contribution to the Millennium Development Goals: Some Key Results from European Commission Programmes. European Commission, Brussels.

76. Van Reisen M. (2010) 2015 Watch, Report 6/2010. Alliance 2015, Copenhagen. Available at http://erd.eui.eu/about-2/mobilizing-european-research-for-development-policies/.

77. Institute for Health Metrics and Evaluation. (2011) Financing Global Health 2011: Continued Growth as MDG Deadline Approaches. IHME, Seattle, WA. Available at http://ec.europa.eu/research/health/public-health/public-health-and-health-systems/index_en.html.

78. Juma C, Lee Y-C. (2005) Innovation: Applying Knowledge in Development — Achieving the Millennium Development Goals. Report of the Task Force on Science, Technology and Innovation of the UN

Millennium Project. Earthscan, London. Available at www.unmillennium-project.org/reports/tf_science.htm.

79. Matlin SA. (2004) The Millennium Development Goals: substance and spirit. In: Matlin SA (ed.), *Global Forum Update on Research for Health 2005: Health Research to Achieve the Millennium Development Goals.* Pro-Brook, pp. 8–12.

80. Stearns BP. (2005) Health Research for the Millennium Development Goals: A Report on Forum 8, Mexico City (16–20 November 2004). Global Forum for Health Research, Geneva.

81. Global Health Technologies Coalition. (2010) Research and the Millennium Development Goals: How Research and Development for New, Innovative Health Tools Can Help Reach Global Health Targets. Global Health Technologies Coalition, Washington, DC. Available at www.ghtcoalition. org/files/MDGfactsheet.pdf.

82. Europa. (2009) The EU Contribution Towards the Millennium Development Goals (MDGs). Europa Summaries of EU Legislation. Available at http:// europa.eu/legislation_summaries/development/general_development_ framework/r12533_en.htm. Available at http://ec.europa.eu/research/ health/infectious-diseases/poverty-diseases/doc/prd-catalogue-fp7_en.pdf.

83. EU €1 billion Millennium Development Goals initiative to support maternal health contribute to fight against child mortality and hunger and improve supply of water and sanitation. (2011) Europa Press Release IP/11/1063, 21 September 2011. Available at http://europa.eu/rapid/press-release_IP-11-1063_en.htm.

84. European Council. (2010) Council Conclusions on the Millennium Development Goals for the United Nations High-Level Plenary Meeting in New York and Beyond. (2010) 3023rd Foreign Affairs Council Meeting, Luxembourg, 14 June 2010. Council of the European Union, Brussels. Available at www.hivresourcetracking.org/sites/default/files/RTWG%20 Advancing%20the%20Sciencefinal.pdf.

85. The European Commission's Technical Assistance for HIV/AIDS, Tuberculosis, and Malaria. Available at www.donortracker.org/sites/default/ files/SEEK%20TA%20Profile%20EC%20January%202012_0.pdf. Available at www.hivresourcetracking.org/sites/default/files/Public_ sector_investment_in HIV_vaccines_and_microbicides_0l.pdf.

86. European Commission. (2012) Mobilizing European Research for Development Policies. European Commission Directorate-General for

Development and Cooperation, Brussels. Available at www.euco-net.eu/fileadmin/euconet/Downloads/OpenAccessJournal/Supplement.pdf.

87. International Public Health and Health Systems. (2013) European Commission Directorate-General for Research and Innovation: Health. European Commission, Brussels. Available at http://www.policycures.org/downloads/DSWreport.pdf.

88. International Public Health and Health Systems: Projects. EC DG Research and Innovation: Health. (2013) European Commission, Brussels. Available at http://ec.europa.eu/research/health/public-health/public-health-and-health-systems/projects_en.html. www.policycures.org/downloads/GF2012_Report.pdf.

89. European Commission Research and Innovation: HIV/AIDS, TB and Malaria. Available at http://ec.europa.eu/research/health/infectious-diseases/poverty-diseases/index_en.html.

90. European Commission. (2012) About FP5 Funding: European Research Programme on HIV/AIDS, Malaria and Tuberculosis (1998–2002). European Commission, Brussels. Available at http://ec.europa.eu/research/health/infectious-diseases/poverty-diseases/fp5projects_en.html.

91. European Commission. (2012) About FP6 Funding: European Research Programme on HIV/AIDS, Malaria and Tuberculosis (2002–2006). European Commission, Brussels. Available at http://ec.europa.eu/research/health/infectious-diseases/poverty-diseases/fp6projects_en.html. Available at http://ec.europa.eu/research/health/poverty-diseases/doc/catalogue-3rdcall_en.pdf.

92. European Commission. (2010) EU Research Fighting the Three Major Deadly Diseases: HIV/AIDS, Malaria and Tuberculosis. First edition: EU Projects 2007–2010. European Commission, Brussels.

93. Investing to End the AIDS Epidemic: A New Era for HIV Prevention. Research & Development. (2012) HIV Vaccines and Microbicides Resource Tracking Working Group, July 2012. Available at www.hivresourcetracking.org/sites/default/files/July%202012%20Investing%20to%20End%20the%20AIDS%20Epidemic%20A%20New%20Era%20for%20HIV%20Prevention%20Research%20&%20Development.pdf. Available at www.edctp.org/fileadmin/documents/our_work/EDCTP project_portfolio.pdf.

94. HIV Vaccines and Microbicides Resource Tracking Working Group. (2010) Advancing the Science in a Time of Fiscal Constraint: Funding for

HIV Prevention Technologies in 2009. Available at www.edctp.org/fileadmin/documents/Final_IER_report.pdf.

95. HIV Vaccines and Microbicides Resource Tracking Working Group. (2006) Public and Philanthropic Investments in Preventive HIV Vaccines and Microbicides: 2000 to 2005. Preliminary Report, May 2006, pp. 1–6. Available at http://ec.europa.eu/research/health/infectious-diseases/poverty-diseases/doc/iee-report-edctp-programme_en.pdf.

96. Giehl C. (2011) Supplementary information on global and European funding on HIV/AIDS and *M. tuberculosis*/TB. *The Open Infectious Diseases Journal* **5(Suppl 1-M8):** 89–90.

97. Saving Lives and Creating Impact: EU Investment in Poverty-Related Neglected Diseases. (2012) DSW/Policy Cures, Hannover/London. Available at http://ec.europa.eu/commission_2010–2014/geoghegan-quinn/headlines/speeches/2012/documents/20121105-opening-address_en.pdf.

98. Moran M, Guzman J, Henderson K, *et al.* (2012) Neglected Disease Research and Development: A Five-Year Review. Policy Cures, Sydney, p. 80. Available at www.msps.es/profesionales/saludPublica/prevPromocion/promocion/desigualdadSalud/PresidenciaUE2010/conferencia Expertos/docs/haciaLaEquidadEnSalud_en.pdf.

99. Available at Innovative Medicines Initiative. www.imi.europa.eu/content/home.

100. Available at IMI Ongoing Projects. http://www.imi.europa.eu/content/ongoing-projects.

101. Combatting Deadly Diseases. (2007) EU-Funded Projects on Poverty-Related Diseases HIV/AIDS, Malaria, Tuberculosis. Third edition (all FP6 calls). European Commission, Brussels. Available at http://www.consilium.europa.eu/uedocs/cms_data/docs/pressdata/en/er/97496.pdf.

102. European & Developing Countries Clinical Trials Partnership (EDCTP). Available at www.edctp.org. Available at http://ec.europa.eu/research/iscp/pdf/policy/call_fp7_africa.pdf.

103. EDCTP. (2014) EDCTP Project Portfolio: A compendium of clinical trial, capacity building and networking projects. The Hague: EDCTP June 2014. Available at www.edctp.org/fileadmin/documents/our_work/EDCTP_project_portfolio.pdf.

104. W Van Velzen, *et al.* (2007) Independent External Review Report: European and Developing Countries Clinical Trials Partnership (EDCTP

Programme). Final Report 12 July 2007, 64 pp. Available at www.edctp. org/fileadmin/documents/Final_IER_report.pdf.

105. W Van Velzen, *et al.* (2009) Independent External Evaluation Report of the European and Developing Countries Clinical Trials Partnership (EDCTP Programme). Final Report 14 December 2009. Available at http://ec.europa.eu/research/health/infectious-diseases/poverty-diseases/ doc/iee-report-edctp-programme_en.pdf. Available at http://cordis.europa. eu/eu-funding-guide/home_en.html.

106. Technopolis. (2014) Assessment of the performance and impact of the first EDCTP programme. Technopolis Group, 18 September 2014. Available at www.edctp.org/publication/asscssment-performance-impact-first-edctp- programme/.

107. EDCTP. (2015) EDCTP: European Union Contribution. The Hague: EDCTP. Available at www.edctp.org/get-know-us/.

108. Ministry of Health & Social Policy. (2010) Moving Forward Equity in Health: Monitoring Social Determinants of Health and the Reduction of Health Inequalities. Ministry of Health & Social Policy, Madrid.

109. Garay J. (2012) Global Health (GH) = GH Equity = GH Justice = Global Social Justice. The Opportunities of Joining EU and US Forces Together. Newsletter of the European Union of Excellence at UC Berkeley, Winter 2012. Available at http://eucenter.berkeley.edu/newsletter/winter12/garay.html. Available at http://graduateinstitute.ch/files/live/sites/iheid/files/sites/global- health/shared/1894/Publications/GHEResearchPaperFinalNov2011.pdf.

110. Garay J. (2012) *Global Health Equity and the Challenge for a New Global Health Framework: The US and EU Policies and Opportunities to Improve Global Health.* UC Berkeley.

111. Council of the European Union. (2007) The Africa–EU Strategic Partnership: Lisbon, 9 December 2007: 16344/07 (Presse 291).

112. European Commission Directorate-General for Research and Technical Development. (2009) Africa Call: Call FP7-Africa 2010 (Fab-Env-Health). European Commission, Brussels.

113. EC. (2012) Europe 2020. Brussels: European Commission 2012. Available at http://ec.europa.eu/europe2020/index_en.htm.

114. EC. (2013) One trillion euro to invest in Europe's future — the EU's budget framework 2014–2020. EC Press Release, Brussels, 19 November

2013. Available at http://europa.eu/rapid/press-release_IP-13-1096_en.htm.

115. Rabesandratana T (20L5) EU trims Horizon 2020 but spares European Research Council Science, 29 May 2015. Available at http://news.sciencemag.org/europe/2015/05/e-u-trims-horizon-2020-spares-european-research-council.

116. EC. (2013) Factsheet: Horizon 2020 budget. Brussels: EC, 19 November 2013. Available at www.ec.europa.eu/research/horizon2020/pdf/press/fact_sheet_on_horizon2020_budget.pdf.

117. Battams S, Matlin SA, Jahn A, Kickbusch I. (2011) The Case for Europe as a Leader in Research and Innovation for Global Health. Geneva: Global Health Europe, Nov 2011. Available at www.globalhealtheurope.org/images/stories/ghe/GHEResearchPaperFinalNov2011.pdf.

118. Global Health Advocates. (2013) Poverty-Related and Neglected Diseases in Horizon 2020 — Gaps and Challenges. Global Health Advocates. Available at www.ghadvocates.eu/wp-content/uploads/2013/09/20130114_PRNDs-in-Horizon-2020-Gaps-and-Challenges-.pdf.

119. EC. (2012) Report of a joint European Commission/Alliance for Biomedical Research in Europe conference: "the Future of Health Research and Innovation in Europe: the need for strategic action" held at the Belgian Royal Academy of Medicine, Brussels 23 May 2012. Available at www.esc-crt.org/news/Pages/EU-Policy-News.aspx.

120. European Report on Development. Available at www.erd-report.eu.

121. Overcoming Fragility in Africa. (2009) European Report on Development 2009. Robert Schuman Centre for Advanced Studies, European University Institute, San Domenico di Fiesole.

122. Social Protection for Inclusive Development. (2010) European Report on Development 2010. Robert Schuman Centre for Advanced Studies, European University Institute, San Domenico di Fiesole. Available at www.ema.europa.eu/docs/en_GB/document_library/Other/2009/12/WC500016817.pdf.

123. ODI. (2012). Confronting Scarcity: Managing Water, Energy and Land for Inclusive and Sustainable Growth. European Report on Development 2011/2012. Overseas Development Institute (ODI), European Centre for Development Policy Management (ECDPM), German Development Institute/Deutsches Institut für Entwicklungspolitik (GDI/DIE).

Available at https://ec.europa.eu/europeaid/sites/devco/files/consca-report-erd-2011_en.pdf.

124. ODI. (2013) Post-2015: Global Action for an Inclusive and Sustainable Future. European Report on Development 2013. Overseas Development Institute (ODI), German Development Institute/Deutsches Institut für Entwicklungspolitik, (DIE), European Centre for Development Policy Management (ECDPM). Available at www.erdreport.eu/erd/report_2012/documents/FullReportEN.pdf.

125. ODI. (2015) Financing and other means of implementati on in the post-2015 context. European Report on Development 2015, Overseas Development Institute (ODI), German Development Institute/Deutsches Institut für Entwicklungspolitik, (DIE), European Centre for Development Policy Management (ECDPM), Brussels, 2015 in preparation. http://jica-ri.jica.go.jp/event/assets/ERD20I5%20note.pdf.

126. European Medicines Agency. Available at http://www.ema.europa.eu/ema/index.jsp?curl=pages/home/Home_Page.jsp&mid=.

127. European Medicines Agency. (2008) EMEA Strategy Paper: Acceptance of Clinical Trials Conducted in Third Countries, for Evaluation in Marketing Authorisation Applications. Doc. Ref. General-EMEA/228067/2008. EMEA, London.

128. European Medicines Agency. (2011) Draft Reflection Paper on Ethical and GCP Aspects of Clinical Trials of Medicinal Products for Human Use Conducted in Third Countries and Submitted in Marketing-Authorisation Applications to the EMEA. Report of an International Workshop, 6–7 September 2010. EMEA, London.

129. European Medicines Agency. (2012) Reflection Paper on Ethical and GCP Aspects of Clinical Trials of Medicinal Products for Human Use Conducted Outside of the EU/EEA and Submitted in Marketing Authorisation Applications to the EU Regulatory Authorities. EMEA, London, 2012.

130. Schipper I, Weyzig F. (2008) Ethics for Drug Testing in Low and Middle Income Countries. Considerations for European Market Authorisation. Centre for Research on Multinational Corporations (SOMO), Amsterdam.

131. European Medicines Agency. (2007) European Commission–European Medicines Agency Conference on the Operation of the Clinical Trials Directive (Directive 2001/20/EC) and Perspectives for the Future,

3 October 2007. Conference Report. EMEA, London. Available at www. who.int/bulletin/volumes/90/1/11-092007/en/.

132. European Medicines Agency. (2010) Road Map to 2015: The European Medicines Agency's Contribution to Science, Medicines and Health. EMEA, London. Available at http://journals.plos.org/plosmedicine/article? id=l0.1371/journal.pmed.l001115. Available at www.ema.europa.eu/docs/ en_GB/document_library/Report/2011/01/WC500101373.pdf.

133. Paediatric European Network for Treatment of AIDS (PENTA). Available at www.pentatrials.org. Available at www.health-policy-systems.com/ content/9/1/11.

134. Paediatric European Network for Treatment of AIDS (PENTA). (2009) Available at www.ema.europa.eu/docs/en_GB/document_library/ Presentation/2009/11/WC500007138.pdf.

135. Moran M, *et al.* (2011) Registering New Drugs for Low-Income Countries: The African Challenge. *PLoS Medicine* 8(2): e1000411. doi:10.1371/ journal.pmed.l000411. Available at www.plosmedicinc.org/article/info% 3Adoi%2F10.1371%2Fjournal.pmed.1000411.

136. Battams S, Matlin SA. (2012) Research Policies and Global Health. Symposium Report: World Health Summit: Research for Health and Sustainable Development, Berlin, 21–24 October 2012. Global Health Europe, Geneva. Available at www.globalhealtheurope.org/images/stories/ event_report_berlin_Final.pdf.

137. Pratt B, Loff B. (2012) Health research systems: promoting health equity or economic competitiveness? *Bulletin of the World Health Organization* **90(1):** 55–62. Available at www.who.int/bulletin/volumes/90/1/11-092007/en/.

138. Ostlin P, *et al.* (2011) Priorities for research on equity and health: towards an equity-focused health research agenda. *PLOS Medicine* **8(11):** 2. Available at http://journals.plos.org/plosmedicine/article?id=10.1371/ journal.pmed.1001115.

139. Frenk J, Chen, L. (2011) Overcoming gaps to advance global health equity: a symposium on new directions for research. *Health Research Policy and Systems* **9(11).** Available at www.health-policy-systems.com/ content/9/1/11.

140. Frenk J, Moon S. (2013) Governance challenges in global health. *The New England Journal of Medicine* **368:** 936–942. Available at www.nejm.org/ doi/full/10.1056/NEJMra1109339.

141. Roos R. (2013) Scientists Seek Ethics Review of H5N1 Gain-of-Function Research. CIDRAP. Available at www.cidrap.umn.edu/cidrap/content/influenza/panflu/news/mar2913ethics.html.
142. Connor S. (2013) Leading scientists urge President Obama's advisers to investigate ethical issues raised by creating highly infectious strain of bird-flu. *Independent*, 1 April 2013. Available at www.independent.co.uk/news/science/leading-scientists-urge-president-obamas-advisers-to-investigate-ethical-issues-raised-by-creating-highly-infectious-strain-of-birdflu-8556082.html.
143. Roos, *ibid*.
144. HAI Europe & Oxfam. (2014) Trading away access to medicines — revisited: How the European trade agenda continues to undernlitle access to medicines. Hal Europe & Oxfam. Available at www.oxfam.org/sites/www.oxfam.orglfiles/file_attachments/bp-trading-away-access-medicines-290914-en.pdf.

8

Humanitarian Aid, the Global Health Communication and the Council Conclusions on the EU Role in Global Health[a]

*Jorge Castilla**

"Health is a core sector of humanitarian aid. Indeed it has a particularly broad application across all humanitarian sectors because humanitarian aid needs and impact are largely measured in terms of human health".[1]

Health in humanitarian emergencies is exceptional in that a population endures acute excess mortality, morbidity and suffering or the risk of it, typically due to a conflict, epidemic, acute or slow onset natural disaster, or chemical/nuclear event. The increased risk of acute mortality frequently relates to warfare, displacement and overcrowding, insufficient nutrients, communicable diseases with epidemic potential, proliferation of vector diseases, rupture of water/sanitation/hygiene systems, toxic or

* ECHO's Health Sector Global Advisor, Avenue Appia 20; 1211 Geneva 27, Switzerland.
[a]The views expressed in this article are the personal views of the authors and in no way constitute the official views of the institution.

215

radiation poisoning, or the breakdown of vaccination and health services.

The Humanitarian Regulation (1996) established the basis of EU humanitarian aid: "Humanitarian aid, the sole aim of which is to prevent or relieve human suffering, is accorded to victims without discrimination on the grounds of race, ethnic group, religion, sex, age, nationality or political affiliation and must not be guided by, or subject to, political considerations"; "Humanitarian aid decisions must be taken impartially and solely according to the victims' needs and interests."[2]

The European Consensus on Humanitarian Aid (2008) set the vision of the 27 EU Member States together with the European Commission, on common principles aimed at improving the coherence, effectiveness and quality of its humanitarian response.[3]

The Lisbon Treaty, which entered into force in December 2009, established that "The Union's operations in the field of humanitarian aid shall be conducted within the framework of the principles and objectives of the external action of the Union." and "Humanitarian aid operations shall be conducted in compliance with the principles of international law and with the principles of impartiality, neutrality and non-discrimination."[4]

Through ECHO — the European Commission Directorate-General for Humanitarian Aid and Civil Protection — funding, millions of people are helped each year in more than 70 countries through 200 partners (international NGOs, the Red Cross and Red Crescent movements, and specialized UN agencies.[5]

In 2012, ECHO's total expenditure was €1.3 billion. Health expenditure varies from year to year, with a mean of around 20% recorded. This 20% does not include the 148 million spent on nutrition-related activities in 2012, which could be summed together with health.

Humanitarian Aid in the Global Health Communication and the Council Conclusions

The Commission's Global Health Communication (GHC)[6] highlights "the importance of access to health services for populations under stress in fragile contexts, humanitarian crisis and in peace and stabilization processes" (GHC 4.3). Furthermore, the Communication states that the EU needs to cater for "the special needs of people in humanitarian crisis situations" (GHC 3.2).

The subsequent Council Conclusions (CC) on the EU role in global health[7] affirm that the EU should "seek to ensure optimal access to health services for populations in fragile contexts, emergency and/or humanitarian situations and in peace and stabilization processes" (CC 16.c).

The Global Health Communication defines four sets of objectives to be applied by the Commission as a whole. These objectives promote the application of common values and principles of solidarity in order to reach equitable and universal coverage through quality health systems, in the frame of joint and coherent EU actions:

- Governance, supporting a stronger leadership by the WHO at the global and national levels for normative and guidance functions and full participation of all stakeholders.
- Equity of effective aid commitment to health based on programs and country health systems, ensuring that their main components — health workforce, access to medicines, infrastructure, logistics and decentralized management — are effective enough to deliver basic equitable and quality healthcare for all.
- Coherence, particularly in the aspects of trade and finance (including quality medicines), migration and brain drain, security (in particular the prediction of, detection of and response to global health threats) and food security.
- Global health knowledge, including evidence based decisions.

However, equitable and universal coverage through quality health systems does not fully capture the specificity of impartial humanitarian aid. Humanitarian aid aims to save lives and alleviate suffering for populations in acute need, based solely on the assessment of those needs.

When people are affected by conflicts or natural disasters, they are likely to suffer an increase in illnesses and deaths well above the usual levels, or they face a higher risk of death, if effective interventions do not mitigate the mortality. Fast effective health interventions can reduce mortality and morbidity via the delivery of services to the people affected. To do so the interventions must assure predictable means, which usually include autonomous supplies and separate human resources to ensure the response and that this response is fast and effective in saving lives, alleviating suffering and minimizing disability during the emergency phases.

Health is a core sector of humanitarian aid, absorbing a substantial part of funds. Nutrition in emergencies is an element of paramount importance in improving survival and it is inextricably linked to health. The Global Health Communication and the Council Conclusions on the EU's role in global health do not introduce novelties to the basics of humanitarian aid; they reaffirm the purpose of the Humanitarian Regulation of 1996 and of the Humanitarian Consensus of 2008. The regulation and the consensus frame the basis of humanitarian aid. Both the Commission's communication and Council Conclusions are essentially a reaffirmation of principles, stating that access to health services should be "optimal" for populations in fragile contexts, emergency and/or humanitarian situations as well as in peace and stabilization processes. "Optimal" is a term that may need some precision: disasters create gaps between needs and capacities, and also frequently destroy or reduce capacities and create obstacles to providing health services. So the term may be interpreted as "as good as possible" given the context, in order to initially lower mortality and under-nutrition to beneath emergency thresholds, and later to pre-emergency levels.

Conversely, there are many elements of the Global Health Communication and the Council Conclusions which are not specific to emergency and/or humanitarian situations, but do apply in the frame of emergency aid. These elements deserve analysis because specific evolutions can be reported, even if those evolutions advanced independently of the Communication and Council Conclusions themselves.

The GHC and CC Elements related to Humanitarian Aid

While humanitarian health actions are delivered mainly via community outreach, primary, secondary or higher care, medicine supplies, outreach response and temporary infrastructure interventions, the specific main causes of mortality in poor tropical settings are an exacerbation of the base pathology: respiratory diseases, diarrhea, neonatal/maternal mortality, malaria and tuberculosis. Injuries are frequent in conflict settings and in acute natural disasters. Disease and death in emergencies are accelerated by conditions that decrease immunity such as undernutrition and vulnerability to infectious diseases like HIV and measles. The typical epidemics that require immediate mass response are meningitis, yellow fever, other oral viral hemorrhagic fevers (Ebola, Marburg…) and cholera. Physical and mental disabilities are common sequels of violence and trauma. Some other common field pathologies and conditions seen in emergencies are neglected tropical diseases, chronic non-communicable diseases, dengue and pandemic risks.

Among the different emergencies, some can extend beyond borders, such as disease outbreaks, conflicts, toxic spills and nuclear events. The Commission Communication states that the EU should contribute to early prediction detection of, and response to global health threats, under the International Health Regulations (GHC 4.3). Here, ECHO contributes by funding early warning and surveillance systems inside health programs and via permanent contact with the WHO-hosted Global Outbreak Alert and Response Network and its members, including the ECDC.

Other related elements of the GHC are the references to food security ("d. Strengthen the links between food security, nutrition and health, with particular support to the most vulnerable groups, *inter alia* children under five and women in pregnancy and lactating period"; "On food security, food assistance and nutrition the EU should ensure that its policies work to increase access to food and link with national health strategies that include nutrition services and monitoring of nutritional status in the population") (GHC 4.3) and climate change ("e. Include consideration of health issues in the adaptation and mitigation strategies in developing countries in environmental and climate change policies and actions").

One can say that in relation to both issues, ECHO works on disaster preparedness, disaster risk reduction, and resilience experiences (AGIR — *Alliance globale pour l'Initiative Résilience*; SHARE — Supporting the Horn of Africa's Resilience). West Africa's recurrent nutritional crisis has led to the aim of creating links between nutrition and health, but this is an ongoing task and not a specificity that would link emergency, relief and rehabilitation with global health very much.

There are other elements of the GHC Council Conclusions that have a clear application in humanitarian settings such as in the Council Conclusions:

- To monitor the EU distribution of direct and indirect health aid.
- To support an increased leadership of the WHO at global, regional and country level, in its normative and guidance functions.

Currently the WHO is undergoing a major change in its emergency response role and structure at central level linked to the humanitarian reform. These changes are still to be reflected in field practice.

- The Council acknowledges the International Health Partnership (IHP+) principles. This last part relates to LRRD — "Linking relief, rehabilitation and development.
- Flexibilities for the protection of public health provided for in TRIPS agreements, in order to promote access to medicines.

The aim of ECHO partners is to save lives; this includes the provision of medical supplies. Sometimes intellectual property rights may pose a challenge to access to life-saving treatments for populations that cannot afford them. One example is the access to antiretrovirals in South Africa. Some of the ECHO partners have built advocacy operations to request using flexibility and exceptions allowed in the TRIPS (intellectual property) Agreement.

- Respecting the principle of evidence-based approach when setting normative action of food, feed, products, pharmaceuticals and medical devices.

The GHC emphasizes that "the EU should also work at global and regional level to eliminate trade in falsified medicines," which is indeed a main concern in emergencies, as the impact of an intervention is the result of the effectiveness multiplied by the coverage: falsified or substandard medicines make interventions ineffective, and ineffective treatments lead to death.

In its field operations, contractually ECHO requires partners to guarantee and prove the quality of the medical supplies. Easier said than done, medicine quality assurance requires know-how, people with competencies which are not that easy to find, and funding. Therefore, less than a handful of organizations are able to do this, at a very high cost and with a complex setup. To help in this, ECHO audits a number of procurement centers — an audit based on documented proof of steps, giving assurance to partners on the quality of supplies. Nevertheless, partners sometimes buy elsewhere for different reasons (such as a piece of legislation that precludes importation or a drive to support local production), but they do not have the capacities to assure quality. In the previous years (2012, 2013), ECHO has supported a coalition of more that 15 NGOs — called QUAMED — that pools NGO and academic resources to provide medicine quality assurance services to the member partners (http://www.quamed.org/en/home.aspx).

The EU Communication on Resilience COM (2012) 586, of 3rd October 2012,[8] gives ground to build on the articulation of emergency and development by jointly focusing on the resilience of communities and on service provision.

There are thus multiple elements from the more global frame provided by the GHC and the CC that apply in specific aspects of humanitarian aid.

Outlook: What is Ahead of Us?

As survival at a young age improves globally in times of peace, acute excess mortality continues to be associated with conflicts which are not ending any time soon, and with natural and man-made disasters, whose effects are increasing. The typical interventions implemented during humanitarian assistance are strongly influenced by trends[9,10] that will also affect the larger global health agenda, such as changes in demography (aging, change of the disease pattern toward chronic noncommunicable diseases, more urban populations), technology and science (mobile phones, social transfer modalities, geographical information systems, information drones), economics (inequality, uneven growth, unemployment, safety nets), political power (emerging donors, stronger and more assertive countries, weaker and fragile states, dynamic civil societies, new actors), climate change (vector-borne diseases, zoonosis, water scarcity, insufficient food, environment deterioration, resilience) and patterns of conflict (prolonged, simmering, urban and internal conflict; terrorism, use of robotic, automated and distance killing; risk of biological, chemical or nuclear events).

To end this chapter, a quote from Article 214 of the Lisbon Treaty: "Humanitarian aid operations shall be conducted in compliance with the principles of international law and with the principles of impartiality, neutrality and non-discrimination." This is in line with the 1996 Humanitarian Regulation, the legal basis of ECHO.

References

1. Matthew Sayer.
2. Council Regulation 1257, 20 June 1996, http://mcaf.ee/hce8r.
3. Council Declaration, 30 January 2008/C 25/01, http://mcaf.ee/6cd9w.
4. Chapter 3, Humanitarian Aid, Article 214, as published in 2010, http://mcaf.ee/07bfs; previously Article 188j.
5. http://mcaf.ee/okrqy.
6. COM (2010) 128, http://mcaf.ee/bes3z.
7. http://mcaf.ee/lbvk4.
8. http://mcaf.ee/w8sr2.
9. http://mcaf.ee/v54km.
10. http://mcaf.ee/k6fba.

Council of the European Union. (1996) Council (Humanitarian) Regulation 1257/96. Available at http://eurlex.europa.eu/LexUriServ/LexUriServ.do?uri=CONSLEG:1996R1257:20090420:EN:PDF.

Council of the European Union. (2008) Joint Statement by the Council and the Representatives of the Governments of the Member States Meeting Within the Council, the European Parliament and the European Commission. The European Consensus on Humanitarian Aid. Brussels, 30 January, 2008. 2008/C 25/01. Available at http://eurlex.europa.eu/LexUriServ/LexUriServ.do?uri=OJ:C:2008:025:0001:0012:EN:PDF.

European Commission. (2012) Communication from the Commission to the European Parliament and the Council — The EU Approach to Resilience: Learning from Food Security Crises. COM (2012) 586 final. European Commission, Brussels.

European Commission. (2013) Communication from the Commission to the European Parliament, the Council, the European Economic and Social Committee and the Committee of the Regions — A Decent Life for All: Ending Poverty and Giving the World a Sustainable Future. COM (2013) 92 final. European Commission, Brussels.

European Commission — Humanitarian Aid and Civil Protection. (2014) European Consensus on Humanitarian Aid: ECHO Factsheet. Available at http://ec.europa.eu/echo/files/aid/countries/factsheets/thematic/consensus_en.pdf.

Lisbon Treaty, Chapter 3, Humanitarian Aid, Article 214, as published in 2010; previously Article 188j. http://eur-lex.europa.eu/LexUriServ/LexUriServ.do?uri=OJ:C:2010:083:0047:0200:en:PDF.

The future of humanitarian action. (2011) *International Review of the Red Cross* **93(884)**.

European Commission (2013) Communication from the Commission to the European Parliament and the Council: The EU Approach on Resilience: Learning from Food Security Crises. COM(2012) 586 final. European Commission, Brussels.

European Commission (2011) Communication from the Commission to the European Parliament, the Council, the European Economic and Social Committee and the Committee of the Regions: An EU Budget for 2020. Delivering Investment Growth and Strengthening. COM(2011) 500 final. European Commission, Brussels.

European Commission (2012) Humanitarian Aid and Civil Protection: ECHO. European Commission's Humanitarian Aid. <http://ec.europa.eu/echo/index_en.htm> (accessed ...).

FAO, IFAD, & WFP (2013) The State of Food Insecurity in the World 2013. The Multiple Dimensions of Food Security. Rome: FAO.

Food and Agriculture Organization (2011) ... last updated 2011. <http://www.fao.org/ ... >

9

The Consideration of Health in EU Financial Programmes

Von Thea Emmerling[*][a]

The EU budget is one of the major instruments the EU has at its disposal to support and pursue specific policies. The other instruments are legislative instruments (regulations, directives, etc.), "soft law" (Recommendations, Council conclusions etc.) and political instruments (Declarations, statements etc.). The EU budget has a yearly volume of around 130 billion Euros, which constitutes approximately 1% of EU GNI.

Every five to seven years, the EU embarks on a major round of planning of its political priorities and future budgets, the so-called financial perspectives or financial framework. In its Communication "A Budget for Europe 2020"[b] the European Commission stressed, that "the next financial framework 2014–2020 is "tied in with the Europe 2020 strategy for smart, sustainable and inclusive growth"[c] and empasized that "the optimal achievement of objectives in some policy areas — including climate

---

[*]Thea Emmerling, Minister Counselor, Head of the Health, Food Safety, and Consumer Affairs Section, Delegation of the European Union to the United States, Washigton DC, USA.
[a]The views expressed in this article are the personal views of the author and do in no way constitute the official views of the institution.
[b]A Budget for Europe 2020 — COMMUNICATION FROM THE COMMISSION TO THE EUROPEAN PARLIAMENT, THE COUNCIL, THE EUROPEAN ECONOMIC AND SOCIAL COMMITTEE AND THE COMMITTEE OF THE REGIONS, COM (2011) 500 final PART I of 29.6.2011, http://ec.europa.eu/health/programme/docs/maff-2020_en.pdf.
[c]A Budget for Europe 2020, p. 2.

action, environment, consumer policy, health and fundamental rights — depends on the mainstreaming of priorities into a range of instruments in other policy areas".[d]

This chapter analyzes whether the mainstreaming of health into the different financial instruments of the EU was really done for the period 2014–2020. It screens all major EU financial instruments for the term "health" or other health-related activities. It also looks at the relative weight of health-related expenditure in the future EU financial framework.

It comes to the conclusion that the present situation as regards health-related expenditure from the EU budget does not seem to have much further evolved for the new period 2014–2020 as compared to 2007–2013. Although health actions are eligible under a considerable number of financial instruments, the intended mainstreaming of health does not yet follow a consistent nor strategic approach. However, in the light of continued financial austerity and the re-orientation of the EU budget towards economic growth, a status quo on health financing could already be considered an achievement.

The EU Budget and Financial Perspectives

Every five to seven years, the EU embarks on a major round of planning of its political priorities and future budgets, the so-called financial perspectives or multi-annual financial framework. The financial perspectives specify maximum amounts that are intended to be spent in a given year for a certain broad policy area as well as the planned maximum amounts for the yearly overall budgets over five to seven years. Or, to say it in budgetary terms, the multi-annual financial framework sets the maximum amount of commitment appropriations in the EU budget each year for broad policy areas ("headings") and fixes an overall annual ceiling on payment and commitment appropriations.[e]

This multi-annual financial framework is unanimously adopted by the European Council (of Heads of State) in the form of a Council Regulation, with the consent of the European Parliament (Article 312). It is important

---

[d] A Budget for Europe 2020, p. 22.
[e] http://ec.europa.eu/budget/biblio/documents/fin_fwk1420/fin_fwk1420_en.cfm.

to note that the financial perspectives are financial planning figures for a certain period of time. The yearly EU budgets that follow the agreement on the financial perspectives are then drawn up and decided within these overall maximum amounts agreed upon. The yearly EU budgets are adopted by the two arms of the Budgetary Authority (Council of Ministers and European Parliament — Article 314) and executed by the Commission, which is responsible and accountable for the implementation of the EU budget (Article 17, para 1).

This medium-term financial planning has brought peace to the EU budgetary and financial system, which had been paralyzed over several years, especially in the 1970s due to constant fights between the two arms of the Budgetary Authority.[f] It also allows a proper planning for the years ahead and therefore gives stability to the whole system.

So far, the EU had four of these financial packages (Delors I, Delors II, Agenda 2000, Financial Perspectives 2007–2013), with five to seven years of duration each. The EU has just finalized its fifth multi-annual financial framework 2014–2020: The process started with the Commission Communication "A Budget for Europe 2020"[g] and related proposals. The package was heatedly discussed in the Council in November 2012 and February 2013 and the broad budgetary figures were agreed upon between Heads of State in a "night of long knives" during the European Council 7–8 February 2013[h]: They decided to cut the budget from its previous level for the first time in EU's history. An agreement with the European Parliament, that had to give its consent, was reached on 2 December 2013 and formalized in the Council Regulation 1311/2013 on 20 December 2013.[i] Parliamentarians had insisted on a real system of own resources

---

[f] More information on the background of these budgetary struggles between the Council and the European Parliament see European Commission, European Union Public Finance, fourth edition, Luxemburg 2008, pp. 23–34, http://ec.europa.eu/budget/library/biblio/publications/public_fin/EU_pub_fin_en.pdf.

[g] "A Budget for Europe 2020", Communication from the Commission to the European Parliament, the Council, the European Economic and Social Committee and the Committee of the Regions, COM (2011) 500 final of 29 June 2011; The communication and all related documents can be found under: http://ec.europa.eu/budget/reform/index_en.htm.

[h] http://www.consilium.europa.eu/uedocs/cms_data/docs/pressdata/en/ec/135344.pdf.

[i] http://eur-lex.europa.eu/LexUriServ/LexUriServ.do?uri=OJ:L:2013:347:0884:0891:EN:PDF.

for the EU, and the compromise reached was to set up a high level group to look at the issue.[j]

Normally, the negotiations around the financial perspectives take two to three years, because they need unanimity between Member States and agreement between the two Arms of the Budgetary Authority. Most of the financial packages also include changes in the financing of the budget, which are difficult to agree upon. In addition, with each multi-annual financial framework most of the financial instruments and some-times whole policy areas are overhauled and reformed and their legal bases being renewed — to bring them through the process alone takes one and a half to two years. This was also done this time in parallel with the financial negotiations.

Whereas the first three financial packages were structured mainly around agriculture and structural funds, the two biggest spending blocks in the EU budget, the Financial Perspectives 2007–2013 tried to group the spending programmes on the basis of political priorities, starting with the major political priority of creating growth.[k] The fifth package largely followed that logic.

Table 9.1 gives a brief overview of the main policy changes in the different financial packages, combined with a short appreciation and the policy context.

Specific Health Programme and Mainstreaming of Health Activities

As regards health activities, the above-mentioned Commission Communication on the budget for Europe 2020 puts all its emphasis on "smart and inclusive growth." Health is one of the policy sectors that is being mainstreamed into different financial instruments rather than ring-fenced with a specific amount: "The optimal achievement of objectives in

---

[j] http://register.consilium.europa.eu/doc/srv?l=EN&f=ST%2015997%202013%20 ADD%201.

[k] For a thorough discussion of the different financial packages, see European Commission, *European Union Public Finance*, Luxemburg 2008, pp. 35–118, http://ec.europa.eu/ budget/library/biblio/publications/public_fin/EU_pub_fin_en.pdf.

Table 9.1 Main Elements of the Five Financial Packages

	Agricultural Policy	Structural Policy	Own Resources	Special Remarks
Delors I 1988–1992	• Agricultural guideline • Production reduction by stabilizers and set aside • Early warning system	Fundamental reform: • European approach: • Three objectives • Four principles: — concentration — partnership — complementarity — programming • Doubling of structural funds	• Introduction of new own resource (GDP) • Introduction of ceiling • Interinstitutional Agreement	• European Single Act (internal market research, cohesion further developed); • Southern Enlargement
Delors II 1993–1999 Rural Development	Fundamental reform (McSharry) one year ahead of FP: from price policy to income policy: • Introduction of direct payments to compensate for price reductions	• Increase of structural funds • Introduction of Cohesion fund	• Lifts own resources ceiling to 1.27% of GDP	• Maastricht Treaty (TEN, education, industry, culture, 2nd and 3rd Pillar developed) • Northern Enlargement

(Continued)

Table 9.1   *(Continued)*

	Agricultural Policy	Structural Policy	Own Resources	Special Remarks
Agenda 2000 2000–2006	• Stabilization of GAP budget in real terms • Differenciation and ceilings for direct payments • Continuation of McSharry Reform	• Stabilization of structural funds • 4% absorption capacity • Simplification, concentration, phasing-out	• Stabilization of EU expenditure in real terms; • Financing of enlargement within 1.27%	• Amsterdam Treaty • Eastern Enlargement • Special instrument for accession countries
Financial Perspectives 2007–2013	• Nominal stabilization of agricultural budget	• Stabilization of structural funds (SF)	• Financing of enlargement within existing ceilings	• Lisbon Treaty — strengthining of external action — restructuring of headings according to political priorities (growth); new heading citizenship
Financial Perspectives 2014–2020	• Slight nominal decrease but some agricultural expenditure outside heading • Greening, capping of direct payments to large farms	• Continued stabilization of SF • 2.5% absorption capacity • Conditionality linked to economic governance (partnership contracts)	• New own resource (financial transaction tax) to reduce GNI contribution was proposed, but not decided, High-Level Group set up	• Nominally constant, but relative decrease of EU budget to about 1% of EU GNI • 5 instruments outside financial perspectives

some policy areas — including climate action, environment, consumer policy, health and fundamental rights — depends on the mainstreaming of priorities into a range of instruments in other policy areas."[l]

The mainstreaming itself can be derived from Treaty article 168(1) which specifies: "A high level of human health protection shall be ensured in the definition and implementation of all Union policies and activities."

Nevertheless, a specific public health and a food safety programme are being maintained. The third public health programme 2014–2020[m] is included in Heading 3 "Security and Citizenship" for the FP 2014–2020 (see Table 9.2). A constant amount of 449 million € is foreseen over the next seven years. As regards food, feed, animal and plant health, the nearly 1.9 billion € for the next seven years constitute a decrease. This is not exceptional; the negotiators cut the financial allocation of a lot of policy areas as compared to the year 2013 as well as compared to the Commission's proposal, as the negotiations fell into a time of economic crisis and budgetary austerity in the EU. Also, several important payer Member States were eager to push the EU budget to even below 1% of EU GNI.

Mainstreaming Health — Financial Instruments for Internal Policies

The specific health programme and the food safety programme are nevertheless by far not the only health spending in the EU budget, which has currently an overall yearly volume of around 130 billion €, thus representing around 1% of the EU Gross National Income. Other policies contribute higher amounts to health, especially the financially important instruments of research and cohesion:

---

[l] http://ec.europa.eu/budget/library/biblio/documents/fin_fwk1420/MFF_COM-2011-500_Part_I_en.pdf, pp. 22.

[m] Proposal for a Regulation of the European Parliament and of the Council on establishing a Health for Growth Programme, the third multi-annual programme of EU action in the field of health for the period 2014–2020, COM (2011) 709 final of 9 November 2011, http://ec.europa.eu/health/programme/docs/prop_prog2014_en.pdf.

Table 9.2   Multi-annual Financial Framework (Eu-28) 2014–2020*

(EUR million — 2011 prices)

Commitment Appropriations	2014	2015	2016	2017	2018	2019	2020	Total 2014–2020
1. Smart and Inclusive Growth	**60 283**	**61 725**	**62 771**	**64 238**	**65 528**	**67 214**	**69 004**	**450 763**
1a: Competitiveness for growth and jobs	15 605	16 321	16 726	17 693	18 490	19 700	21 079	125 614
1b: Economic, social and territorial cohesion	44 678	45 404	46 045	46 545	47 038	47 514	47 925	325 149
2. Sustainable Growth: Natural Resources	**55 883**	**55 060**	**54 261**	**53 448**	**52 466**	**51 503**	**50 558**	**373 179**
of which: Market related expenditure and direct payments	41 585	40 989	40 421	39 837	39 079	38 335	37 605	277 851
3. Security and citizenship	**2 053**	**2 075**	**2 154**	**2 232**	**2 312**	**2 391**	**2 469**	**15 686**
4. Global Europe	**7 854**	**8 083**	**8 281**	**8 375**	**8 553**	**8 764**	**8 794**	**58 704**
5. Administration	**8 218**	**8 385**	**8 589**	**8 807**	**9 007**	**9 206**	**9 417**	**61 629**
of which: Administrative expenditure of the institutions	6 649	6 791	6 955	7 110	7 278	7 425	7 590	49 798
6. Compensations	**27**	**0**	**0**	**0**	**0**	**0**	**0**	**27**
Total Commitment Appropriations	**134 318**	**135 328**	**136 056**	**137 100**	**137 866**	**139 078**	**140 242**	**959 988**
as a percentage of GNI	1.03%	1.02%	1.00%	1.00%	0.99%	0.98%	0.98%	1.00%
Total Payment Appropriations	**128 030**	**131 095**	**131 046**	**126 777**	**129 778**	**130 893**	**130 781**	**908 400**
as a percentage of GNI	0.98%	0.98%	0.97%	0.92%	0.93%	0.93%	0.91%	0.95%
Margin available	0.25%	0.25%	0.26%	0.31%	0.30%	0.30%	0.32%	0.28%
Own Resources Ceiling as a percentage of GNI	1.23%	1.23%	1.23%	1.23%	1.23%	1.23%	1.23%	1.23%

*Official Journal, 20.12.2013, L347/891: http://eur-lex.europa.eu/LexUriServ/LexUriServ.do?uri=OJ:L:2013:347:0884:0891:EN:PDF.

The biggest financial contribution to health activities — ring-fenced with nearly 7.5 billion € until 2020 — will come from the new research programme Horizon 2020. Health, demographic change and well-being and food security are important own sub-objectives under the Horizon 2020 priority "societal challenges." The specific objective to improve lifelong health and well-being of all, explicitly mentions, among others, health promotion, determinants of health, healthcare, surveillance and preparedness and health data for future research. Under the specific objective "to secure sufficient supplies of safe and high quality food and other bio-based products" research for healthy and safe food and plant and animal health are mentioned. Health-related research is also looked at in some subsections of the priority industrial leadership for certain industrial technologies, like nanotechnologies (including its impact on health and environment) or biotechnology (including producing innovative industrial, health and environmental applications). The European and Developing Countries Clinical Trials Partnership (EDCTP2) for medical interventions against HIV, malaria and tuberculosis will be renewed and research on rare diseases will continue.

Another important policy area that traditionally includes health spending is regional policy. The European Regional Development Fund will continue to be able to co-finance investments in health and social infrastructure within the EU, especially for underdeveloped regions. This was so far the largest EU funding source for investments in health infrastructure. The European Social Fund specifically mentions active and healthy ageing and enhancing access to affordable, sustainable and high-quality services, including healthcare, under its eligibility rules. E-health activities are pre-listed for the new "Connecting Europe Facility" and are contained in several other financial programmes.

The agricultural funds and the European Maritime and Fisheries Fund set public health, animal and plant health as one of the criteria for cross-compliance. They continue to contain market support measures related to animal diseases and loss of consumer confidence due to public health, animal or plant health risks; the agricultural spending continues to cover a school fruit scheme to promote healthy eating habits of children. Health-enhancing physical activity shall be promoted under the Erasmus + programme. The Programme for the Environment and Climate Action

(LIFE) focuses on one specific policy action at the link between environment and health.

The Justice programme foresees to "support initiatives in the field of drugs policy as regards judicial cooperation and crime prevention" in so far as they are not covered by the Internal Security Fund or the Health Programme. The new Asylum, Migration and Integration Fund allows for certain health-related expenditure. The Union Civil Protection Mechanism mentions acute health emergencies under its general objectives. The Internal Security Fund identifies health infrastructure as critical infra-structures of which disruption or destruction would have a serious impact on the well-being of people, or of the functioning of the Union or its Member States. The anti-fraud programme Hercule continues to finance the fight against cigarette smuggling.

For a detailed and complete overview of the "mainstreaming" of health into the financial instruments for internal policy, please see (Table 9.3).

This overview of the internal policy financial instruments shows that health is being looked at in most programmes, with the research pro-gramme being the financially most important one and even ring-fencing a specific amount for health-related research. Also the two major structural policy instruments, the European Regional Development Fund and the European Social Fund, continue to mention health. How much health-related activities the latter will generate in the field is, however, unclear, as this depends on whether and how the regions in the Union will use their structural funds and on which activities exactly they will focus their funds. Several other financial instruments also mention health or health-related activities, but in a patchy manner and according to the needs of these policy areas rather than health needs.

Mainstreaming Health — Financial Instruments for External Policies

As regards the external policy financial instruments, the strongest health references, as in the past, are contained in the Instrument for Development Cooperation (DCI) and the European Development Fund (EDF). The DCI forms part of the EU-Budget, while the EDF is still outside. Both of these instruments, which stand for a big part of health spending in the external

Table 9.3 EU Financial Instruments in the Field of Internal Action 2014–2020[†]

Name and Source	Amount	Overall Objective	Mentioning of Health
1a: Competitiveness for Growth and Jobs			
Programme for the Competitiveness of Enterprises and small and medium-sized enterprises (2014–2020) (Regulation 1287/2013)	2.298,000,000 €	Improve the competitiveness of enterprises, with special emphasis on small and medium-sized enterprises (SMEs)	Health not mentioned specifically, but, like any other industry, health companies can benefit from the program if they qualify as SME
Horizon 2020 — The Framework Programme for Research and Innovation (2014–2020) (Regulations 1291/2013, 1290/2013, 1292/2913, Decision 13/12/2013)	79,402,000,000 €	Determines the framework governing Union support to research and innovation activities The general objective shall be pursued through three mutually reinforcing priorities dedicated to: (a) excellent science (b) industrial leadership (c) societal challenges	• Health, demographic change and well-being and food security as important own sub-objectives under priority societal challenges (Part 3 of Annex 1), • Applies a wide approach to health questions and consumer protection, including disease prevention, healthcare, e-health, health workforce, healthy diets, safe food, also mentions health effects of some technologies (e.g. bio, nano); continues European and Developing Countries Clinical Trials

(Continued)

[†]All the financial programmes for 2014–2020 that are available on the European Commission's website http://ec.europa.eu/budget/mff/programmes/index_en.cfm were screened by the author whether or not they use the term "health" in the main body of the legal text. This analysis does not include the programmes Copernicus, Creative Europe, Europe for Citizens, Galileo, ITER, the nuclear decommissioning assistance programs and the rights equality and citizenship program as they do not mention health in their core legal text.

Table 9.3   *(Continued)*

Name and Source	Amount	Overall Objective	Mentioning of Health
			Partnership (EDCTP2) • Ring-fencing of 7,472,000,000 € for health, demographic change and well-being • The European Institute of Innovation agenda has healthy living and active ageing as one focus
Erasmus + (Regulation 1288/2014)	14,775,000,000 €	Aims at boosting skills and employability; provides funding for the professional development of education and training staff, youth workers and for cooperation between universitites, colleges, schools, enterprises and NGOs	Physical activity mentioned as one of the specific objectives under "sport" chapter ("to promote voluntary activities in sport, together with social inclusion, equal opportunities and awareness of the importance of health-enhancing physical activity through increased participation in, and equal access to, sport for all")
Connecting Europe Facility (Regulation 1316/2013)	21,934,000,000 €	Promotes projects of common interest within the framework of the trans-European networks policy in the sectors of energy, transport and telecommunications	The telecom regulation 284/2014 covers interoperable cross-border e-health services as eligible actions. This refers to interaction between citizens/patients and healthcare providers, and/or health professionals and institutions. The services shall comprise cross-border access to electronic health records and electronic prescription services as well as remote health/assisted living teleservices, etc.

with $D_{\tau,dR}(V) = (V \otimes_{\tau,L} B_{dR})^{G_L}$; which is an E vector space of dimension $\dim_E V$. The τ in the notation signifies that we view V as a vector space over L via the embedding $\tau : L \to E$.

If (r, V) is de Rham, then for each of the embeddings $\tau : L \to \overline{\mathbb{Q}}_p$, we define a multiset of size $\dim_E V$ in which the integer j appears with multiplicity $\dim_E \text{gr}^j D_{\tau,dR}$. Here $\text{gr}^j D_{\tau,dR}$ is the jth graded component of the filtration on the module $D_{\tau,dR}$ induced by the filtration on D_{dR}. This multiset is denoted by $\text{HT}_\tau(r, V)$ and its elements are called the Hodge-Tate weights of (r, V) with respect to τ.

We know that every de Rham representation (r, V) is potentially semistable, see [1]. That is, there exists a finite Galois extension L' of L, such that $D_{st}(V) := (V \otimes_{\mathbb{Q}_p} B_{st})^{G_{L'}}$ is a free $E \otimes_{\mathbb{Q}_p} L'_0$-module of rank $\dim_E V$. Here L'_0 is the maximal unramified subextension of $L'/\mathbb{Q}_p$. As before for any embedding $\tau : L'_0 \to \overline{\mathbb{Q}}_p$ define $D_{\tau,st}(V) = (V \otimes_{\tau,L'_0} B_{st})^{G_L}$ which is a E-vector space of dimension $\dim_E V$. For any $w \in W_L$ lying above Frob_k^m for any $m \in \mathbb{Z}$, define

$$\rho(w) = r(w) \otimes (w\varphi^{m[k:\mathbb{F}_p]})$$

as an element of $\text{GL}(D_{\tau,st}(V))$.

Finally define, $\text{WD}(r, V)_\tau = (\rho, D_{\tau,st}(V), 1 \otimes N)$. This is the Weil-Deligne representation associated to (r, V). It is independent up to isomorphism on the choices involved in its definition, hence we drop τ from the notation.

In a similar manner, we can associate a Weil-Deligne representation to a (r, V) that is crystalline. A representation (r, V) is called crystalline, if $D_{cris}(V) = (V \otimes_{\mathbb{Q}_p} B_{cris})^{G_L}$ is free as an $E \otimes_{\mathbb{Q}_p} L_0$-module of rank $\dim_E V$. Note that any crystalline representation is also semistable. The module $D_{cris}(V)$ is a filtered φ-module and it can be recovered from the filtered (φ, N)-module $D_{st}(V)$ by the formula

$$D_{cris}(V) = D_{st}(V)^{N=0}.$$

For any embedding $\tau : L_0 \to E$ define $D_{\tau,cris}(V) = (V \otimes_{\tau,L_0} B_{cris})^{G_L}$ which is a E-vector space of dimension $\dim_E V$. The associated Weil-Deligne representation $\text{WD}(r, V)$ is given by the same action as above on $D_{\tau,cris}(V)$. It is again independent of the choice of τ.

3.4.2. Galois representations associated to cusp forms on definite unitary groups

We now recall the contruction of Galois representation associated to cusp forms on definite unitary groups.

Let $r : G_K \to \mathrm{GL}_n(\overline{\mathbb{Q}}_p)$ be a Galois representation. Let $c \in \mathrm{Gal}(K/F)$ be the non-trivial element in the Galois group of K/F. Choose any lift $\tilde{c} \in G_F$ of c. Define the conjugate representation

$$r^c : G_K \to \mathrm{GL}_n(\overline{\mathbb{Q}}_p) \qquad \text{by sending} \qquad g \mapsto r(\tilde{c}g\tilde{c}^{-1}).$$

We fix an isomorphism $\iota : \overline{\mathbb{Q}}_p \to \mathbb{C}$. Let Π be a RACSDC, irreducible, admissible representation of $\mathrm{GL}_n(\mathbb{A}_K)$. The following theorem associates a Galois representation to Π.

Theorem 3.30. *Let Π be a RACSDC automorphic representation of $\mathrm{GL}_n(\mathbb{A}_K)$ of weight λ. Associated to Π, there exists a Galois representation*

$$r_{p,\iota}(\Pi) : G_K \to \mathrm{GL}_n(\overline{\mathbb{Q}}_p)$$

such that

- $r_{p,\iota}(\Pi)^c \simeq r_{p,\iota}(\Pi)^\vee \otimes \epsilon^{1-n}$, *where ϵ is the p-adic cyclotomic character.*
- *For all w of K above p, the representation $r_{p,\iota}(\Pi)|_{G_{K_w}}$ is de Rham and it is crystalline if Π_w is unramified. Moreover, let $\tau : K \to \overline{\mathbb{Q}}_p$ be an embedding corresponding to w, the Hodge-Tate weights are*

$$\mathrm{HT}_\tau(r_{p,\iota}(\Pi)|_{G_{K_w}}) = \{\lambda_{\iota\tau,1} + n - 1, \ldots, \lambda_{\iota\tau,n}\}.$$

- *For all places w of K above p, we have*

$$\iota \mathrm{WD}(r_{p,\iota}(\Pi)|_{G_{K_w}})^{F-ss} \simeq rec_{K_w}(\Pi_w^\vee \otimes |\det|^{\frac{1-n}{2}}).$$

Here $\mathrm{WD}(r_{p,\iota}(\Pi)|_{G_{K_w}})^{F-ss}$ denotes the Frobenius semi-simplication of the Weil-Deligne representation associated to $r_{p,\iota}(\Pi)|_{G_{K_w}}$.

Proof. The proof of this theorem is contained in [42],[16],[11],[5],[12]. $\square$

Let π be a cuspidal automorphic representation for G. If $v \notin S_p$ and v splits as ww^c in K, then $\pi_w := \pi_v \circ i_w^{-1}$ is an admissible irreducible representation of $\mathrm{GL}_n(K_w)$. By local Langlands, we associate a Weil-Deligne representation $rec_{K_w}(\pi_w^\vee \otimes | \;|^{(1-n)/2})$ of W_{K_w}. We denote by $r_p(\pi_w)$, the p-adic Galois representation associated to this Weil-Deligne representation, as discussed in the previous section. We then denote by $r_p(\pi_w)^\vee(1-n)$ the Tate twist, $r_p(\pi_w)^\vee \otimes \epsilon^{1-n}$, of $r_p(\pi_w)^\vee$ by a power of the p-adic cyclotomic character. The following theorem associates a Galois representation to π.

Theorem 3.31. *[26, Proposition 2.7.2] Let λ be a dominant weight for G and let π be an irreducible constituent of the $G(\mathbb{A}_F^\infty)$-representation $S_\lambda(\overline{\mathbb{Q}}_p)$. Then there exists a continuous semisimple representation*

$$r(\pi) : G_K \to \mathrm{GL}_n(\overline{\mathbb{Q}}_p)$$

with the following properties.

Programme	Budget	Description	Health consideration
Customs 2020 (Regulation 1294/2013), **Fiscalis 2020** (Regulation 1286/2013), **Pericles 2020** (Regulation 331/2013), **Hercule III** (Regulation 250/2013)	908,000,000 €	Improve the operation of the taxation systems in the internal market and the functioning of the Customs Union	Health not specifically mentioned, however, it covers excise duties on alcohol and alcoholic beverages and tobacco taxation; also the fight against cigarette smuggling and counterfeiting is included
Employment and Social Innovation Programme (Regulation 1296/2013)	919,000,000 €	Aims to contribute to the implementation of the Europe 2020 Strategy, supports employment and social policies across the EU	Health stressed in recitals; in the eligible actions health and safety at work is mentioned, also healthier work-life balance; other actions could be subsumed under "adequate, accessible and efficient social protection systems"
1b: Economic, social and territorial cohesion **Regulation laying down common provisions of the structural funds** Regulation 1303/2013	185,374,000,000 € + 55,780,000,000 € + 35,701,000,000 € + 1,563,000,000 €	Lays down the common rules applicable to the European Regional Development Fund, the European Social Fund, the Cohesion Fund, the European Agricultural Fund for Rural Development and the European Maritime and Fisheries Fund, which are operating under the Common Strategic Framework	Health not mentioned in core text, can be subsumed under "promoting social inclusion." In the Annex, certain health actions mentioned

(Continued)

Table 9.3 (*Continued*)

Name and Source	Amount	Overall Objective	Mentioning of Health
European Regional Development Fund (Regulation 1301/2013)		Support with regard to the investment for growth and jobs and the European territorial cooperation goals	Investments in social, **health** and educational infrastructure, e-health eligible; use of a health indicator; specifically excludes the support of manufacturing, processing and marketing of tobacco and tobacco products
European Social Fund (Regulation 1304/2013)		Overall objective is to promote high levels of employment and job quality, mobility of workers, enhance social inclusion and combat poverty	Health mentioned in several investment priorities: Active and healthy ageing, enhanced access to affordable and sustainable services including healthcare, reduction of health inequalities also mentioned
Cohesion Fund (Regulation 1300/2013)	74,928,000,000 €	The Cohesion Fund helps Member States whose GNI per inhabitant is less than 90% of the EU average in making investments in TEN-T transport networks and the environment	No mentioning of health at all

European Territorial Cooperation (Regulation 1299/2013)	10,229,000,000 €	Helps regions across Europe to work together to address shared problems	Mentions cooperation among universities or health centers as examples in a recital and uses a health indicator in the Annex, but health not specifically mentioned in core legal text; however, it could be thought to be subsumed under "promoting social inclusion"
2. Sustainable Growth: Natural Resources			
Common agricultural policy (pillar I) (Regulatios 1306/2013, 1307/2013, 1308/2013)	312,735,000,000 €	Supports farmers' incomes in the form of direct payments and market-support measures	• contains market support measures related to animal diseases and loss of consumer confidence due to public, animal or plant health risks • covers school fruit scheme to promote healthy eating habits of children • contains rules to ensure that products comply with hygiene and health standards and to protect animal, plant and human health, including restrictions to free circulation resulting from the application of measures intended to combat the spread of animal diseases

(Continued)

Table 9.3 (*Continued*)

Name and Source	Amount	Overall Objective	Mentioning of Health
Rural Development Fund (Regulation 1305/2013)	95,577,000,000 €	Aims at boosting development in rural regions	Mentions health aspects of animal husbandry, new economic activities related to healthcare in rural areas, compensation for animal diseases, food quality, food safety and healthy diet
Common Fisheries Policy and European Maritime and Fisheries Fund (Regulations 508/2014, 1379/2013 and 1380/2013)	7,405,000,000 €	Sets rules for managing fishing fleets and conserving fish stocks, Fisheries Fund aims at promoting fishing industry and coastal communities	• Common Fisheries Policy should pay full regard, to animal health, animal welfare, food and feed safety • mentions health in promotion of aquaculture having a high level of environmental protection, and the promotion of animal health and welfare and of public health and safety • improve hygiene, health, safety and working conditions for fishermen • compensation to mollusc farmers for public health reasons

Programme	Amount		
Programme for the Environment and Climate Action (LIFE) (Regulation 1293/2013)	3,457,000,000 €	Aims at improving EU environment and climate policy and legislation	Link between environment and health mentioned in one specific policy action; also defines thematic priorities for environment and health, including chemicals and noise
3. Security and Citizenship			
Public Health Programme (Regulation 282/2014)	449,000,000 €	The EU Health Programme is about fostering health in Europe by encouraging cooperation between Member States to improve health policies	All objectives cover health; aims at complementing Member States' health policies by promoting health, encouraging innovation in health, increasing sustainability of health systems and protecting citizens from cross-border health threats
Food chain, animal health and welfare and plant health programme (Regulation 652/2014)	1,892,000,000 €	Aims at contributing to a high level of health for humans, animals and plants along the food chain and in related areas and a high level of protection for consumers and the environment; aims also at strengthening enforcement	Most of the specific objectives cover health-related measures related to animal and plant health Covers programmes for the eradication, control and surveillance of animal diseases and zoonoses and plants, veneterinary measures and purchase of vaccines/antigen, emergency measures, laboratories, alert systems, data collection, training programmes for safer food

(Continued)

Table 9.3   *(Continued)*

Name and Source	Amount	Overall Objective	Mentioning of Health
Consumer Programme (Regulation 254/2014)	189,000,000 €	Helps citizens to enjoy their consumer rights and actively participate in the single market; the programme will do so by contributing to protecting the **health**, safety and economic interests of consumers	Health mentioned under objective 1 — safety: scientific advice and risk analysis relevant to consumer health and safety regarding non-food products and services; Supports also NGOs that have as their primary objectives the promotion and protection of health, safety, economic and legal interests of consumers in the EU
Justice Programme (Regulation 1382/2013)	378,000,000 €	Aims to make sure that EU legislation in civil and criminal justice is effectively applied, also supports EU actions to tackle drugs and crime	One of four specific objectives is to "support initiatives in the field of drugs policy as regards judicial cooperation and crime prevention aspects" in so far as they are not covered by the Internal Security Fund or the Health Programme
Asylum, Migration and Integration Fund (Regulation 516/2014)	3,137,000,000 €	Contributes to an effective management of migration flows in the Union	Certain health spending possible, its eligibility mentioned under specific chapters of the programme, f.ex. provision of health and psychological care for asylum seekers, pre-departure health assessments and medical treatment, medical screening, medical escorts, providing advice and assistance in health, psychological and social care as integration measures

Internal Security Fund (External border management and visa, as well as police cooperation, preventing and combating crime, crisis management) (Regulations 515/2014, 513/2015)	3,800,000 €	The Fund promotes the implementation of the Internal Security Strategy, law enforcement cooperation and the management of the Union's external borders. The ISF is composed of two instruments, ISF Borders and Visa and ISF Police	Health not specifically mentioned, but Regulation 513/2014 also includes health infrastructure as "critical infrastructure"; health also mentioned when it comes to "measures increasing the Union's resilience to crisis and disaster, ... supporting an effective and coordinated response to crisis linking up existing sector-specific capabilities, expertise centers and situation awareness centers, including those for health, civil protection and terrorism
Union Civil Protection Mechanism (Decision 1313/2013)	224,000,000 € + 145,000,000 €	Coordinates the EU response to natural and man-made disasters within and outside the EU, covers prevention, preparedness and response	Mentions acute health emergencies under general objectives; no more specific health mentioning later in the text when eligible actions are defined
EU Aid Volunteers Initiative (Regulation 375/2014)	148,000,000 €	Provides practical training for humanitarian volunteers and ensures their deployment in EU funded humanitarian aid operations worldwide	Health not specifically mentioned, but as it covers humanitarian work health is normally part of it

policies, aim at poverty reduction and traditionally have a relatively consistent overall approach to the development of the social as well as the
health sector. Health systems development is at the center of future EU
health activities in the external field. The DCI also specifically mentions
MDGs and global public goods. It ring-fences 25% of the new "global
public goods and challenges thematic programme" for human development, of which 40% are devoted to health.

Several of the other external instruments mention health in a patchy
manner, depending on their own policy needs, or one can assume that
health actions could be eligible under "social" actions, although they are
not specifically set out in the legal text. It is noteworthy that neither the
pre-accession instrument (the instrument to support the future accession
countries), nor the Partnership Instrument (instrument to address major
global challenges) mentions health specifically as being eligible.

For a detailed and complete overview of the "mainstreaming" of health
into the financial instruments for external policies, please see Table 9.4.

How Much Money for Health in the EU Budgets for 2014–2020?

Overall, one can say that there are two specific health-related financial
instruments for use in the EU, the public health and the food and feed
safety programme, but, compared to other financial programmes, they are
relatively small (about 64,000,000/270,000,000 €/year). The big bulk for
health spending within the EU will continue to come from the new
research framework programme Horizon 2020 which ring-fenced nearly
7,500,000,000 € for health-related research and the European structural
funds. The structural funds (ERDF and ESF) explicitly mention health
activities as eligible, but the amounts finally dedicated to health will
depend on the priorities that receiving regions define themselves and one
can therefore not say in advance how much of these funds will be used for
health.

In the external policies, the EDF and the DCI will continue to support
health activities outside the EU in a consistent manner. DCI also ring-
fenced a certain amount for health. The EDF and the geographic programmes under the DCI at the country level follow the same logic as the

Table 9.4 EU Financial Instruments in the Field of External Action 2014–2020[‡]

		Overall Objective	Mentioning of Health
Pre-Accession Instrument (Regulation 231/2014)	11,699,000,000 €	Financial support to enlargement countries in their preparations for EU accession (8 countries)	Health not mentioned in body of legal text; some health activities could be subsumed under "social and economic inclusion"
European Neighbourhood Instrument (Regulation 232/2014)	15,433,000,000 €	Strengthens relations with 16 partner countries to the East and the South, all EU policies, with a focus on human rights, the rule of law, sustainable development	Funds can be used to promote public health, in cross border programs public health is also mentioned as eligible

(Continued)

[‡]All the financial programmes for 2014–2020 that are available on the European Commission's website http://ec.europa.eu/budget/mff/programmes/index_en.cfm were screened by the author whether or not they use the term "health" in the main body of the legal text. This analysis does not include the Guarantee Fund for External Actions nor the Macro-financial assistance facility as they do not mention health at all.

Table 9.4   (*Continued*)

	Overall Objective	Mentioning of Health
Instrument for Development Cooperation (DCI) (Regulation 233/2014)	19,662,000,000 € Covers geographic programs with developing countries that are included in the list of recipients of ODA (official development assistance) by OECD/DAC (with some exceptions), thematic programs, a Pan-African Program; poverty reduction as prime objective	Substantial explicit mentioning of health; • the instrument shall also contribute to "fostering sustainable economic, social and environmental development" (Article 2) • "global public goods and challenges" as a specific thematic programme under the DCI and health also one of the objectives • Cooperation under geographical programmes include "health, social protection," and culture, also "food and nutrition security" • MDGs mentioned as specific activity • Ring-fencing: 25% of funds of **"Global public goods and challenges thematic programme"** go into human development, out of which 40% into health
Partnership Instrument (Regulation 234/2014)	955,000,000 € Advance and promote EU and mutual interests and to address major global challenges; all third countries, regions and territories may be eligible	Health not mentioned in body of legal text nor in the annex that specifies thematic priorities, but Commission can change the annex via comitology procedure

Instrument for Stability (Regulation 230/2014)	2,339,000,000 €	Addresses conflict prevention and peace-building, crisis response and security threats	EU technical and financial assistance can be provided to ensure "an adequate response to major threats to public health, including sudden epidemics with a potential transnational impact"; also mentions as eligible international cooperation relating to problem of drugs and enhanced safety practices in civilian facilities that handle chemical, biological, radiological and nuclear material
Instrument for Democracy and Human Rights (Regulation 235/2014)	1,333,000,000 €	Aims at enhancing the respect of human rights and fundamental freedoms and supporting democratic reforms in third countries	Does not mention health at all; certain health activities could, however, be interpreted into the instrument under the promotion of economic, social and cultural rights
Instrument for Nuclear Safety Cooperation (Regulation (EURATOM) 237/2014)	225,000,000 €	Aims at promotion of a high level of nuclear safety, radiation protection and safeguards of nuclear material in non-EU countries	Supports measures for ensuring safety of nuclear installations, protective measures to reduce radiation risks for workers and of the general public
Humanitarian Aid (Regulation 1257/96)	6,622,000,000 €	Provide assistance, relief and protection to victims of natural or man-made disasters outside the EU	The legal text does does not mention health at all, there is also only one mentioning of the term "social". However, the definition of eligibility is very wide and it is clear that humanitarian operations aim at alleviating social suffering which can include health

(Continued)

Table 9.4   (*Continued*)

	Overall Objective	Mentioning of Health
European Development Fund (outside EU Budget) As a framework, the Second Revision of the Cotonou Agreement 11th March 2010 is valid until 2020: http://ec.europa.eu/ development/icenter/ repository/second_ revision_cotonou_ agreement_20100311.pdf Cotonou Agreement: http://eur-lex.europa.eu/ LexUriServ/LexUriServ. do?uri=CELEX:22000A 1215(01):EN:HTML	34,276,000,000 € European Development Fund (EDF) is the main instrument for providing EU assistance for development cooperation under the Cotonou Agreement; poverty reduction and elimination, sustainable development and progressive integration of ACP countries into world economy as main objectives; Development cooperation, economic and trade cooperation and political dimension with Afrcan, Caribbean and Pacific countries (Cotonou Agreement); centers around poverty eradication	Social sector development includes health: • "Cooperation shall support ACP States' efforts at developing general and sectoral policies and reforms which improve the coverage, quality of and access to basic social infrastructure and services and take account of local needs and specific demands of the most vulnerable and disadvantages, thus reducing the inequalities of access to these services. … In this context, cooperation shall aim at. … "improving health systems, in particular equitable access to comprehensive quality and healthcare services, and nutrition, eliminating hunger and malnutrition, ensuring adequate food supply and security, including through supporting safety nets" • MDGs explicitly mentioned in second revision • Acknowledgmnt that **pandemics** need to be addressed • "Systematic account shall be taken in mainstreaming into all area of cooperation the following … themes: …, communicable and non communicable diseases, …" • Cooperation in the area of regional policies shall support the priorities of ACP countries, "in particular … **health**, education and training… • New article on HIV/AIDS

structural funds: It is the receiving country that decides on its priorities and therefore the use of the funds. In principle, health activities are eligible, but how much EU money will finally flow into health, is not predetermined in these financing instruments.

Although health-related elements are mentioned in most of the other financial instruments for the EU's external policy, one would go too far to characterise this as a "coherent mainstreaming" of health, as no consistent overall approach can be observed. This is all the more astonishing, as — in addition to the Treaty basis on mainstreaming and in addition to the explicit reference to mainstreaming in the Commission Communication "A budget for Europe 2020" — the EU also has a "Health in all policies approach" which can be interpreted as including the integration of health into all other policies, including financial programmes.

Conclusion

The present situation as regards health-related expenditure from the EU Budget does not seem to have been much further developed for 2014–2020 as compared to the period 2007–2013. As regards EU internal policies, health research, health investments, e-health and food safety continue to be important elements of EU support. In the EU's external policies, health systems development remains at the center of financing health activities. However, the mainstreaming of health into the different EU financial instruments does not yet follow a consistent approach. For the next financial perspectives, a clear strategy and reasoning should be developed. Nevertheless, the EU can continue to use its financial instruments to push its internal health and the global health agenda also in the new planning period. In light of the continued financial austerity and the re-orientation of the EU budget towards economic growth, this status quo on health financing could already be considered an achievement.

10

Law and the EU Role in Global Health Strategies: The Case of the FCTC

*Lourdes Chamorro**

The FCTC

The World Health Organization Framework Convention on Tobacco Control (WHO FCTC)[1] was the first treaty under Article 19 of the WHO constitution[2] and it has given a new legal dimension to international health cooperation. It was adopted by the World Health Assembly in May 2003[3] and came into force in February 2005. Its objective is "to protect present and future generations from the devastating health, social, environmental and economic consequences of tobacco consumption and exposure to tobacco smoke by providing a framework for tobacco control measures to be implemented by the Parties at the national, regional and international levels in order to reduce continually and substantially the prevalence of tobacco use and exposure to tobacco smoke."[4] The FCTC is one of the most quickly ratified and most widely embraced treaties in United Nations history. To date, only 17 out of the 194 WHO Member States have not ratified or acceded to it.[5]

---

*Political Officer, Delegation of the European Union to the United Nations and other International Organisations, Geneva, Switzerland.

When the idea of a convention that utilizes international law to further public health was born in 1993, it constituted a revolutionary new approach to health. Since then, particularly during the actual negotiation of the FCTC text in 1999–2003, the full potential of such a tool has become truly evident, and even more so when defining the multisectoral approach required in the fight against the tobacco epidemic. In 1999, the World Health Assembly called for work on the Framework Convention to begin, and to that end it created a Technical Working Group and established an Intergovernmental Negotiating Body (INB).[6] The Working Group met twice and the INB held six sessions between 2000 and 2003. Apart from achieving consensus on a text for the Convention and submitting it to the World Health Assembly for adoption, this intensive process served to raise awareness, educate and engage countries and relevant stakeholders around a common goal under the umbrella of the WHO Tobacco Free Initiative. The process itself constituted a strong advocacy tool against tobacco. Although it was not a formal participant in the negotiations, the role of the Framework Convention Alliance (FCA), a civil society alliance which advocates global tobacco control, should be given due recognition as an important and constructive non-state actor throughout the process.

Currently, the FCTC's implementation is fully underway. The Conference of the Parties (COP) has adopted seven guidelines[7] for implementation of different provisions of the Convention and at its fifth session, held in Seoul in November 2012, it adopted the first FCTC Protocol to Eliminate Illicit Trade in Tobacco Products.[8] The Secretariat assists the COP and implements its decisions as appropriate, and it is funded through "voluntary assessed contributions" (VACs), according to a scale of assessment based on the WHO's scale, and through "extrabudgetary funds" coming from the Parties.[9] The total budget adopted for 2014–2015 is US$17.3 million.[10]

The EU and the FCTC

The EU (formerly the European Community), as a regional economic organization (REIO), is a contracting party to the convention and it is the only signatory that is not a nation state. Article 1 of the FCTC, on the use of terms, defines a REIO as *"an organization that is composed of several sovereign states, and to which its Member States have transferred competence over a range of matters, including the authority to make decisions binding on its Member States in respect of those matters."* It adds as footnote clarifying that, where appropriate, the term "national" will refer equally to REIOs. On the right to vote, the Convention[11] states that REIOs, in matters within their competence, shall exercise their right to vote with a number of votes equal to the number of their Member States that are Parties to the Convention, and that they shall not exercise their right to vote if any of their Member States exercises their right, and vice versa.

While membership in a wide range of UN platforms is mostly limited to individual states, the participation of other actors became possible through a variety of means, such as UN resolutions granting observer or full participant status or the inclusion of a REIO, or more recently, a regional integration organization (RIO) clause in international conventions. The inclusion of the REIO clause in an international agreement is an additional overture, enabling REIOs to participate in the UN system. A REIO is commonly defined in UN protocols and conventions in the same way as mentioned above with respect to the FCTC.[b]

These provisions give the basis for the full recognition and participation of the EU in the FCTC implementation. This recognition was the culmination of the EU's strong commitment to tobacco control at both EU and global level.[12] Tobacco regulation has a long tradition in the EU; the community *acquis* includes myriad directives addressing warning labels, advertising and promotion bans, maximum tar yields, workplace air quality and safety, protection from environmental tobacco smoke, and recommendations to reduce tobacco use, among others.[13,14] In 1989 the Commission presented its first proposal for a directive to ban tobacco

---

[b] For REIO, the FAO Constitution Article XIV 3(b), the United Nations Framework Convention on Climate Change Article 1(6), Statute of The Hague Conference on Private International Law Article 3(2). For RIO, see the United Nations Convention on the Rights of Persons with Disabilites Article 44. Articles 216–219, Treaty on the Functioning of the European Union, *OJ C* **326**, 26 October 2012.

advertising.[15] Unfortunately, after a lengthy process, the Court of Justice annulled this first text[16] in 2000, and a new proposal,[17] which took on board the ruling, was presented in 2001 and finally adopted in 2003. In addition, in 1999 the Commission had presented a proposal for a directive that recast three internal market directives existing at that time that dealt with the tar content of cigarettes, oral tobacco, and labeling of tobacco products, and aimed at updating and completing these provisions taking as a basis a high level of public health protection. This proposal was finally adopted in 2001 and was known as "the tobacco products directive."[18] Four more nonbinding texts[19] were adopted between 1993 and 2003, in order to make recommendations to Member States when developing their tobacco control policies. Parallel initiatives took place in the area of taxation and the fight against smuggling also from the early 1990s, even if they did not incorporate a health-related dimension until very recently.

In this context of evolving tobacco control regulation, in 1999 the Council of the EU adopted by qualified majority a decision authorizing the Commission to open negotiations with the WHO on an international FCTC and related protocols with regard to matters within the EU competence, and provided it with agreed negotiating directives. Two preparatory working group meetings and a first session of the INB had taken place on that basis when the need to extend the negotiating mandate to areas requiring unanimous decision, such as taxation, became apparent. The Council therefore extended the mandate in 2001. Importantly enough, the negotiating directives included, *inter alia*, a provision specifying that the FCTC and its protocols should allow the EU to become a contracting party.

The convergence of (1) the legal basis for tobacco control regulation, (2) substantial ongoing legislative processes within the EU, (3) strong commitment to tobacco control by the Commission, European Parliament, Council and EU Member States, which often went beyond the EU minimum requirements at national level, and (4) international political momentum and a supportive environment from civil society, led to decisive EU involvement in the FCTC negotiations.

The Dynamics of the Decision-Making Processes to Define the EU Negotiation Positions

According to the mandate, the negotiations were to be conducted in consultation with a special committee, and the Council appointed the Public Health Working Party (PHWP) to take up this role. This was instrumental in forging the very specific dynamics that would accompany the negotiation process and would continue beyond the adoption of the Convention.

The FCTC negotiations were always based on the "Chair's text,"[20] which was released by the Chair of the INB prior to each negotiating session. This text, like the finally adopted text, covered a wide range of areas, such as health, development, research, agriculture, taxation, financing or illicit trade. The first relevant discussion that took place in the PHWP referred to who (the Commission or the EU rotating Presidency) should lead the negotiations on the different items covered by the draft text. Intense scrutiny of the related EU's and Member States' competences was carried out at that time in the Council. It soon became clear that most of the issues covered by the Chair's text fell under areas of shared competences and that establishing a strict division of the draft articles based on competences would be quite challenging. Finally, a pragmatic *ad hoc* approach was adopted, and preference was given to a division of tasks rather than a strict division of competences. The articles in the draft FCTC text were informally divided into those "under predominantly EU competence" and those under "predominantly Member States competence": the Commission and the Presidency would lead the negotiations on the two groups of articles, respectively. For example, labeling and advertising largely involve issues for which the EU had legislated, while education, communication, training and public awareness mainly fall under Member States' responsibilities. In addition, it was agreed that the EU position for both types of articles would be agreed by consensus in the PHWP. Only if discussions were exhausted and such a consensus proved to be impossible at that level would the issue be taken to COREPER or the Council, guided by the principle of unity of representation. That was for example the case for the provisions dealing with tobacco advertising, where the uncertain status of the directive at that stage was interpreted by a few Member States as the lack of a sound EU basis for negotiation.

Within the Commission, once the "Chair's text" was made available, the Directorate-General for Health and Consumers (DG SANCO) led a wide-reaching interservice consultation process with other Directorates-General (agriculture, trade, development, taxation and customs union, enterprise, justice, legal service). An *ad hoc* interservice group was created and the proposed positions were defined and agreed among the Commission services before presenting them for discussion in the PHWP. The Commission also engaged in frequent consultation with technical experts and civil society (the NGO community became particularly active and relevant at this stage) to develop its proposals.

Within the Council, while the PHWP systematically kept the "*chef de file*" role, it was decided that some parts of the text would be prepared beforehand by other Council configurations (for example, the illicit trade article was initially discussed in the Customs Union Group) or by other instances (for example, the budgetary and institutional aspects were prepared by the EU Delegation and EU Member States based in Geneva). This fact represented an additional layer of internal coordination.

Coordination in the PHWP was intense and sometimes difficult. The negotiating stance of the EU was based both on its existing legislation and on a shared position agreed between the EU Member States in areas where there was no such legislation. A common understanding among the EU Member States in the PHWP was built over time and the level of trust in the European Commission rose. Confidence and a spirit of teamwork were fostered during the negotiations. The working relationships between the Commission and the Member States throughout the process were largely based on trust and finally went beyond the strict interpretation of the division of roles and legal competences. The Commission and the PHWP traveled and held on-the-spot coordination meetings during all the negotiation sessions, and the EU and its Member States' joint effort was particularly intense during those periods, with up to three coordination meetings per day. The Commission and the rotating Council Presidency were in charge of the EU representation and actual negotiation of the agreed positions. Aside from the EU Member States, a number of countries with special relations with the EU (such as the accession countries) systematically aligned themselves with the EU's positions, making the EU and its Member States an even stronger force during the negotiations.

During the FCTC negotiations the EU faced two main criticisms. The first one referred to the defined positions: some non-EU countries and civil society felt that the EU's positions, as limited by the existing *acquis communautaire*, represented an obstacle to establishing more progressive health-oriented obligations in the Convention. It was often interpreted that existing legislation, or similarly agreed positions, would necessarily reflect the lowest common denominator among EU Member States. In addition, the EU was then somehow perceived as not willing to change its own *status quo*. The consequences of this perception were not major since the EU legislation was considered to be quite progressive at that time when compared to other strong international partners.

The second issue referred mainly to the negotiation process itself and it was more a "time issue." The need to systematically revert to the EU group before the negotiators were able to accept a given compromise was often perceived as a lack of flexibility or as inadequate EU adaptation to the rhythm of international negotiations. Non-EU actors complained about a certain level of rigidity that the EU internal working methods imposed on the process. It should also be mentioned that, as the negotiations progressed and the EU red lines became progressively clearer, the EU gained in effectiveness and got better at adapting to the required pace. This was also when alliances with non-EU actors and various outreach activities proved to be most effective.

Overall, and despite several difficulties in defining specific positions, the EU and its Member States negotiated during the six INB sessions with a single voice, and its visibility and level of influence throughout the process was considered to be very high. Its performance improved over the course of the process, as the negotiating positions became clearer within the EU group and the level of trust in the negotiators progressively increased. Overall, the EU was widely recognized as a leading and reliable international partner and negotiator whilst constituting a new institutional setting for national and international actors.

Approval or Ratification and FCTC Implementation in the EU

Once the World Health Assembly unanimously adopted the text in May 2003, it was open for signature, and 28 countries and the EU signed the treaty on the first day (16 June).

The Commission presented a proposal for a decision to the Council for the European Communities to adopt the FCTC. The Council adopted the decision[c,d] and the European Communities (the EU after the Treaty of Lisbon) became a contracting party to the Convention at the same level as any other country. Apart from this decision to adopt the Convention, the legal obligations included in the FCTC did not require any change in the existing *acquis communautaire*.

Once the FCTC entered into force on 27 February 2005 (90 days after the deposit of the 40th instrument of ratification, acceptance, approval, formal confirmation or accession), the first session of the Conference of the Parties (COP) was convened in Geneva in February 2006. At that session 18[e] EU Member States and the EU were already Parties to the Convention. At that meeting the COP requested the Health Assembly, to be held in May that year, to establish the Convention Secretariat[21] and in June 2007 Dr. Haik Nikogosian was appointed as the first head of the Convention Secretariat. The follow up to the implementation of the Convention at international level could now be fully developed. It is now nine years since the Convention entered into force, and a total of five sessions of the COP have taken place. The EU, as a full party, still plays an active role in implementing the Convention at international level.

As regards technical issues, the COP has developed a number of guidelines (seven so far) on the different articles of the Convention.[22] They are considered to be non-binding recommendations and they aim to help Parties in their implementation efforts. The guidelines have been drafted by different working groups under the leadership of two or three Parties acting as facilitators. Once finalized, they are submitted to the

---

[c] 2004/513/EC of 2 June 2004.
[d] Council Decision 2004/513/EC, *OJ L* **312**, 15 June 2004.
[e] List of participants, A/FCTC/COP/1/DIV/2Rev.1.

COP for adoption. The EU has taken up the role of key facilitator for the guidelines on tobacco contents and emissions (Articles 9 and 10), tobacco advertising (Article 13), packaging and labeling (Article 11), and partly on tobacco taxation — currently in preparation (Article 6). In addition, it has participated in most of these working groups of the other guidelines. A number of EU Member States have also played an active role in the working groups, as either facilitators or participants. The EU position on the final texts of the guidelines to be adopted by the COP, as well as other technical points under discussion during the COP session, has been coordinated in the Council (PHWP or Customs Union Group) based on the same approach adopted when negotiating the text of the Convention itself. This also applies to the decision on who takes the lead in proposing the initial position (the Commission or the Presidency), depending on the article. After eight years of implementation of the Convention, the EU has consolidated its position as a strong actor on tobacco control in international fora and it is widely recognized as a key player when working on the FCTC implementation. The fact that the EU was able to speak with one single voice during the whole process has been essential to that recognition.

On financial issues, every two years the COP adopts a work plan and a budget.[23] Interestingly, when comparing to other organizations within the UN system, the budget clearly differentiates the use of the "voluntary assessed contributions" (VACs) from the extra-budgetary contributions collected from different donors.[24] Traditionally, VACs are assigned to core functions of the Secretariat (structure and staff, monitoring and reporting, organizing COPs and priority working groups), while the extra-budgetary contributions are allocated to developing activities for which additional funds need to be raised for implementation. The EU and its Member States contribute almost 45% of the total VACs.[25] While the PHWP establishes the EU and its Member States' final positions for a COP session, EU coordination on the institutional and budgetary matters to be discussed by the COP is initially prepared by the EU and Member States representatives to the WHO based in Geneva.

With regard to the extra-budgetary contributions, it is worth mentioning two main issues: (1) the European Union's grant part of the "Investing in People" program and (2) the support given to the drafting and negotiation of the Protocol on illicit trade in tobacco products, which will be presented below.

The grant that the European Commission signed with the FCTC Secretariat in 2012[26] provided €5.2 million to support low- and middle-income countries in their tobacco control efforts through effective implementation of the WHO FCTC. The funding was aimed at helping the Convention Secretariat to scale up the work already undertaken on joint needs assessments, capacity building and enhancement of international cooperation, in line with the provisions of the Convention and decisions of the COP. This grant is a reflection of the EU's commitment to global tobacco control and of its commitment to supporting those developing countries willing to work further on the FCTC implementation.

Within the EU, as mentioned above, the legal obligations included in the Convention did not require any change in existing EU legislation, and this fact was one of the criticisms the EU faced as a negotiator. Nevertheless, the Convention not only does not prevent any Party from going beyond the legal obligations but also encourages parties to do so in many provisions. In fact, several EU Member States have very often gone beyond the EU requirements. Such encouragement became even clearer through the development of the implementation guidelines. Consequently, and since the guidelines have been adopted by consensus by the COP, they are considered to reflect the "best practice" or the gold standard. This not only helps Parties when they are developing their national policies but also represents an additional pressure on them should they diverge from the adopted recommendations. The Commission has also taken this into account when drafting a proposal, for example on the revision of the tobacco products directive. As such, there continue to be links between the international and European levels as they evolve together. Another example to be mentioned is the review of the tobacco taxation directive[27] and the influence which the FCTC article had on the Commission's proposal. In line with the FCTC text, the Commission's proposal and related impact assessment considered for the first time the direct relation between tobacco taxation (due to its impact on tobacco price) and health. The fact that a binding, worldwide ratified treaty clearly sets out that relationship constituted a strong basis for the EU legislator and had an impact on the final revised legislative text.

Finally, another significant impact of the FCTC implementation at EU level, apart from the impact at national level in the EU Member States, is the political impact. The negotiation and implementation of the FCTC has kept tobacco control on the political agenda of the Council and other political fora for more than ten years. Tobacco control was systematically on the agenda of the Health Council Ministers during the 1990s. This has significantly "educated" leaders and decision-makers, maintained the interest of different stakeholders, facilitated a wider permeation of tobacco control in sectors other than health, allowed for a more intersectoral approach, and has built a solid tobacco control community at national, European and global level. Collaterally, it has increased the cohesion of the EU and Member States around common positions and policies on tobacco control.

The FCTC Protocol on Illicit Trade in Tobacco Products

In 2007, at its second session in Bangkok, the COP opened negotiations on the first protocol to the Convention, on illicit trade in tobacco products.[28] It aims to eliminate all forms of illicit trade in tobacco products by requiring Parties to take measures to ensure effective control of the tobacco products supply chain and to cooperate internationally on a wide range of matters. The INB in charge of drafting and negotiating this protocol held a total of five sessions from 2008 to 2012, and the COP adopted the text at its fifth session in Seoul in 2013. Like the FCTC, it will enter into force 90 days after the deposit of the 40th instrument of ratification.

The process and methods of work have been very similar to those followed during the negotiations of the FCTC itself. Nevertheless, there are some particular points that can be mentioned.

One major achievement of the EU was to hold the chairmanship of the INB during the whole process. A Commission official, Ian Walton-George, Director at the European Anti-Fraud Office (OLAF), was elected to chair the process and to prepare the subsequent "Chair's texts."[29] This was quite a unique achievement, since the role of the EU in the UN system remains quite limited and it was a reflection of the leading role that the EU had played during the FCTC negotiations.

One interesting aspect of the protocol negotiations was the necessary combination between the health and the customs and enforcement experts. Although the health experts had been following the FCTC negotiations, they lacked expertise on the technical aspects of the protocol, and the opposite case was true for the customs experts. The challenge of finding common ground added to the difficulties of the negotiations. It proved to be a real intersectoral process. As in the case of the FCTC, it evolved and improved along the way. NGO participation in the process was less significant, though not inexistent, than during the FCTC negotiations, probably due to the specific technical expertise required.

Within the EU, the mandate from the Council to the Commission to negotiate the Protocol had already been included in the original mandate to negotiate the FCTC. Only a minor review was required to specify the concrete Protocol to be negotiated. In terms of coordination, the Council attributed the *"chef de file"* role to the Customs Union Group. While this group had followed the negotiations of one of the articles or the FCTC (Article 15), it was nevertheless quite new to the negotiation dynamics and to the broadly health-led environment in the WHO. In addition, due to the change of Working Party in the Council, the relationship between the Commission and the Member States needed to be rebuilt and the approaches taken differed somewhat from those of the PHWP.

Within the Commission, OLAF was designated *chef the file* due to its high level of specific expertise on fighting tobacco smuggling and counterfeiting built up over more than 10 years. OLAF was in charge of leading the coordination among the different services within the Commission, supported by DG SANCO, and of preparing the proposals for the Council. One of the parts of the protocol, considered to be the core of the text, deals with the control of the supply chain of tobacco products, and it is precisely this part that is directly related to OLAF's competence and experience. OLAF led the negotiations and represented the EU on this issue. In addition, the Commission provided significant financial support to the negotiation process.[30]

The EU has been very significantly involved in this process. It held the Chairmanship, had a strong and effective voice during the negotiations, and supported it financially. It has consolidated its role as international partner and negotiator. It also constitutes a precedent for any similar future process.

The FCTC as a Success Story

The FCTC process can be considered a success story from different perspectives, including the EU one. It has defined the main principles and best policies and practices on tobacco control to be implemented at national and local level, and has substantially contributed to enhancing international collaboration at global level in this area. The process itself has had a transformative and capacity building effect. It had a significant impact in keeping tobacco control high on the political agendas and in promoting a global movement against tobacco at different levels, notably among civil society. The FCTC negotiations have been largely health-led with a relatively low influence from foreign affairs, in line with the current trend of global health negotiations.

From the EU perspective, the FCTC can also be considered a success story. The EU is a full signatory party to the Convention, the first and only REIO, and the EU positions can be found widely in the adopted text. It has a central role to play in accelerating progress on global health issues, including tobacco control, through its commitment to protect and promote the right of everyone to enjoy the highest attainable standard of physical and mental health. The FCTC negotiations and its further implementation are fully in line with this commitment.

From an institutional point of view, the EU and its Member States are committed to speaking with a stronger and more coherent voice at the global level, including on global health initiatives, and this has been the case during this process. The EU's leadership and effectiveness throughout the process can be considered to be extremely significant and the EU has bolstered its position as a sound and reliable international partner in global health. The international community has become more familiar with this specific institutional context by virtue of having the EU as a negotiator and a legal contracting partner.

As already mentioned, one of the EU's particularities is that it has sometimes been perceived as having a limited capacity to react quickly to new proposals or compromises emerging on the table. The need to systematically coordinate EU positions with the EU Member States was, especially early in the process, not always well understood by third countries. Nevertheless, this issue and perception have been significantly reduced throughout the process as the EU positions became progressively clearer and firmer, and the trust in the negotiators grew. Overall, it did not constitute an obstacle but, as mentioned, a new environment for third countries. The fact that the negotiators, both within the EU and in third countries, remained relatively stable throughout the process and allowed for the establishment of longer relationships also significantly contributed to enhancing the dynamics of the negotiations over time. Clear definition of EU positions, defined red lines and trust in the negotiators are essential for enhancing the EU's role in international negotiations.

Internally, the strong EU and Member States' political commitment to tobacco control and the existing EU legislation were key factors in forging the EU's strong commitment to the FCTC process. Effective coordination in the Council PHWP and progressive consolidation of a common understanding of the EU positions between the Commission and the Member States have also been essential. The methods of work correspond to a pre-Lisbon era, tailored to the specific process stretching sometimes formal institutional boundaries. There was similar inertia after the Lisbon Treaty entered into force. Nevertheless, some adjustments have already been introduced. During the fifth session of the COP in 2012,[31] the European External Action Service chaired the EU's on-the-spot coordination meetings. In addition, the Commission represented the EU when dealing with all technical matters. That was not the case for institutional and financial issues, for which the rotating Presidency was in charge of the EU representation.

Finally, while the adoption of the FCTC by the EU did not require any change of the existing legislation, it has had an impact on the EU and Member States' policies and activities, and also on subsequent legislative proposals on tobacco control. The EU's engagement in the process has had an impact at both global health and EU levels.

Conclusion

The FCTC process, the first binding public health treaty under the auspices of the WHO, can be considered a success story at global level from the public health perspective, and it has also served as a mechanism for the EU to contribute to the achievement of its global health objectives. It constitutes an excellent example of a strong and effective EU voice in the global health arena thanks to the common effort made by the Commission and the EU Member States to work together so that real added value could be achieved. In addition, it has exposed the international community to a new institutional setting, having a REIO as a partner, adding a new factor to the already complex multi-actor global diplomacy.

References

1. World Health Organization. (2003) WHO Framework Convention on Tobacco Control. World Health Organization, Geneva.
2. World Health Organization. (1946) Constitution of the World Health Organization (consolidated version). New York.
3. World Health Organization. (2003) WHA Resolution 56.1, WHO Framework Convention on Tobacco Control. WHO Doc. WHO/PMA/21/5/2003.
4. World Health Organization. (2003) Article 3, WHO Framework Convention on Tobacco Control. Geneva, 21 May 2003.
5. Available at http://www.who.int/fctc/signatories_parties/en/ (accessed on 13 February 2014).
6. World Health Organization. (2003) OP 8-9, WHA Resolution 56.1, WHO Framework Convention on Tobacco Control. WHO Doc. WHO/PMA/21/5/2003.
7. Guidelines for implementation of the WHO FCTC, Article 5.3 | Article 8 | Articles 9 and 10 | Article 11 | Article 12 | Article 13 | Article 14 (consolidated version 2013).
8. FCTC. (2012) Decision on the Protocol to Eliminate Illicit Trade in Tobacco Products. FCTC/COP5(1). Seoul, 12 November 2012.
9. World Health Organization. (2003) Article 26, WHO Framework Convention on Tobacco Control. Geneva, 21 May 2003.
10. FCTC. Proposed workplan and budget for the financial period 2014–2015. FCTC/COP/5/23. Available at http://apps.who.int/gb/fctc/PDF/cop5/FCTC_COP5_23-en.pdf (accessed on 13 February 2014).

11. World Health Organization. (2003) Article 32(2), WHO Framework Convention on Tobacco Control. Geneva, 21 May 2003.

12. European Union Key Documents on Tobacco Policy. Available at http://ec.europa.eu/health/tobacco/key_documents/index_en.htm#anchor1 (accessed on 13 February 2014).

13. Studlar DT, Christensen K. (2009) The Impact of Tobacco Control Policies in the EU: Comparing Old and New Member States. Paper for EUSA Conference, Los Angeles.

14. Council Directive 89/552/EEC, Council Directive 89/654/EEC, Council Directive 92/85/EEC, Council Regulation (EEC) No. 2075/92, Council Directive 92/85/EEC, Council Resolution 96/C 374/04, Council Resolution 96/C 374/04, Directive 97/36/EC, Commission Regulation (EC) No. 1648/2000, Directive 2001/37/EC, Directive 2003/33/EC.

15. European Parliament, Council of the European Union. (1998) Directive 98/43/EC of the European Parliament and of the Council of 6 July 1998 on the approximation of the laws, regulations and administrative provisions of the Member States relating to the advertising and sponsorship of tobacco products. *Official Journal L* **213**.

16. Case C-376/98. (2000) Advertising and sponsorship of tobacco products. E.C.R. I-08419.

17. European Parliament, Council of the European Union. (2003) Directive 2003/33/EC of the European Parliament and of the Council of 26 May 2003 on the approximation of the laws, regulations and administrative provisions of the Member States relating to the advertising and sponsorship of tobacco products. *Official Journal L* **152**.

18. European Parliament, Council of the European Union. Directive 2001/37/EC of the European Parliament and of the Council of 5 June 2001 on the approximation of the laws, regulations and administrative provisions of the Member States concerning the manufacture, presentation and sale of tobacco products. *Official Journal L* **194(26)**.

19. Communication from the Commission COM/99/407/final, Council Conclusions 2000/C 86/03, Council Resolution 2000/C 218/03, Council Recommendation 2003/54/EC.

20. Chair's text of a framework convention on tobacco control. (2003) Geneva, 13 January 2013. Available at http://apps.who.int/iris/bitstream/10665/75493/1/einb62.pdf?ua=1 (accessed on 13 February 2014).

21. Resolution A/FCTC/COP/1/5, on the designation of the permanent secretariat and arrangements for its functioning.
22. Guidelines for implementation of the WHO FCTC, Article 5.3 | Article 8 | Articles 9 and 10 | Article 11 | Article 12 | Article 13 | Article 14 (consolidated version 2013).
23. FCTC. (2012) Proposed workplan and budget for the financial period 2014–2015, FCTC/COP/5/23. Available at http://apps.who.int/gb/fctc/PDF/cop5/FCTC_COP5_23-en.pdf.
24. World Health Organization. (2003) Article 26, WHO Framework Convention on Tobacco Control. Geneva, 21 May 2003.
25. FCTC. (2013) Status of payments of voluntary assessed contributions (VAC) as of 15 November 2013. Available at http://www.who.int/fctc/cop/VAC_15_November_2013.pdf?ua=1 (accessed on 13 February 2014).
26. Operating Grant No. 20123206 under EU Health Programme 2008–2013.
27. Council Directives 92/12/EEC and 2008/118/EC.
28. FCTC. (2014) Negotiations of the Protocol to Eliminate Illicit Trade in Tobacco Products, Sessions of the INB. Available at http://www.who.int/fctc/protocol/about/inb/en/index.html (accessed on 13 February 2014).
29. Intergovernmental Negotiating Body document FCTC/COP/INB-IT/1/5, Officers of the Intergovernmental Negotiating Body on a protocol on illicit trade in tobacco products.
30. European Commission. (2012) Commission welcomes positive outcome of WHO conference with signature of a protocol to stop illicit trade on tobacco. Press release, IP/12/1223.
31. Documentation of the fifth session of the COP in 1212. Available at http://apps.who.int/gb/fctc/E/E_cop5.htm (accessed on 13 February 2014).

11

The EU's Role in the International Health Regulations and the Pandemic Influenza Preparedness Framework Agreement

Didier Houssin*

Introduction

In order to clarify the point of view from which the EU role in two global health instruments is analyzed in this chapter, it is necessary to give some details about the author. DH is a citizen of the EU with a favorable opinion about the process which has led to the construction of the EU. As a representative, over several years, of the health authorities of France, he was involved to some extent in these agreements. As a Member, since 2011, of the international group of advisors to the Director-General of the World Health Organization (WHO) about the implementation of the Pandemic Influenza Preparedness Framework Agreement, he is directly concerned with the implementation of this framework.

*President, High Council for the Evaluation for Research and Higher Education. 20, rue Vivienne, 75002 Paris, France.

Background and Brief Description of the Two Global Health Security Instruments

The International Health Regulations

Europe has a long history of being at the forefront of international health security. It started with the Republic of Venice inventing the quarantine for ships a few years after the Black Death — the plague — had struck Europe in the middle of the 14th century. That was followed by the negotiation of the first International Health Convention in Paris, in 1851, after several epidemics of cholera in Europe, and then by the creation of the *Office International d'Hygiène Publique,* which was established in Paris in 1907. Under the auspices of the United Nations (UN), it ended in 1948 with the creation of the WHO, which was established in Geneva.

Gathering, in 1951, the existing rules that pre-existed to the creation of the WHO, the International Health Regulations were revised for the first time in 1969, with a larger ambition for disease prevention. The new Regulations adopted by the Member States aimed at applying epidemiological methods for the detection and eradication of sources of infection, at implementing hygiene measures at harbors and airports, at combatting some insect vectors, and at reinforcing epidemiological activities in each Member State. However, these Regulations applied only to a short list of six quarantine diseases: plague, cholera, smallpox, recurrent fever, typhus and yellow fever. The only real obligations for Member States were to notify cases of these diseases to the WHO and to maintain capacities of public health at harbors and airports.

These Regulations were modified in 1973, and then in 1981, but only to reduce the list of diseases under investigation. Due to its eradication, smallpox was removed from the list in 1981. The list then had only three diseases: plague, cholera and yellow fever.[1] For 20 years, these Regulations were felt adequate for facing the major epidemics without frontiers.

The emergence of a new infectious disease transmitted mainly through sexual contact at the beginning of the 1980s, followed by its pandemic dimension at the end of the century, created a world shock. The AIDS epidemic was a demonstration that surveying only a limited number of diseases was not appropriate for coping with new infectious agents.

However, the need to revise the Regulations had other motives: the observation that, in some countries, well-known epidemics of cholera or plague were not notified, and that, in many countries, particularly in Africa, means of detection and alert were extremely weak. In 1995, it was decided to revise the Regulations again. These most important changes in international law about public health aimed at focusing the revision on the concept of public health emergency with an international dimension, on a syndrome approach to notification — cases presenting similar and unusual clinical signs had to be notified even before the precise nature of the infectious agent was identified — and on the reinforcement of the capacities to detect and alert in all the Member States. The negotiations went on slower than expected and, in 2001, the revision, which should have taken place in 2000, was not implemented. Two events had a tonic effect on the process of revision: firstly, the attacks on September 11, 2001, which, conjoined to the bioterrorist attacks using anthrax, increased cooperation in health security among the countries feeling the most threatened, and that included the EU; secondly and foremost, the outbreak of severe acute respiratory syndrome (SARS), in March 2003, which struck several European countries (France, Germany, Ireland, Italy, Romania, Spain, Sweden, Switzerland and the UK). An earlier notification, nationally and internationally, of the first cases observed in the south of China could possibly have limited or delayed the rapid diffusion of an epidemic which caused nearly 800 deaths among the 8000 cases identified.

The risk of troubling commercial exchanges, stopping the flow of tourists or, simply, giving a bad image of the governance or public health condition in a country can explain the reticence of a regional or national political entity to notify early a public health emergency of international dimension, such as an uncontrolled epidemic. With regard to neighboring countries and, in fact, to the whole world, the SARS epidemic was the demonstration that such a notification had to become an obligation.

In 2003, the human and animal densities had also grown considerably in the world. The circulation of persons and goods had increased in a spectacular manner, due to the development of the air traffic and globalization. The possibilities of contact between wild and domestic animal species and the human species had also increased, because of deforestation and new techniques of animal husbandry. Besides early notification, the risk of emergence of new infectious threats required much stronger measures than those permitted by the existing International Health Regulations. It was time to make happen the revision of the International Health Regulations decided by the World Health Assembly (WHA) in 1995! Even if they were qualified as "important preliminary works," the initial lengths of this revision were thus accelerated "due to the dynamic created by the emergence of the SARS (the first public health world emergency of the twenty-first century)."[2]

In May 2005, the 193 Member States of the WHO adopted new global rules to enhance national, regional and global public health security: the International Health Regulations 2005. "Key milestones for the countries include the assessment of their surveillance and response capacities and the development and implementation of plans of action to ensure that these core capacities are functioning by 2012."[3]

The main innovations were the notions of a public health emergency of international dimension, and of shared responsibility. Transmissible diseases remained the main target, but without a limitative list in order to be able to address new infections and other diseases. To allow early notification of the events possibly qualified as public health emergencies of international concern to the WHO, a network of corresponding officers dedicated to the tasks of collecting and transmitting information, and functioning permanently, had to be installed in all Member States and at the level of the WHO.

As for the creation of the quarantine in 1380, prevention of the international propagation of diseases remained nuanced by the necessity to keep the reaction proportionate and limited to the risks presented for public health in order to "avoid creating unnecessary obstacles to international traffic and commerce."[4]

The Pandemic Influenza Preparedness Framework Agreement

As soon as the revised International Health Regulations were adopted in spring 2005, a new threat was identified, arising from the same region of the world. The spread of the avian influenza virus (H5N1) was immediately there to test these new international Regulations. In April, epizootic outbreaks diffused to Cambodia and Vietnam. At the beginning of May, they multiplied in China and, in July, they extended to Indonesia and the north of China. At the end of the summer and during the autumn, the outbreaks rapidly extended westward from Southeast Asia to Europe, and then Africa. Human cases concerning people in contact with these outbreaks were more and more frequent. In some cases, inter-human transmission of the virus was suspected.

Together with the extension of the epizooty, the fear grew of the possible occurrence of a pandemic influenza in humans. Recalling the souvenir of the 1918–1919 influenza pandemic, which had caused more than 50 million deaths in the world, such a threat led the WHO to ask Member States to accelerate the implementation of the Regulations recently adopted, and gave an impulse to major efforts of preparation for pandemic flu all around the world.

In some countries like Indonesia, severely stricken by the epizooty, such a message was the occasion of a bitter observation. H5N1 viruses, which were collected in Indonesia from animals or human cases, were sent to the WHO Global Influenza Surveillance Network, made up of national influenza laboratories and of a small number of laboratories technically able to define the genetic characteristics of new influenza viruses. These viruses, the corresponding information and seeds for the elaboration of adapted vaccines were then sent by the laboratories to vaccine producers all over the world. The health authorities of Indonesia discovered that viruses with pandemic potential, collected in Indonesia, were the source of the production of pre-pandemic or pandemic vaccines, most of which were, however, pre-empted or bought by developed countries as a component of their pandemic preparedness plan. Even if it had wanted to, Indonesia could not buy the vaccines, at the origin of which were the viruses sent to the Global Influenza Surveillance Network by Indonesia, as the markets were empty.

In December 2006, the Ministry of Health of Indonesia decided[5] not to send virus samples to the network anymore if a fair compensation was not offered to the countries contributing to the network. Just two years after the revision of the International Health Regulations, which had placed an accent on the cooperation between countries for the purpose of international health security, and at a moment when the threat of a pandemic flu was perceived as imminent, such a decision had to find a solution through negotiation. Launched under the auspices of the WHO, and marked by difficult technical aspects, the negotiation, which concerned the 193 Member States, industry and other stakeholders, lasted approximately four years.

The Pandemic Influenza Preparedness Framework Agreement for the sharing of influenza viruses and access to vaccines and other benefits was approved on 16 April 2011, and it was adopted on 24 May by the WHA. "This agreement brings together Member States, industry, other key stakeholders and the WHO to implement a global, Member State developed, approach to pandemic influenza preparedness and response. The Pandemic Influenza Preparedness Framework Agreement aims to improve the sharing of influenza virus with pandemic potential, and to achieve more predictable, efficient and equitable access for countries in need, to life-saving vaccines and medicine during future pandemics."[6]

The EU Role in the Two Global Health Security Agreements

The WHO is the directing and coordinating authority for health within the UN system. Any country that is a member of the UN may become a member of the WHO. Today, the WHO has 193 Member States. The EU is an observer in the governing bodies of the WHO and as such can only speak after all the Member States have spoken. Therefore, during a debate, EU interventions are usually made by the country that holds the Presidency of the Council of the EU at any given time.

In intergovernmental negotiating bodies or other fora, to which regional economic integration organizations (REIOs) (the EU is an REIO) are invited, the Member State that holds the Presidency of the Council of the EU usually speaks on national competence matters and the EU delegation speaks on matters of EU competence. The new Lisbon Treaty has reinforced the role of the EU delegation in the preparatory work and the EU internal coordination, as well as in the external representation.

The EU role was studied in two global health security instruments: the International Health Regulations, which is a directly applicable regulation, and the Pandemic Influenza Preparedness Agreement, which is a framework adopted by a WHA resolution.

The EU Role in the International Health Regulations

During the nearly 10 years of the negotiation phase for the revision of the International Health Regulations under the leadership of the WHO, the EU acted as a facilitator of coordination between EU Member States. Because the SARS epidemic had struck several European countries in 2003, the role of the EU was intensified during the accelerated post-SARS negotiation. Sessions of the WHO Executive Board and the WHA were usually preceded by coordination meetings chaired by the Member State that held the Presidency of the Council of the EU. The negotiations took place between Member States; the European Commission was involved as an observer.

The Regulations refer to REIOs in only two articles: Article 47 (REIOs can propose experts for the IHR Roster) and Article 57(3) (State Parties that are members of an REIO shall apply in their mutual relations the common rules in force in that REIO).

However, the EU, as such, is not a party to the International Health Regulations. Retrospectively, the important role of the EU during the implementation phase of the Regulations suggests that it would have been justified for the EU to be a party to them.

In 2005, when the International Health Regulations were agreed on, Europe was immediately under the pressure of the H5N1 avian epizooty and the threat of a pandemic flu. Therefore, the necessity-driven and functionally complex implementation of the Regulations led the EU, through the European Commission, to play a more important role at this stage, on several aspects:

- Contribution to coordination of the relationships between the headquarters of the WHO, the European region of the WHO, and the EU and its Member States, about the inflow and outflow of information through the national focal points imposed by the Regulations on all WHO Member States.

- Coordination of the position of the EU and its Member States about the reserves to be made to the Regulations and about the definition and characterization of the points of entry.
- Initiatives about the implementation of the application of the Regulations: in September 2006, considering the risk of a pandemic influenza and following the proposal made by the WHA in June 2006, the EU adopted a communication calling for an anticipated application of the specific dispositions of the Regulations applicable to this risk. It described the European context in order to encourage a common position within the EU. Each Member State was encouraged to elaborate, but also share, its own measures to implement these essential Regulations.
- Creation of an electronic bridge between the community system of alerts for communicable diseases (Decision 2119/98) and the alert system of the Regulations.
- Organization of annual contact meetings between the Regulations contact points in EU Member States and the officials responsible for the operation of the EU communicable disease control system.

The occurrence of the pandemic flu H1N1 in April 2009 was an opportunity to test the role of the EU in the situation of a public health emergency of major international concern. Daily coordination of the Member States by the EU, using audio conferencing between all the members of the European Health Security Committee, was conducted. This coordination, which included the participation of the European agencies, focused on epidemiological assessment, expert analysis about candidate vaccines and antivirals, public health recommendations, harmonization of communication messages within the EU and interaction with the WHO. These were among the most visible aspects of the practical role of the EU in the implementation of the International Health Regulations.

The lessons drawn from this experience as shown in several evaluations and an impact assessment,[7,8] have led recently to the elaboration of a project of European law about trans-frontier threats.[9] This health security package emphasizes the role of the EU in coordinating several actions, such as alert sharing, exchange of information, a mechanism for common procurement of vaccines and other medical countermeasures, and reinforces the role of the health security committee.

The EU Role in the Pandemic Influenza Preparedness Framework Agreement

The negotiation for the Pandemic Influenza Preparedness Framework started two years after the end of the 10-year long negotiation of the International Health Regulations, i.e. at a time when the Member States of the EU and the Commission had more experience in negotiating together and more human resources on the ground in Geneva, and when the EU was more recognized as an REIO. As a consequence, REIOs were already invited to participate fully in the negotiations on the PIP Framework.

A challenge for this negotiation process was, at the same time, "to ensure a thorough technical understanding (how viruses behave, how they are identified, the role of the laboratories and the WHO, how antivirals and vaccines are manufactured by the industry and what is required to do so, how the industry functions, etc.) and to establish a government-led multistakeholders-inspired process."[10]

The ultimate phase of the negotiation, which was diplomatic, was conducted under the leadership of two ambassadors — one from Norway, a non-EU European state, and the other from Mexico. The EU role at this stage was important due to the EU competence concerning economic questions, medical products, intellectual property, and matters regarding the Nagoya protocol. For the EU, what was at stake in this negotiation was important: on the one hand, to stay in line with the values supported by the EU about global health (strengthening global health security, promoting global health equity, enhancing good governance for global health[11]), which are exemplified by the EU being the world's largest provider of development and humanitarian aid[12]; on the other hand, to ensure its integration role among the EU Member States and to take into account that a large part of the industry concerned with the production of influenza vaccines and antivirals is Europe-based. During the negotiation, the EU spoke on matters of EU competence, whereas the country holding the Presidency of the Council of the EU spoke on matters of national competence.

In the context of the recent H1N1 influenza pandemic, a public health emergency of major international concern, the EU declared, in its statement before the International Health Regulations review committee in March 2011, that it remained keen to conclude negotiations of the Open-ended Working Group on Pandemic Influenza Preparedness.

Contrary to the International Health Regulations, the EU is also being directly addressed by the Pandemic Influenza Preparedness Framework Agreement: WHA resolution 64/5, which adopted the framework, urges not only Member States to implement it and to support its wide implementation, but also REIOs. This is done via a footnote in the resolution, which specifies that it applies, where applicable, also to REIOs.

However, whereas the EU has been rather active during the negotiation phase of the PIP Framework, regarding the implementation of this recent agreement it has been less involved, and there may be areas of overlap with the joint procurement exercise underway at EU level, which may be significant.

Conclusion

If one considers that public health is largely a competence of Member States, and not of the EU, and, for this reason, that Member States of the EU, and not the EU itself, are Member States of the WHO, the role of the EU in global health agreeements should be quite limited.

However, if responsibility and emulation are potent motors for initiative among EU Member States with regard to global health, the necessity of coherence, solidarity, burden sharing and coordination, required by global health security problems, points to a major role for the EU.

In fact, in the field of global health, global health security requires a special treatment. Cross-border events, the necessity of a high situational awareness, the need often for an intersectoral treatment of the event, the critical coherence of communication messages across frontiers, the importance of mutualization of capacities — all these factors argue for a coordinated EU approach at a higher level than is necessary for facing other public health problems. If global health security is also seen as combining animal and human health security, the role of the EU in this context is closer to the situation regarding animal health, a truly European competence, than to what it is usually the case concerning human health.

Paraphrasing the prediction of Jacques Delors made in the foreword to this book, it is clear that, with regard to the two global health security agreements presented in this chapter, the EU becomes an "unusual political object." In fact, in the context of its contribution to global health security, the role of the EU was unusually important, during the implementation phase of the revised International Health Regulations and during the negotiation phase of the Pandemic Influenza Preparedness Framework Agreement. In the coming years, the role of the EU in the just starting implementation phase of the Pandemic Influenza Preparedness Framework Agreement will be interesting to follow.

Acknowledgment

The author thanks John F. Ryan, Acting Director, Public Health Directorate, Health and Consumer Directorate General, European Commission, for reviewing the manuscript.

References

1. World Health Organization. (2005) *International Health Regulations*, second edition, p. 8.
2. *Ibid.*, p. 8.
3. www.who.int/ihr/en.
4. World Health Organization. (2005) *International Health Regulations, op. cit.*, p. 9.
5. Supari SF. (2008) *It's Time for the World to Change*. PT Sulaksana Watinsa, Jakarta, p. 24.
6. www.who.int/influenza/pip/en.
7. European Commission. (2010) Commission Staff Working Document on Lessons Learnt from the H1N1 Pandemic and on Health Security in the European Union. SEC (2010) 1440 final. European Commission, Brussels.
8. European Commission. (2011) Commission Staff Working Paper Executive Summary of the Impact Assessment, Accompanying the Document: Decision

of the European Parliament and of the Council on Serious Cross-Border Threats to Health. SEC (2011) 1520 final. European Commission, Brussels.

9. European Commission. (2011) Proposal for a Decision of the European Parliament and of the Council on Serious Cross-Border Threats to Health. COM (2011) 866 final. European Commission, Brussels.

10. Gomez Camacho JJ. (2012) Improving the negotiating process in preparing for an influenza pandemic. *Global Health.* Newsdeskmedia, London, p. 46.

11. Kickbusch I. (2006) The need for a European strategy on global health. *Scandinavian Journal of Public Health* **34**: 561–565.

12. Dalli J. (2012) The European Union and global health. *Global Health.* Newsdeskmedia, London, p. 12.

12

The EU Voice in the UN System Related to Health and Other Health Actors

*Lourdes Chamorro**

The European Union's Mandate in Global Health

The Treaty on the Functioning of the European Union[1] (hereafter TFEU), in its Articles 9 and 168, stipulates that a high level of human health protection shall be ensured in the definition and implementation of all the European Union (hereafter EU) policies and activities. The Charter of Fundamental Rights[2] further stipulates in its Article 35 that everyone has the right of access to preventive healthcare and the right to benefit from medical treatment under the conditions established by national law and practices.

The TFEU states that the EU action, which shall complement national policies, shall be directed toward improving public health, preventing physical and mental illness and diseases, and obviating sources of danger to physical and mental health. Such action shall cover the fight against the major health scourges, by promoting research into their causes, their transmission and their prevention, as well as health information and education, and monitoring, early warning and combating of serious cross-border threats to health.

---

*Political Officer, Delegation of the European Union to the United Nations and other International Organisations, Geneva, Switzerland.

When it comes to the division of competences, Article 6 TFEU states that the EU shall have competence to carry out actions to support, coordinate or supplement the actions of the Member States in the area of protection and improvement of human health, among others. However, according to Article 4 TFEU, common safety concerns in public health matters are an area where competence is shared between the EU and the Member States. In this framework of division of competences, Article 168 TFEU reflects the different types of measures that the EU can take:

- Adopting measures setting high standards of quality and safety for organs and substances of human origin, blood and blood derivatives, medicinal products and devices for medical use, and also measures in the veterinary and phytosanitary fields.
- Adopting incentive measures in other matters pertaining to the protection and improvement of human health, i.e. for fighting major cross-border health scourges, and monitoring, early warning and combating of serious threats to health as well as measures which have as their direct objective the protection of public health regarding tobacco and the abuse of alcohol.
- Finally, the EU can encourage and support cooperation between the Member States in the area of public health through the so-called "open method of coordination."

EU legislation in this field is enacted by the Council and the European Parliament in accordance with the ordinary legislative procedure (as defined by Article 294 TFEU). The Council may additionally adopt recommendations on a Commission proposal on the basis of a qualified majority.

Finally, the TFEU acknowledges that the Member States remain responsible for the definition of their health policy and the organization and delivery of health services and medical care, including the management of health services and medical care and the allocation of resources assigned to them.

At international level, it is worth remembering that the Lisbon Treaty introduces a single legal personality for the EU that enables it to conclude international agreements and join international organizations, and it is therefore able to speak and take action as a single entity.

Particularly with regard to health, Article 168 TFEU states, *inter alia*, that the EU and the Member States shall foster cooperation with third countries and competent international organizations in the sphere of public health.

The Treaty of the European Union[3] (hereafter TEU) states the common values of the EU, such as combating social exclusion and discrimination, promoting social justice and protection, equality between women and men, etc., and that, in its relations with the wider world, the EU shall uphold and promote those values. Furthermore, the EU has agreed on the shared values of solidarity toward equitable and universal coverage of quality health care.[4] In addition, Article 21 TEU states, *inter alia*, that the EU shall ensure consistency between the different areas of its external action and between these and its other policies. Addressing global health requires coherence of all the internal and external policies and actions based on agreed principles. This becomes particularly relevant since multisectoral efforts are needed to tackle the variety of social, economic and environmental determinants of health. The EU systematically endorses the "Equity and Health in All Policies" approach.[a]

In May 2010, the Council of the European Union adopted its Conclusions on the EU Role in Global Health[5] ("the Conclusions" hereafter) recognizing the need to take action to improve health, reduce inequalities and increase protection against global health threats. The Conclusions stress that health is central to people's lives, including as a human right, and a key element of equitable and sustainable growth and development including poverty reduction.

The Council gives the EU the political mandate to play a central role in accelerating progress on global health challenges, including the health-related Millennium Development Goals and non-communicable diseases, through its commitment to protect and promote the right of everyone to enjoy the highest attainable standard of physical and mental health. The common agreed values of solidarity toward equitable and universal coverage of quality health services serve as basis for the EU policies in this area.

---

[a] Council Conclusions on Health in All Policies (HiAP) of 30 November 2006 and Council Conclusions on Equity and Health in All Policies: Solidarity in Health of 8 June 2010, among others.

At global level, the Conclusions seek for the EU to endeavor to defend a single EU position and voice within the UN agencies. The EU should work to cut duplication and fragmentation, and to increase the coordination and effectiveness of the UN system. It should support stronger leadership by the WHO in its normative and guidance functions to improve global health. The EU should seek synergies with the WHO to address global health challenges and decrease the fragmentation of funding to the WHO, and gradually shift toward funding its general budget.

Apart from the specific references to health in the EU legislative or political acts, other areas are indirectly linked to public health, such as free movement of goods (restrictions based on the protection of the health and life of humans, animals or plants), the internal market (legislation on tobacco products or tobacco advertising, and pharmaceutical legislation), the environment, agriculture, taxation, development, transport, etc., in line with the mandate to ensure a high level of human health protection in the definition and implementation of all EU policies and activities.

World Health Organization

Cooperation between the European Commission and the WHO

The World Health Organization (WHO hereafter) has been the directing and coordinating specialized agency for health within the United Nations system since 1948, the year in which the World Health Assembly approved its Constitution.[6] Currently 194 countries are members of the WHO. It is organized in three different levels: the headquarters in Geneva, six highly autonomous regional offices on the different continents, and 150 country offices around the world. The WHO's governing bodies are the World Health Assembly, where the full membership meets yearly in May, and the Executive Board, which is composed of 34 members that are elected for three-year terms and that come from the different WHO regions. The Executive Board meets at least twice a year and its main functions are to give effect to the decisions and policies of the World Health Assembly, to advise it and generally to facilitate its work.

The WHO is responsible for providing leadership on global health matters, shaping the health research agenda, setting norms and standards, articulating evidence-based policy options, providing technical support to countries, and monitoring and assessing health trends. Its objective, as referred in its Constitution,[b] is the attainment by all peoples of the highest possible level of health. As is widely the case in the UN system, the EU shares common values and principles with the WHO and, given that, a broad range of common grounds for mutual collaboration could be easily identified by both entities.

The EU is an increasingly important actor in global and international affairs beyond Europe and a strong supporter of the UN system, particularly with regard to global security, development and humanitarian assistance. This includes strong support for health and for the WHO's work, both globally and within Europe. The European Commission has long-standing bilateral relations with the WHO. The cooperation between the European Commission (the former European Communities) and the WHO dates back to the exchange of letters between the two organizations in the year 1982. At that time both organizations underlined the importance of effective coordination on matters of common interest. With this objective, they committed themselves to encourage and facilitate reciprocal participation in their meetings, and to exchange pertinent information and documentation. Some years later, due to changes that had occurred in the WHO and in the EU, a revised framework governing the cooperation between them was set out by a new exchange of letters in the year 2000. The Memorandum[7] attached to that exchange of letters addresses the principles, objectives, areas of cooperation, priorities and procedures for the conduct of their activities. It identifies a number of priority areas — including health information, communicable diseases, tobacco control, environment and health, sustainable health development, health research — and outlines practical procedures for cooperation. It embraces the global dimension of the cooperation, as well as the benefits that enhanced, focused and coherent EU–WHO cooperation brings for the common EU–WHO Member States.

Since then, at the political level, regular high-level meetings have taken place between the EU Health Commissioner and the WHO Director-General, as well as Senior Official Meetings (SOMs hereafter), where high-level and senior officials of the two organizations meet periodically

---

[b]Article 1, WHO Constitution; see *supra* note 10.

to discuss health and cooperation issues. On the Commission side the SOMs are usually attended by the Directorates-General Health and Consumers, Development Cooperation, Research, Humanitarian Aid and Information Society. The European External Action Service (EEAS hereafter) also participates, as well as the European Centre for Disease Prevention and Control (ECDC hereafter). On the WHO side, the participants usually include the WHO Director-General, the Directors of the WHO European and African Regions and the WHO Pan-American Health Organization as well as senior managers and representatives of other regions.

In practical terms, cooperation takes place at three geographic levels: with the WHO HQ in Geneva on issues of global concern, with the WHO Regional Office for Europe (based in Copenhagen) on European issues, and country-level cooperation around the world. The ECDC also works closely with the WHO on a range of issues related to communicable diseases.

At the regional level, the Commission also keeps working relations with the WHO European regional office in Copenhagen. Such collaboration has been going on for years and has addressed a number of areas. In this sense, it is worth mentioning the Moscow Declaration,[8] on which the WHO European office and the Commission agreed in 2010. It seeks to strengthen the policy dialogue and the technical cooperation on public health between the two. It outlines a five-year framework and envisages the development of joint systems for health surveillance, alert and information, and stronger collaboration at the country level. The Moscow Declaration aims at achieving a cohesive effort to improve health security and join forces to help improve public health surveillance and strengthen alert and response systems so as to allow quicker and more efficient responses to disease outbreaks and pandemics, and for tackling existing challenges across the 53 countries in the WHO European Region.

At the country level, EU Delegations in third countries around the world and WHO country offices are called on to cooperate with each other to optimize the efficacy of the health assistance they both provide to their hosts.

In addition to the collaboration, the Commission is a donor to the WHO. The WHO budget comprises assessed contributions from WHO

Member States[c] and voluntary contributions from WHO Member States and third parties, which may or may not be earmarked for specific tasks or projects. The EU and its Member States, individually and collectively, account for about one-third of the total WHO annual income. Most of this financing comes under the category of voluntary contributions. The contribution from the EU budget administered by the European Commission is not negligible. At about €100 million per biennium, averaged over the last 10 years, the EU ranks high among the major voluntary nonstate contributors to the WHO.

As a contributor, the European Commission systematically aims at supporting the priorities common to the EU and the WHO. The EC–ACP–WHO Partnership on Pharmaceutical Policies, the EU–WHO Universal Health Coverage Partnership Programme, or projects on improving access to medicines and effective health services through innovation and technology transfer, and the major contributions to the humanitarian activities of the WHO can be mentioned as some of the main examples. It is also worth mentioning that the EU budget is a public budget, managed and executed under strict financial rules and which only allows for earmarked funds. The financial modalities of EU assistance are based on the Financial and Administrative Framework Agreement, which the Commission concluded with the UN system and which is applied across the UN system.

The EU's Participation in the WHO

The EU is not a member of the WHO, yet it holds an observer status in the organization and, since the Lisbon Treaty introduced a single legal personality for the EU and dropped the European Community, sits behind the nameplate "European Union" (previously it sat behind "European Community"). According to Article 3 of the WHO Constitution,[d] membership in the WHO is open to all states. This means that only "states" (and not other types of entities) are and can become members of the WHO. So, even if the EU, as a regional economic integration organization (REIO hereafter), is composed

---

[c] The assessed contributions to the WHO are a type of "membership fee" based on the latest available UN scale of assessments.

[d] See *supra* note 10.

of several sovereign states which have transferred to it competence over a range of matters, including the authority to conclude binding decisions, it still cannot apply for membership without meeting the requirement of the WHO Constitution.

On the contrary, the 28 EU Member States of the EU are members of the WHO (14% of the overall membership), and all of them are part of the WHO European Region, which is composed of a total of 53 states. Therefore, the EU Member States represent 53% of the membership of the WHO European Region.

The WHO Rules of Procedure[9] establish the rights and duties that observers hold within the Organization. Plenary meetings of the World Health Assembly are, by default, open to attendance by observer inter-governmental and non-governmental organizations admitted into relation-ship with the Organization. In addition, on the basis of the exchange of letters in 2000, the EU Delegation to the World Health Assembly or to the Executive Board sessions is invited, after prior *ad hoc* request at the beginning of each governing body meeting, to attend and participate (without a vote) also in the deliberations of the meetings of subcommi-ttees or other such subdivisions. Such invitations significantly facilitate the coordination toward defining EU common positions.

The EU and its Member States attach great importance to the WHO and to its ongoing processes: the overall contributions of the EU Member States and the Commission represent one-third of the income of the WHO, and the EU and the Member States devote a significant amount of resources, both in capitals and in Geneva, to this specific matter.

The vast majority of EU Member States' Permanent Missions in Geneva follow the WHO processes with a different degree of intensity, through a diplomat from the foreign affairs services, or through a repre-sentative from the relevant national health services, or sometimes through two representatives coming from both services. In some cases those rep-resentatives focus exclusively on health processes, while in other cases they are responsible for different organizations based in Geneva.

Additionally, there is often another representative who follows the humanitarian activities, including those conducted by the WHO in its role as the health cluster lead in humanitarian crises of the UN Department for the Coordination of Humanitarian Action (OCHA hereafter). The Global

Health Cluster aims to strengthen system-wide humanitarian preparedness by ensuring sufficient capacity in information management; surge, normative guidance and tools, development of the capacities of national stakeholders, and advocacy and resource mobilization. Over 30 partners are working together in the Cluster, under the leadership of the WHO. This is a particularly relevant area for the EU and its Member States, as together they are the most important donor in this field.

In the EU Delegation in Geneva, there are currently two professionals dedicated full-time to health issues, namely the ongoing processes in the WHO. Their role focuses mainly on the relations between the Commission/ EEAS and the WHO, on the coordination of the EU and its Member States' common positions, on the outreach to third countries and parties, and on the representation of the EU when the rules of procedure allow it.

Without prejudice to the division of competences, the EU and its Member States currently tend to coordinate in order to reach common positions on many of the priority issues discussed in the WHO, both at the headquarters in Geneva and at regional level. As will be mentioned below, such positions can then be expressed differently, depending on the specific settings and processes.

While the common institutional framework for the EU institutions is clearly defined, local coordination and representation practices are still diverse among the multilateral EU Delegations, or even among the different areas within the same Delegation. This fact can be explained by several factors, including previous consolidated practices, different rhythms toward full implementation of the Lisbon Treaty, and the different statuses or interests of the EU in the different international organizations. Locally in Geneva, the EU coordination related to the WHO in Geneva is organized around two practical tools: (1) a common web portal used to share information and discuss among the EU institutions and the 28 Member States, and (2) face-to-face meetings chaired by the EU Delegation (with the periodicity according to needs, usually daily during the governing bodies' sessions and once or twice a week during the intersessional periods; approximately 120 meetings per year).

Considering the intense work involved in preparing the final EU positions to be expressed, some Member States volunteer to "burden-share" part of the work related to EU statements and EB/WHA resolutions.

In addition to the coordination within the EU, and usually only for the sessions of the WHO's governing bodies, a number of countries in special relations with the EU (currently the 14 potential or official candidate countries) are invited *ad hoc* to align themselves with the agreed positions of the EU and its Member States expressed in the form of statements during the meetings. This alignment procedure could potentially place a total of 42 countries around one common position coordinated by the EU (28 EU Member States plus, currently, the 14 additional countries), representing altogether more than 20% of the WHO membership. Also in this sense, it is worth highlighting the role that the EU plays — or, more accurately, could potentially play — within the 53 countries of the WHO European Region, considering that 28 EU Members, with the possible additional 14 countries, can act on the basis of a common coordinated position.

While such wide representation provides the EU and its Member States with a prominent position, it is worth considering the decision-making dynamics currently in place in the WHO. Unlike other organizations within the UN system, decision-making in the WHO is systematically based on consensus. Voting methods are usually not used (except for the resolution on the health conditions in the occupied Palestinian territory and for the election of the Director-General at the headquarters level) and, even more, are considered undesirable and are actively avoided by the WHO's membership. This reality implies that, apart from a greater influence in decision-making processes, one major advantage of the wide EU representation relies more on its increased capacity for intelligence gathering and outreach to third countries than on its actual majority within the membership. Particularly at regional level and aware of the impact that the common EU positions could have on the governance of the region, the EU and its Member States are politically committed to systematically outreach to the non-EU members in the region when preparing for the sessions of the Regional Committee.

In addition to the governing bodies' sessions and the intersessional processes, the EU participates actively in a number of more informal contacts around the WHO to further develop the EU political agenda on global health: meetings with the different departments of the WHO Secretariat, bilateral contacts with other countries or groups (such as the African Union), like-minded or Western European and Others Group (WEOG hereafter) informal meetings, outreach exercises at Ambassador level, meetings with NGOs and civil society, etc.

Overall, it could be concluded that, while the EU holds an observer status in the WHO, the participation of the EU at the different levels, settings and processes of the Organization is widely developed and recognized at this stage. The EU and its Member States are progressively being recognized in the WHO fora and negotiations as a sound and reliable partner.

EU representation at the WHO

As already mentioned, the EU and its Member States endeavor to speak with a stronger and coherent voice at global level and in dialogue with third countries and global health initiatives.

In 2011, the Council agreed on the General Arrangements regarding EU Statements in multilateral organizations[10] as a result of a significant institutional crisis. They recalled that the Treaty of Lisbon[e] enables the EU to achieve coherent, comprehensive and unified external representation and that the EU Treaties[f] provide for close and sincere cooperation between the Member States and the Union. Given the sensitivity of representation and potential expectations of third parties, the Council deemed it essential that the preparation of statements relating to the sensitive area of competences of the EU and its Member States remained internal and consensual. Therefore, if an agreed EU position exists, it is for an EU actor (i.e. the President of the EU Council, the High Representative, the Commission or the EU Delegations) to represent the EU and its Member States as appropriate, and express it in the international fora, provided that the rules of procedure of the specific setting allow an effective EU representation. It is to be noted that the General Arrangements are a guidance document only and that the Commission has annexed a declaration, recalling that according to the relevant provisions of the treaties, it is for the President of the European Council, the Commission, the High Representative of Foreign Affairs and Security Policy and the EU Delegations to ensure the external representation of the EU, regardless of the categories and areas of competence conferred upon the EU.

---

[e] See *supra* note 4.
[f] TEU, see *supra* note 4; TFEU, see *supra* note 2.

In the case of the WHO, observers such as the EU may make a statement on the subject under discussion upon the invitation of the President and with the consent of the World Health Assembly or the committee. The established practice is then that observers are invited to take the floor at the end of the discussion, once all the Member States have intervened, or that one Member asks the President to let the EU Delegation speak on a particular subject (which was done two or three times before the Lisbon Treaty came into effect). Speaking from the observer seat after the discussion is over was not considered as being an influential voice. Therefore, the EU is represented by an EU Member State in the WHO governing body official meetings and this person often speaks early in the debate. During the Executive Board sessions that role is generally given to one of the EU Member States that is a member of the Board, usually the one closest to holding the Presidency of the Council, even if this is not a strict rule. During the World Health Assembly, the role is usually given to the Member State holding the rotating Presidency of the Council. In other words, an almost purely "pre-Lisbon" arrangement for external representation persists in the WHO governing bodies' settings, due to the constraints imposed by the observer status of the EU in the WHO.

On the contrary, for the formal or informal intergovernmental processes that regularly take place between the WHO governing bodies' sessions (intergovernmental meetings, consultations, working groups, etc.), the EU is normally granted access as a REIO on an equal footing to the Members of the Organization. This is now a well-established practice, which is formalized through the systematic addition of a footnote — "*and, where applicable, to REIOs*" — to the relevant references to the "*Member States*" in the WHO resolutions that set up those processes. This development was greatly facilitated by the role of the EU during the negotiations of the WHO Framework Convention on Tobacco Control (FCTC) and by the fact that, as a REIO, the EU became a Party to the convention. The practice of having a REIO as a partner has exposed the WHO international community to a new institutional setting and has, successfully in the case of the FCTC, added a new factor to the already complex multi-actor global health diplomacy.

In these particular processes, the EU Delegation in Geneva can effectively represent the EU and its Member States. This has already been the case for several WHO processes during the last few years, even if decisions in that regard are taken on an *ad hoc* basis after the EU Delegation and the Member States specifically assess each of the processes.

Overall, the EU's voice in the WHO, represented by an EU Member State or an EU actor (usually the EU Delegation), can be considered as widely present and as particularly strong in certain global health processes.

Full EU membership or enhanced speaking rights in line with those granted by the UN General Assembly resolution of May 2011 on the participation of the EU in the work of the UN[11] could further contribute to strengthening the EU's visibility and pursuit of the EU agenda on global health issues.

Joint United Nations Programme on HIV/AIDS

Established in 1994 by a resolution of the UN Economic and Social Council[12] and launched in January 1996, the Joint United Nations Programme on HIV and AIDS (UNAIDS) is the main advocate for accelerated, comprehensive and coordinated global action on the HIV/AIDS epidemic at global level. It is guided by a Programme Coordinating Board (PCB) with representatives of 22 governments from all geographic regions, the UNAIDS Cosponsors, and five representatives of non-governmental organizations (NGOs), including associations of people living with HIV.[13]

The countries participating in the PCB are organized around constituencies, and EU Member States are divided among the different constituencies that group EU and non-EU Member States. In this situation, aiming at establishing or coordinating a common EU position remains extremely challenging. In addition, and linked to political sensitivities around the EU participation in the UN Programmes and Funds, some EU Member States have so far been very reluctant to have any EU voice expressed during the meetings of the PCB even in the form of a statement at a more general or principles level.

So, even if since the late 1980s the HIV/AIDS epidemic has been a major health concern and a high priority for the EU and a large number of different types of initiatives have taken place at both EU and neighboring countries level and under most of the developing countries health cooperation activities, such a voice is not raised in the main HIV/AIDS advocacy UN Programme.

Cooperation between the European Commission and UNAIDS is established at technical level when organizing joint activities/conferences or punctually at country level when coordinating efforts in the fight against HIV/AIDS, as was for example the case in Benin or Nigeria, through the respective Memorandums of Understanding. No further intervention from the EU takes place at political level at the UNAIDS headquarters in Geneva. The EU Member States participate actively on an individual basis at the PCB on a national basis within their constituencies.

Global Fund to Fight AIDS, Tuberculosis and Malaria

The Global Fund (GF) is a public–private partnership and a global financial instrument designed to make available and leverage additional financial resources to fight HIV/AIDS, tuberculosis and malaria.[14]

It is estimated that as of December 2012, GF grants have provided antiretroviral (ARV) treatment for AIDS to more than 4.2 million people, 250 million counseling and testing sessions have been made available, 4.2 billion condoms have been distributed, 1.7 million HIV-positive pregnant women have been provided with Prevention of Mother to Child Transmissions treatment, 9.7 million people with new cases of infectious tuberculosis have been detected and treated, 290 million people have been given malaria treatment, and more than 310 million insecticide-treated mosquito nets have been provided to families. By December 2012, the GF had approved a total of US$26 billion to finance more than 1000 programs in 151 countries and had disbursed US$18.5 billion to grant recipients. Of the approved grants, 54% were committed to AIDS programs, 17% to tuberculosis and 28% to malaria.

The EU and its Member States have been proud to be associated with the GF since its inception 11 years ago. The EU collectively (Member

States and EU funds managed by the Commission) has been the biggest contributor to the GF, with 51% of all contributions received. The US, as the biggest single donor, contributed 30%, followed by France (13%), the UK (8%) and Germany (7%). The European Commission managed EU funds accounted for 6%. However, the pledges for 2011–2013 see a drop in the collective EU share of pledges to 42%, as important European donors of the past are currently not pledging resources due to domestic financial constraints. Conversely, the US has considerably increased its pledged contributions, now representing 38% of all pledges.

The GF promotes certain values that are close to the aid effectiveness principles strongly defended by the EU and its Member States, such as partnerships among governments, civil society, the private sector and affected communities — the most effective way to help reach those in need. This innovative approach relies on country ownership and performance-based funding, meaning that people in countries implement their own programs based on their priorities and the GF provides financing where verifiable results are achieved.

The GF is guided by a Board which is composed of representatives from donor and recipient governments, civil society, the private sector, private foundations, and communities living with and affected by the diseases. The Board is responsible for the organization's governance, including establishing strategies and policies, making funding decisions and setting budgets. The EU Member States participating in the GF are well represented on the Board. Of the 20 Board Members with voting rights, eight represent donor government constituencies. The Board representation is assigned on the basis of the financial contributions made to the GF. The EU Member States and the Commission occupy five of those eight seats. Two EU Member States occupy a seat on their own (DE, FR), two other seats include also a non-EU country (the UK with Australia, or Ireland–Denmark–Luxembourg–The Netherlands–Sweden with Norway), and the Commission (DG DEVCO as *chef de file*) holds a seat with Belgium–Finland–Italy–Portugal–Spain. Such representation gives the EU and its Member States the possibility of exercising an influential position in decision-making, including the possibility of exercising a "blocking minority."

Formal coordination of the EU position does not take place in this case. Nevertheless, where the EU has shared principles like the ones on aid effectiveness or those expressed in the Council Conclusions on the new development policy "Agenda for Change," a coordinated EU approach can have a large impact. This was for example the case in September 2012 for the Board decision on the principles that a new funding model should have, which was not only welcome as it helped break an important impasse on the way to a more aid-effective funding model, but also let the EU appear more than the sum of its Member States. This was appreciated not only by the Commission and the EU Member States but also by the main interlocutors from the US, Japan, the Gates Foundation, the representatives of civil society and the implementing partner countries.

This case constitutes a particular one for which the European Commission occupies, with five EU Member States, a seat on the Board, ensuring that the EU policies and interests are in any case present in the Board discussions and decision-making processes.

In addition, even if there is no formal EU coordination and the EU Member States act primarily on a national basis, the existence of common principles and related policies, and the participation of the Member States in an open exchange of views and information, have led in some cases to greater effectiveness in defending common interests and to higher EU visibility in this particular international setting. Currently, informal exchanges of information and views among the Commission and the EU Member States are held on a regular basis, mainly with a view to preparing the Board meetings.

Conclusions

While the political mandate from the Treaties and the Council clearly states that the EU and its Member States will endeavor to speak with a stronger and coherent voice at global level and in dialogue with third countries and global health initiatives, the implementation of such a mandate varies greatly from one organization to another.

In the WHO, given the nature of many of the issues addressed there and their relation to the EU priorities, the EU and its Member States usually coordinate and define common positions on the main issues in discussion to be presented and defended during the sessions of the governing bodies of the Organization. This is also often the case for *ad hoc* or specific processes happening in the intersessional periods.

However, as the EU holds an observer status in the WHO, representation in the governing bodies of the Organization (EB and WHA) is done by an EU Member State instead of by an EU actor. This is not the case for some intergovernmental intersessional processes, where the EU and its Member States decide to coordinate and to be represented by the EU Delegation in line with the Lisbon Treaty and on the basis of a WHO resolution including REIOs.

In any case and independently of who holds the representation, the EU is progressively gaining presence and playing a significant role in the WHO. Ongoing efforts within the EU to (1) maximize the strategic added value and effectiveness of the EU positions and (2) enhance outreach activities in third countries are positively contributing toward enhancing the EU's voice and visibility in the WHO. In addition, the enhancement of speaking rights in the WHO by a specific resolution, following the example of the one in the UN General Assembly, could constitute a step forward to further enhance that visibility.

In contrast to what happens in the WHO, the EU voice is non-existent in UNAIDS. The unfeasibility of coordinating EU positions within mixed constituencies of EU and non-EU countries, and the political reluctance of some EU Member States to have the EU voice raised in the UNAIDS PCB, limit the relation between the EU and UNAIDS to specific and *ad hoc* activities or projects at the margins of the UNAIDS governing body.

Finally, the example of the GF presents a different situation. The participation of the EU Member States is defined by their financial contribution to the Fund, and they are currently either occupying a Board seat on their own, or organized around constituencies including EU and non-EU countries. In this context, formal EU coordination among EU Member States does not take place, but the European Commission (with its constituency) occupies one of the voting seats and therefore its voice is clearly heard in the Board (one vote out of the eight attributed to donors).

In addition, participating EU donors in the GF recognize their commitment to shared values and principles of aid effectiveness and development cooperation and had benefited from such common grounds to have them effectively defended in the Board. Regular informal exchanges of views on the GF issues take place among EU Member States and a certain degree of alignment of national positions with a shared "EU position" is not uncommon, even if ever formulated or formalized as such.

When one is considering the three presented cases together, it becomes clear that the status of the EU in each organization, the functioning of its structures and, more importantly, the political will of the EU Member States, as expressed by the Council and/or on a case-by-case basis for the different health related processes and organizations, play a critical role in the ongoing efforts toward the Lisbon Treaty implementation in the areas of external action. Such political will constitutes in itself a dynamic element that strongly shapes the EU voice in global health, going *de facto* beyond the formal mandate from the Treaty or as expressed by the Council.

References

1. European Union. (2008) Consolidated Version of the Treaty on the Functioning of the European Union. *Official Journal C* **115(47)**.
2. European Union. (2010) Charter of Fundamental Rights of the European Union. *Official Journal C* **83(02)**.
3. European Union. (2010) Consolidated Version of the Treaty on the European Union. *Official Journal C* **83(01)**.
4. European Union. (2006)Council Conclusions on Common Values and Principles in European Union Health Systems. *Official Journal C* **146(01)**.
5. Council of the European Union. (2010) Council Conclusions on the EU Role in Global Health of 10 May 2010. 3011th Foreign Affairs Council meeting. Brussels, 10 May 2010.
6. Consolidated version of the Constitution of the World Health Organization. New York, 22 February 1946.
7. European Commission, World Health Organization. (2001) Exchange of Letters between the WHO and the Commission of the EC concerning the

consolidation and intensification of cooperation and Memorandum concerning the framework and arrangements for cooperation between the WHO and the Commission of the EC. *Official Journal C* **1:** 7–11.

8. Joint Declaration of the WHO Regional Office for Europe and European Commission seeking to strengthen policy dialogue and technical cooperation on public health. Moscow, 13 September 2010.

9. Articles 19 and 45, Consolidated Version of the WHO Rules of Procedure, adopted by the Eighth World Health Assembly, Resolutions. WHA8.26 and WHA8.27.

10. Council of the European Union. (2011) EU Statements in multilateral organisations — General Arrangements. 15901/11.

11. Assembly resolution on the participation of the EU in the work of the UN. A/RES/65/276.

12. United Nations Economic and Social Council. (1994) Joint and co-sponsored United Nations programme on human immunodeficiency virus/acquired immunodeficiency syndrome (HIV/AIDS). Resolution 1994/24.

13. Modus Operandi of the Programme Coordinating Board of the Joint United Nations Programme on HIV/AIDS (UNAIDS). (2011) Available at http://www.unaids.org/en/media/unaids/contentassets/documents/pcb/2014/20120301_Revised_Modus_operandi_dec2011_en.pdf (accessed December 2013).

14. The Global Fund to Fight AIDS, Tuberculosis and Malaria. Official website. Available at www.theglobalfund.org/en (accessed December 2013).

13

Germany's Role in Promoting Systems of Solidarity in Healthcare[a]

*Jean-Olivier Schmidt**

Why is Social Health Protection[b] an Issue in Global Health?

One hundred million. This figure stands for the number of people that fall into poverty every year[1] due to so-called catastrophic healthcare expenditure. This makes ill health and the healthcare spending that follows the biggest single risk factor leading to impoverishment worldwide. Beyond the individual tragedies that are hidden behind the statistics, this figure also illustrates how critical disease and its relationship to poverty is in hindering and affecting overall economic and social development. As the Commission on Macroeconomics and Health[2] has demonstrated, a vicious circle of poverty and disease exists, not only at the individual level but also at the level of society itself. There are strong macroeconomic repercussions from sickness and the inability of people to afford adequate

---

[a] This article does not represent the opinion of the organization.

[b] In this chapter, "social health protection" (SHP) and "social health insurance" (SHI) will be used interchangeably with universal health coverage (UHC). The main difference in the concept consists in whether income loss will be compensated for (SHP) or not (UHC).

* Head of Section Health and Social Protection, GIZ GmbH, Dag-Hammarskjöld-Weg 1-5, 65760 Eschborn.

healthcare without the risk of falling into poverty. More than one billion people — approximately one out of every seven people on the planet — are not able to get adequate access to health services, partly due to financial constraints. This also makes it a major problem for the world community in achieving the Millennium Development Goals, which were agreed upon internationally in 2000.

Since then, the world has witnessed a lot of change, sometimes dramatic: the last decade has brought unprecedented economic growth to many countries, be it in Asia or sub-Saharan Africa. In turn, this has generated new possibilities in terms of the fiscal space and scope for redistribution policies. At the same time, growth has also widened economic disparities in many countries, thus increasing the risks of social unrest and instability. In part, this is because the awareness has grown, at an international level as well as within countries and among individual citizens, that access to basic healthcare is a human right. As such, it follows that non-access constitutes a violation of essential human rights as laid down in the UN Charter of Human Rights of 1948 (Article 25).[3] A growing number of litigation cases have shown that citizens can claim and demand the fulfillment of these rights from their states.[4] Finally, some elements of access to healthcare can also be understood as global public goods (such as prevention from pandemic diseases as the world has recently again been alerted through the Ebola crisis in 2014), and thus, in addition, one can discuss this issue in terms of an obligation of the international community to promote access to health globally.[5]

The international community has invested a lot of money in global health initiatives over the last decade (hence Chan calls it a "golden decade for health"[6]). The Global Fund on AIDS, TB and Malaria (GFATM), the Global Alliance on Vaccination and Immunization (GAVI), the Clinton Health Access Initiative (CHAI), the US President's Emergency Plan for AIDS Relief (PEPFAR), etc. were created. However, most of these initiatives focus on specific diseases and rather narrow vertical approaches and, as a result, neither always strengthen the long-term implementation of sustainable healthcare systems nor promote social health protection at a country level.

Beyond these developmental and rights perspectives, there are economic aspects: as economies mature, the tertiary sector gains in importance and this has seen the health sector grow into one of the most dynamic branches of many national economies, with a staggering worldwide turnover of US$5.3 trillion.[7] There are many business interests associated with the sector and, as a result, the business community often has a common interest in developing and strengthening healthcare delivery and financing health systems. Finally, a lack of access to quality promotive, preventative and curative healthcare services causes a tremendous loss of productivity for individuals and for society as a whole in low- and middle-income countries. For NCDs alone, there are estimates that cardiovascular disease, chronic respiratory disease, cancer, diabetes, mental health problems, etc., will lead to cumulative output loss at a global scale of US$47 trillion over the next two decades. This loss would represent 75% of global GDP in 2010.[8] The pandemic Ebola crisis has severely impacted on the economy of the affected countries — countries whose weak healthcare systems were not prepared to react swiftly to the first cases. More and more countries have recognized this and are now focusing on social health protection with the aim of including the whole population and strengthening the overall health systems, but also with a view to managing health financing streams in a more efficient way than through unregulated private insurance or direct payments. With the recent decision of the Supreme Court, the last OECD country — the USA — has confirmed its change in direction toward universal health coverage (UHC), signified by the 2010 Affordable Care Act.[9]

I Did it My Way: Germany's Path Toward Social Health Protection for All

More than 125 years ago, under the leadership of the "Iron Chancellor" Otto von Bismarck, Germany took its first steps[c] toward a mandatory and

---

[c]This does not mean that Bismarck invented and created the German social health insurance system. While he initiated the first steps on a nationwide scale, his approach relied on a variety of pre-existing solidarity and mutual aid schemes that had evolved since the Middle Ages in Europe. Moreover, the laws he issued on social insurance had their roots in Prussian social laws, such as the "revised mining decree from Kleve-Markland" of 1776. The decisive contribution of the Bismarck administration was to initiate the implementation of a countrywide regulatory framework for social protection in the then recently created German national state.

social health protection (SHP) system. The result was still a long way from universal coverage. It was mainly a response to the demand for alleviating the negative repercussions on the social fabric of the "great transformation"[10] due to the industrialization, and more particularly by the political will to prevent workers from revolting. In the initial discussions, there were two opposing camps in the parliament. On one side, there were the supporters of a tax-based scheme[d,11] (mostly from among the ruling party). On the other side, the opposition argued for a system based on contributory financing by the beneficiaries. Afraid of the excessive and dominating influence of the national government, the church, (regional) state governments and representatives of corporations voted against a tax-based system. The social health insurance (SHI) system, as implemented in 1883, thus reflects a compromise between the two parties.[12] With this law Germany became the first country in the world to introduce a mandatory nationwide SHI system, spearheading a movement which other countries were soon to follow. The way the German design emerged was a reaction to four factors, namely: (1) That, as discussed above, industrialization and related urbanization led to vast population movements and to the dismantling of more traditional forms of social protection based on local community structures and churches. More formal mechanisms of social protection therefore became necessary to provide some protection against social risks, particularly in the industrial sector. However, industrialization alone was not a decisive factor, as in the European context Germany was a rather late industrializer; thus, other concurrent reasons were (2) the fear of social unrest (laws against socialists) and Bismarck's effort to counter their propaganda; (3) already existing solidarity mechanisms and principles such as the traditional guild or miners' association support systems; and (4) the "subsidiarity principle"[e] of the Catholic church — this principle helped in shaping the relative autonomy of the social insurance bodies.

Originally, the system covered only a section of the working population, such as miners and some industrial workers, but did not include their dependents. Each of these different occupational groups had its own scheme which was later on complemented by funds for certain regions.

---

[d] Interestingly enough, through taxation on nationalized tobacco production and distribution.[11]

[e] The subsidiarity principle refers to leaving decision-making to the lowest possible level.

This meant that in the early years of the new system only 6–10% of the population had access to it and it took Germany quite a long time to achieve the reality (legal and in actuality) of universal population coverage through comprehensive schemes in which membership was open to those outside occupational groups. In fact, the final reforms to achieve total coverage for the entire population date back to as recently as 2007, making it mandatory for every citizen to have health insurance.[f,13] In this way, the German healthcare system is also a prototype for the so-called continental approach to the welfare state,[14] which links entitlements to social protection with the status of employment, rather than the citizens' rights approach common to the Nordic countries.

The model initiated under Bismarck proved to be very stable institutionally and illustrates how significant a role path dependency plays in the approach chosen by countries.[15] As a result, even today Germany's social protection system is characterized, on one side, by a multitude of social insurance funds[g] with mandatory statutory health insurance for employees with incomes below a certain threshold, and voluntary statutory health insurance for people with higher incomes (who can opt out of statutory health insurance) or self-employed; on the other side, there are private health insurance companies that can be contracted by this group (the self-employed and people with incomes above the threshold). Civil servants are normally also privately insured. The German healthcare system has managed to withstand various profound changes to the German political system and even two devastating world wars. Entitlements associated with the benefits of being a member of a specific insurance scheme proved to be so strong that they even survived changes of states: in Alsace-Moselle, which was part of Germany at the end of the 19th century but has now

---

[f]The reforms helped close the last gaps in universal coverage, as people without insurance, among them self-employed people, were required by law to take out health insurance with their last insurer (public or private) and public and private insurers were forced to contract these applicants. As entitlements to healthcare are still linked to membership in a scheme, before that amendment there were cases where, due to default in payment of contributions, people *de facto* dropped out of schemes and were then only entitled to basic care and emergency treatment (this affects around 0.17% of the population).[13]

[g]Reforms in the early 1990s reduced, drastically the number of insurance schemes from over 2000, but there are still more than 200 different insurance companies in the health sector.

belonged to France for decades, the social security institutions remain a *sui generis* "regime" even today and are distinctly different from the other French regions, resembling much more the German SHI system. Moreover, the German SHI system has remained relatively unaffected by several financial crises, and the impact of the European Union rules on healthcare and social protection, most notably the European Court's decision on transborder access to healthcare services.[h,16–19] The German SHP system has thus shown itself to be a powerful instrument that can readily adapt to changes in its environment — it withstood so far two World Wars, financial and economic crsis and demographic changes. It could even be called an "evergreen" in this respect, and certainly not a one-hit wonder!

Together We Stand Strong: Principles Underlying SHP in the German Context

From the outset, the German system was based on the principle of solidarity, and this is still firmly enshrined in the system today. Essentially this means that the contribution to a scheme depends upon one's ability to pay, whereas treatment and medication is given according to needs (i.e. independent of the level of contribution). Contributions are defined as a percentage of income up to a certain ceiling and are paid through salary deductions for all dependent workers. The combination of income-related contributions and needs-based entitlements ensures financial stability through pooling across different population groups, in addition to forming the basis by which the healthy support the sick. The solidarity principle implies cross-subsidization from the rich to the poor, from the young to the old and from single people to families (children are insured with their parents free of contribution).

---

[h]The Amsterdam treaty assures autonomy of Member States in shaping their health and social policies.[17] However, recent trends in the German SHI system, such as the progressive promotion of competition between health insurance funds and the strong focus on market mechanisms,[18] expected to contribute toward containing increasing healthcare expenditures, put under risk the privileges of public SHP funds and might provide the European Court with strong arguments for considering German SHI funds as being like any other company acting in Europe, and thus applying cartel rights to them.[19]

The principle of subsidiarity is reflected in the fact that the social insurance schemes are self-governed bodies ruled by public law. The state delegates some of its responsibilities — namely the obligation to assure health protection for all citizens, including the tasks of collecting the contributions and managing them as a public good — to the social insurance funds and sticks to its regulatory and supervisory functions. This means that financially and administratively the social insurance schemes are autonomous and do indeed face the risk of bankruptcy if improperly managed. Members can participate in the election of the board. Together with introducing competition between public health insurance funds, the state has set up a risk equalization mechanism which ensures that there is some redistribution of funds between schemes according to a list of criteria that relate to the risk profile of members and, more recently, to the morbidity of beneficiaries. This is a precondition for fair competition and was particularly necessary in Germany because of the different risk profiles of health insurance schemes that had originally emerged from funds for different occupational groups, as mentioned above. On the provider side, the corporatist principle also finds its reflection in the fact that the SHI physicians and hospital associations are self-governed corporate entities that negotiate their payment directly with the federal association of the health insurance schemes.

The state stipulates by law the right of members to adequate, effective and efficient medical services.[i,20] The healthcare providers and the insurers have annual negotiations on which services actually to provide and how many of them, with a predefined financial ceiling. In addition, in order to achieve a competitive advantage, several funds opt to cover services beyond the statutory set benefits.

With a Little Help from My Friends: Instruments to Promote SHP Globally

Through its approach to international cooperation, Germany is supporting a whole range of countries worldwide in setting up their own social

---

[i]The insurance schemes have only small margins and provide additional benefits in order to compete for members; hence and despite strong legal restrictions for preventing risk selection, SHI funds apply strategies for achieving a more positive risk mix among their enrollees.[20]

protection systems, often with a strong focus on SHP. The Ministry of Cooperation and Development (BMZ), through its technical and financial cooperation agencies (GIZ and KfW), has supported many countries across the world to improve their healthcare and social protection systems. While in the past there was considerable emphasis on support in Latin America, the focus has now shifted to Asia and Africa. Currently, Germany is supporting health sector and social protection reforms in Asian countries as diverse as Indonesia, India, Vietnam, Cambodia, Mongolia, Nepal, Bangladesh, Pakistan and Yemen. In Africa, the main regional focus is in eastern Africa (Burundi, Kenya, Tanzania, Rwanda, Uganda) and south-eastern Africa (Malawi, Mozambique, South Africa, Namibia). While some countries have real financial limits to what they can afford in terms of healthcare, in many others the primary issue is more about a lack of human and institutional capacities. It will take some time to develop these — especially as it is clear that each country needs to find its own institutional solutions that reflect its specific values and principles.

The Ministry of Health (BMG) also has cooperation agreements with a number of countries in Eastern Europe, Southern Europe and Central Asia. In relation to its European partners, the aim of cooperation has primarily been to support them in the process of becoming members of the *acquis communautaire*, which is the basic prerequisite for becoming a member of the European Union (EU).

While the countries supported by Germany are culturally very different and at very different stages of economic development, their motivation often stems from similar sources. This is because the process of national development, frequently fosters challenges which are similar to those Germany faced during its own industrial transition, albeit often in a much more rapid and drastic fashion. For example, a huge number of labor migrants are moving within and out of many developing countries, cultural patterns are changing quickly, and income distributions and inequity are skyrocketing. This creates internal pressure to find solutions to stabilize society during the process of economic development, while external pressure comes from an international agenda on SHP and human rights that has become truly global as information is now readily available to people in all countries and at every level of society. Many countries therefore find the German approach to providing SHP an attractive option as public goods are delivered partly through private providers and self-administrated funds, i.e. public mechanisms (insurance bodies). Further, the quality of services is generally perceived as excellent, without discriminating between clients based on their socio-economic backgrounds. As the schemes are self-governed and relatively autonomous, they are generally independent of political day-to-day interference while at the same time being under a genuine obligation to guarantee rights to their beneficiaries and through legal codification in the social law.

Imagine All the People …: The Shaping of Discourse and the Promotion of Norms Internationally

Apart from the individual bilateral support at a country level, Germany is a major actor in shaping the international discourse on SHP and UHC respectively, and is using different institutional bodies to do so. After World War II, Germany's foreign policy objective was to become an integral member of the community of nations and therefore, in a deliberate move, it handed responsibility for some of its national rights to supranational bodies (namely the EU through Article 22 of the constitution) and invested financially in multilateral agreements and institutions, notably in the UN system. Germany is supporting the Global Health Agenda with a considerable amount of funds and through its active participation in a range of initiatives and mechanisms. In 2008, Germany, at the initiative of the Federal Chancellor, Angela Merkel, and together with France, launched the "Providing for Health" initiative during the G8 summit in Heiligendamm, Germany. P4H aims to promote SHP and support countries in a coherent way to achieve the objectives of UHC. It is a partnership of bilateral (France, Germany, Switzerland, Spain) and multilateral organizations (WHO, ILO, WB, AfDB) and an instrument for providing support for SHP in a more coordinated and effective way. It can be seen as an interesting new approach to linking bilateral instruments with multilateral agencies. Currently, the P4H partners are supporting more than 20 countries worldwide. Germany is also a co-signatory of the International Health Partnership + and one of the biggest investors in the Global Fund to Fight AIDS, Tuberculosis and Malaria (GFATM).

In the past decade, Germany has promoted and supported many high-level events on the subject of SHP: it started with the international Ministerial Conference on Social Health Insurance in Berlin in 2005 as a way to move forward Resolution 58.33 on Social Health Insurance at WHA 2005. Germany was further instrumental in promoting the topic of UHC within the WHO and produced in 2011 the first draft of the resolution on UHC, which was then put on the table by the EU. As a way to rally support for this resolution, it hosted the launch of the "World Health Report 2010 on Universal Health Coverage: The Role of Health Financing" in Berlin, which assembled more than 50 ministers and state secretaries. Germany has also been supportive of the "Foreign Policy and Global Health" Group, composed of France, Brazil, Norway, Senegal, Indonesia and Thailand, and collaborated actively through an inter-ministerial effort led by the Ministry of Foreign Affairs to the UN General Assembly declaration on UHC in late 2012.

In the framework of EU-coordinated efforts, Germany frequently assumed the role of burden-sharer when preparing inputs to WHO processes. Germany has also been instrumental in developing and presenting the EU Council Conclusions on the EU Role in Global Health,[21] which also contain a strong statement on "EU values of solidarity towards equitable and universal coverage of quality health services." The German Minister of Health made a strong statement at the World Health Summit 2012 in Berlin concerning the future support for UHC worldwide by stating that it must be included in the post-MDG agenda.

Germany has further promoted Global health, especially in 2015. The Ebola crisis of 2014 has promoted the topic of global health and the importance of health systems strengthening. Therefore, the Chancellor of Germany, Angela Merkel has developed a six-point plan of action to address the issue of weak health systems and the threat of pandemics. The G7 summit of Germany had health at its centerpiece. The rationale for doing so has been explained at the opening of the World Health Assembly by the Chancellor herself: [...] the human right to health can only be enforced if a sustainable health system is in place or is put in place in every country on Earth; and secondly, because globalization is tangibly making us all more dependent on one another, so that increasingly the health of one person is also the health of others. In other words, the effectiveness of the health system in one country impacts on the health of other countries, and on security and stablility. The responsibility of individual countries and global shared responsibility are two sides of one and the same coin.

Acknowledgments

The author would like to thank Matthew Walsham for constructive revision of the language and Amelie Stanzel for editorial support. He would also like to expressh his thanks to Dr. Jens Holst for technical comments and literature sources, and to Roland Panea and Viktoria Rabovskaja for review.

References

1. Evans D, *et al.* (2007) Protecting households from catastrophic health spending. *Health Affairs* **26(4):** 972–983.
2. World Health Organization. (2003) CMH booklet: Investing in Health — A Summary of the Findings of the Commission on Macroeconomics and Health. World Health Organization, Geneva.
3. Pogge T. (2005) Human rights and global health: a research program. *Metaphilosophy* **36(1–2):** 182–209.
4. Hogerzeil H, *et al.* (2006) Is access to essential medicines as part of the fulfilment of the right to health enforceable through the courts? *The Lancet* **368(9532):** 305–311.
5. Ooms G. (2011) Global Health: What It Has Been So Far, What It Should Be, And What It Could Become. Working Paper No. 2, S.30f. Available at http://www.itg.be/itg/Uploads/Volksgezondheid/wpshsop/SHSOP%20 WP%202%20Ooms%20Global%20Health.pdf.
6. Chan M. (2012) Best Days for Public Health Are Ahead of Us, says WHO Director-General. Address to the Sixty-Fifth World Health Assembly. Geneva, Switzerland, 21 May 2012. Available at http://www.who.int/dg/ speeches/2012/wha_20120521/en/index.html.
7. World Health Organization. (2010) The World Health Report — Health Systems Financing: The Path to Universal Coverage. World Health Organization, Geneva. Available at http://www.who.int/whr/2010/whr10_en.pdf.
8. World Economic Forum. (2011) The Global Burden of Non-communicative Diseases. Available at http://www3.weforum.org/docs/WEF_Harvard_HE_ GlobalEconomicBurdenNonCommunicableDiseases_2011.pdf.

9. Whitehouse. (2010) Affordable Care Act: The New Healthcare Law at Two Years. Washington, USA. Available at http://www.whitehouse.gov/sites/default/files/uploads/careact.pdf.

10. Polanyi K. (1944/1957) *The Great Transformation: The Political and Economic Origins of Our Time.* Beacon, Boston.

11. Pflanze O. (2008) *Bismarck: Der Reichskanzler.* Beck, Germany.

12. Busse R, Riesberg A. (2004) Healthcare Systems in Transition: Germany. WHO Regional Office for Europe on behalf of the European Observatory on Health Systems and Policies, Copenhagen. Available at http://www.euro.who.int/__data/assets/pdf_file/0018/80703/E85472.pdf.

13. Destatis. (2012): *Weniger Menschen ohne Kranknversicherungsschutz.* Pressemitteilung, Nr. 285. Available at https://www.destatis.de/DE/PresseService/Presse/Pressemitteilungen/2012/08/PD12_285_122.html.

14. Esping-Andersen G. (1990) *The Three Worlds of Welfare Capitalism.* John Wiley & Sons, Cambridge.

15. Pierson P. (2004) *Politics in Time: History, Institutions, and Social Analysis.* Princeton University Press, Princeton.

16. Blankart C, *et al.* (2009) *Das deutsche Gesundheitswesen zukunftsfähig gestalten — Patientenseite stärken — Reformunfähigkeit überwinden.* Springer, Berlin.

17. European Communities. (1997) Treaty of Amsterdam amending the Treaty on European Union, the Treaties establishing the european Communities and certain related acts. *Official Journal C* **340**.

18. Cucic S. (2000) European Union health policy and its implications for national convergence. *International Journal for Quality Healthcare* **12(3):** 217–225.

19. Bechtold R, *et al.* (2010) *Rechtliche Grenzen der Anwendung des Kartellverbots auf die Tätigkeit gesetzlicher Krankenkassen.* Gutachten im Auftrag des AOK-Bundesverbands. Available at http://www.aok-bv.de/imperia/md/aokbv/politik/reformaktuell/gutachten_kartellrecht_amnog.pdf.

20. Höppner K, *et al.* (2005) *Grenzen und Dysfunktionalitäten des Kassenwettbewerbs in der GKV: Theorie und Empirie der Risikoselektion in Deutschland.* ZeS-Arbeitspapier Nr. 4/2005, Zentrum für Sozialpolitik, Universität Bremen.

21. Council of the European Union. (2010) Council Conclusions on the EU Role in Global Health. Article 8, 10 May 2010.

14

The Civil Society Perspective on the EU's Role in Global Health

Remco van de Pas* and Nicoletta Dentico†

Background: Multiple Actor Governance in Global Health

Over the past decade there has been remarkable political momentum for global health, and funding has increased substantially. Health therefore enjoys unprecedented attention on the international level, with its wake of positive and sometimes controversial implications. In a world of multiple power shifts — between states, between states and non-state actors, and within states between sectors — new challenges emerge for what is a vital institution in a more complex global health environment. Priority setting in health and activities related to global health diplomacy demand a fuller range of voices to be considered if these exercises are to be accorded any real legitimacy. This trend reflects more diffuse power allocated to non-state actors, alongside the traditional institutional and government players.[1] For all their intricacies, these are positive trends that mirror the growing complexity of societal dynamics, in Europe and elsewhere.

*Researcher, Department of Public Health, Institute of Tropical Medicine (Antwerp) & Visiting fellow, Netherlands Institute of International Relations 'Clingendael' (The Hague).
†Co-Director, Health Innovation in Practice (HIP, Geneva) Vice-Chair of the Osservatorio Italiano Salute Globale (OISG, www.saluteglobale.it).

The Treaty of the European Union (the Maastricht Treaty) says that a high level of human health protection shall be ensured in the definition and implementation of all EU policies and activities. The Maastricht Treaty further specifies that the EU and its Member States shall foster cooperation with third countries and international organizations on public health. We all tend to agree that active citizenship and sustained engagement throughout any given political process are key ingredients of a "healthy democracy." The democratic interplay cannot be confined to the periodic exercise of formal voting procedures. Of crucial relevance is the function of civil society, which, according to the political philosopher Antonio Gramsci, refers to the public space that societies must cherish to promote political advancement through citizens' engagement and interaction with mandated institutions. This occurs in the form of public dialogues, participatory consultations, and organization of pressure groups demanding transparency and accountability so as to monitor the advancement of a political agenda that they have contributed toward shaping.[2]

The recently coined paradigm of "multistakeholder engagement" has attracted notable attention in current global health debates, as a consequence of the universal promotion of the partnership model within the UN family as the one unquestioned approach to dealing with global policy issues. The mobilizing concept of "partnership," whose definitions remain quite elastic, has raised some concerns about the consequences that it may determine in governance and policy decision-making processes alike. The authors of this chapter have closely followed this debate in relation to the WHO reform.[3,4] New global health initiatives, civil society organizations, private corporate organizations and non-profit philanthropic actors have all gained a high profile in the new scene of global health governance. For example, for over a decade, CSOs have been instrumental in pushing the discussion on the health and trade agenda with Member States at the WHO, particularly in relation to the management of intellectual property rights in the interest of public health, and to the urgency of securing needs-driven innovation for health and access to lifesaving medicines.[5] Similarly, industry-affiliated organizations strive to ensure that they have a role both in policy agenda setting in multilateral organizations and in policy implementation.[6] Their role and legitimacy is highly contested by some civil society organizations, academia and governments.[7]

The Malaise of Corporate Capture

Europe is no exception to the dynamic of corporate capture, a circumstance that is made visible by the massive imbalance between business lobbyists (approximately 15,000 people in Brussels) and those representing social and environmental concerns.[8] The flawed assumption is that what is good for big business is good for Europe — and the rest of the world. But a rather wide range of actors have come by now to reflect the same claim that the EU altogether suffers from a "democratic deficit" due to its highly inaccessible bureaucratic setup, the distance of ordinary citizens from its decision-making processes, and the complexity of its operations.[9,10] Many analysts attribute Europe's current, multifaceted crisis to the market-led model of European unification, which has dominated since the mid-1980s. The ensuing shift from the original core values of responsibility and the social state, as outlined in the Maastricht Treaty, to the dogmatic austerity and the security state we see today is intrinsically linked to the dominant European political philosophy of economic liberalization.[11,12] The need for increased legitimacy has pushed the EU to seek more openness and greater involvement of interest groups through consultation, dialogue and networking,[13] but the model bias and the persisting asymmetries in the power balance still represent a major challenge. In the field of health, for example, CSOs see that they have an explicit role in providing analysis and demanding accountability and improved global governance for health by the EU, its Member States and the European Commission.[14] On the other hand, the resignation of European Commissioner for Health and Consumer Policy John Dalli in October 2012 stands out to indicate how powerful the tobacco industry can be when influencing decision-makers. Civil society, albeit with limited resources, strives to act as a countervailing power against aggressive corporate lobby.[a]

For its part, civil society has to address its own legitimacy and autonomy while working on advocacy and policy dialogue at the EU level. Firstly, civil society consists of heterogeneous interest groups, with their own respective agendas. Secondly, CSO representatives positioned at the EU consultation level should pay due attention toward including their

---

[a]See http://www.epha.org/spip.php?article5386.

national and local constituencies in the development of their analyses and political stands for policy dialogue and consultation in Brussels or Strasbourg.

The Involvement of Public Interest Civil Society in EU Public Health Policies

The European Commission (EC) has actually encouraged civil society engagement in different ways with the aim of increasing its own legitimacy and create a "social constituency" (see box below). However, its interaction with civil society is not as susceptible to political scrutiny or electoral accountability to citizens at this level, unlike at the European Parliament (EP) and the Council of Europe. A challenge and a goal for the EC is to ensure that CSO representatives do correspond to the diverse range of citizens and territories within European society, in line with the Commission's health strategy. The EC, for its part, is inclined to promote a *pluralist* understanding of civil society. This means including not only the organizations that give voice to the concerns of citizens, but also market-related actors present on the EU scene, with a liberal approach that does tend to distance itself from the deliberative democracy with tight connections to the public sphere, as defined by the sociologist Jürgen Habermas.[15]

The EC strongly advocates the Citizens' Agenda with the aim of promoting citizen empowerment and participation in health policies. The Director-General of the European Commission for Health and Consumers has established the practice of a stakeholder dialogue group having balanced experience from both industry and NGOs, with the aim of contributing to policy shaping and consensus building.[b] At the same time, the Lisbon Treaty made applicable the Citizens' Initiative, formally introduced in January 2012.[c] The Citizens' Initiative — through which one million EU citizens are able to invite the EC to make a legislative proposal — could become a highly relevant tool for advancing common goods in the health realm.[16] In February 2013 the European Citizens' Initiative on the human

---

[b] See http://ec.europa.eu/dgs/health_consumer/sdg/index_en.htm.

[c] See http://ec.europa.eu/dgs/secretariat_general/citizens_initiative/index_en.htm.

right to water was for the first time successful in collecting the necessary number of statements for support.[d]

The Commission Communication on the EU Role in Global Health,[e,17] discussed in detail in another chapter of this book, is built upon the conceptual pillars of human rights, health equity, democratic governance, and policy coherence for development. Public interest organizations have played a very active and constructive role in designing the strategic contours of Europe in global health through consultations — both online and face-to-face — at the end of 2009; 105 of them provided inputs.[f] In their watchdog function, CSOs have a major role in holding the EU and its Member States accountable in relation to the commitments made under this Communication. The principles of the EU role in global health are fundamental grounds for several leading European platforms on public health. They provide the basic notions for advancing the international debate on the need to reconfigure global governance for health through the lenses of health democracy.[18,19] The Council Conclusions on the EU role in Global Health have established a common ground (a common *acquis*) when EU Member States for instance define their position at the World Health Assembly. Civil society is then able to hold the Member States accountable to what has been agreed upon in this EU common *acquis* concerning global health.

NGOs and Global Health

Many and diverse organizations have emerged in the field of global health at the European level, as well as within EU Member States. A first actor mapping, although incomplete, was conducted by Global Health Europe in 2010.[g] The mapping includes EuroHealthNet (an alliance of not-for-profit public health entities aiming to support European health and equity policies), CONCORD (a network of European NGOs working in development

[d]See http://europa.eu/rapid/press-release_IP-13-107_en.htm.
[e]See http://ec.europa.eu/development/icenter/repository/COMM_PDF_COM_2010_0128_EN.PDF.
[f]See http://ec.europa.eu/europeaid/how/public-consultations/4765_en.htm.
[g]See http://www.globalhealtheurope.org/index.php?option=com_sobi2&Itemid=144.

cooperation), the European Public Health Alliance (EPHA; this group broadly represents professional, academic, civil society and patient groups affiliated with public health in the EU context) and Action for Global Health (AFGH; a large European NGO network advocating a more proactive role for European institutions in promoting the Health MDGs agenda and its implementation in low-income countries by 2015). The European Forum for Primary Care (EFPC) is another key European network, which pursues the strengthening of primary healthcare in Europe. Finally, Health Action International (HAI) is an independent global network with its original roots in Europe, actively engaged in increasing access to essential medicines and improving drug rational use worldwide.

As mentioned earlier, a number of European NGOs primarily conduct their activities in global health from a national perspective, as they continue to see development cooperation, to a large extent, as part of their sovereign national policies. Historically, many NGOs receive funding from their national Ministry of Foreign Affairs for a considerable portion to conduct development and human rights programs in former colonial areas. By mean of this national lens and existing cooperation, NGOs pursue policy dialogues around global health in their countries, while implementing activities with partners in Southern countries. Many NGOs that receive funding through an EC-financed consortium actually interface with national governments in the EU primarily, with the UN system or with specific global health initiatives (such as the Global Fund to Fight AIDS, Tuberculosis and Malaria), as well as with actors of international civil society networks. Support from European bodies may then take different and indeed complementary routes, beyond the EU institutions. The reality is that only a limited number of NGOs or civil society networks in Europe consider the EC and the European Parliament as relevant players in global health.

Action for Global Health (AFGH), for instance, is engaged in promoting policy dialogue and advocacy work at national, European and global level.[h] Medicus Mundi International (MMI),[19,i] is engaged in national health fora through its respective members; it has official relations with the WHO and is a key player in global health partnerships such as the

---

[h] See http://www.actionforglobalhealth.eu/index.php?id=215.
[i] See http://www.medicusmundi.org/en/mmi-network.

Global Health Workforce Alliance, but has limited interactions with global health initiatives carried out by the EU institutions.[j] In general, actors involved in the EU global health agenda are the large international development NGOs and similar platforms with a representation in Brussels. These include Oxfam International, Médecins Sans Frontières, Save the Children, CONCORD, the European NGOs for Sexual and Reproductive Health and Rights, Population and Development (EuroNGOs), and the organizations that are members of the AFGH network. These organizations meet formally in the global health policy platform (see below); informal cooperation among them also exists. As many organizations have been confronted with financial constraints that led them to focus on fewer thematic priorities, joint discussion on the implementation of the Council Conclusions has been limited.

The EU Role in Global Health and the Global Health Policy Platform

We have already mentioned how public interest civil society organizations have been inspirationally involved in tailoring the EU positioning in global health. Academic evidence coupled with political and motivational leadership inside the Commission succeeded in making a strong case for governance for global health in the EU. Yet, it was through support and involvement by a myriad of civil society actors that such a solid and progressive framework for Europe emerged. An important recognition for this outcome must be attributed to EPHA. At that time (2009–2010) EPHA was coordinating the EU advocacy of the AFGH network, and in this position it effectively mentored interested civil society actors on global health issues in the EU.[20] EPHA managed to seal the linkage between European health policies and European development policies in the field of health. Largely thanks to its policy analysis, active participation in consultations, and sustained advocacy initiatives, principles like health equity, the right-to-health approach,

---

[j]The exception being a recent hearing on social protection and health in EU development cooperation at the European Parliament. See http://www.wemos.nl/files/Documenten%20 Informatief/20120620%20BACKGROUND%20NOTE%20Social%20Health%20 Protection%20in%20EU%20Development%20Cooperation.pdf.

public responsibility for health and policy coherence for development are prominently featured in the final communication on the EU role in global health.[k] The Health Action Partnership International, via the representation of its member EuroHealthNet, also showed a strong voice in advocating coherent EU policies for global health.[21] As for the chapter concerning the EU investment in needs-driven health and biomedical research, Health Action International and Oxfam have contributed a great deal to its framing, together with MSF.[22]

After the release of the EC Communication and the Council Conclusions, a first inspirational, EU high-level forum on global health took place in June 2010.[23] The forum generated interest and raised the profile of global health for policy-makers, NGOs and diplomats working at the EU level and beyond. The event led to a formal EU Policy Forum on global health convened once every three months, open to a multistakeholder group and well attended by public interest civil society actors.[l] A retrospective analysis of the agenda items and presentations streamlined for the forum over the last three years, however, shows that the linkage between European health policies and European health development policies got sorely lost, as the focus on topics of development cooperation and global health has prevailed, somewhat in isolation from the European health policies chapter. The impact of globalization on European and global health, the vision and the policies of the EU on trade issues impacting health (i.e. investments, health services and intellectual property rights, especially when negotiating bilateral trade agreements), Europe's fiscal policies and migration control strategies, as well as the debates associated with the EU position on governance for global health, have remained largely out of the scope of the policy forum throughout 2011 and 2012. Among the main issues addressed were the advancing of universal health coverage; the joint actions on HIV/AIDS, sexual and reproductive health and reduction of child mortality; the role of the International Health Partnership+; the report of the WHO Consultative Expert Working Group on research and development financing and coordination; the international migration of health workers and the global shortage of the health workforce. Hence, the global health policy forum has become

---

[k] See http://www.epha.org/a/3630.
[l] See http://ec.europa.eu/health/eu_world/events/index_en.htm#anchor0_more.

a discussion platform for actors mainly involved in health development cooperation. One of the factors behind this shift is the degree of fragmentation and capacities within the civil society community itself. In late 2011, EPHA stopped being the AFGH bridging organization as coordinator because its lean resources forced it back to its core mandate — European health policies (EPHA notably started to facilitate the European health policy forum at that point). At the same time the main funder of AFGH, the Bill & Melinda Gates Foundation, required AFGH to focus on health development assistance and universal health coverage. The previously sought connection between European and global health actors was *de facto* broken. Also, the rather widespread inclination to depoliticize the root causes of ill health around the world came to prevail in the European debate.

The tension between funding approaches in times of financial crisis and CSOs' quest for autonomy in tackling national or regional advocacy of global health is interestingly described in an overview report on the first five years of the AFGH network.[24] Indeed, partly due to funding requirements, several NGOs have indulged in pragmatism and are narrowed down to their specific expertise again, with the primary focus on a range of specific health themes, rather than the global health agenda and global governance for health. The more so, because the leadership and support from the competent EC directorates toward coherent activities for global health in Europe have notably been reduced, officially due to economic difficulties and austerity policies.

CSOs' Interaction with the European Parliament in Global Health

Civil society has good working relations with members of the European Parliament (MEP) when it comes to global health issues. As the only EU institution democratically elected by its citizens, it is relevant to bring global health under the attention of the parliamentarians. The interaction between civil society and MEP is often structured around specific topics, depending on the political agenda of the EP, or the agenda of the DEVE committee, the most meaningful parliamentary committee for global health.[m]

---

[m] See http://www.europarl.europa.eu/committees/en/deve/home.html.

There are two relevant working groups for global health that focus on the EP. One is the Working Group on Reproductive Health, HIV/AIDS and Development, hosted by Marie Stopes International.[n] The other, the Working Group on Innovation, Access to Medicines and Poverty-Related Diseases was inaugurated in February 2010.[o] This was the result of a strong alliance between CSOs active in this field (among them Médecins Sans Frontiers) and a small group of European members of Parliament who had followed and actively supported the WHO negotiation on the Intergovernmental Working Group on Public Health, Innovation and Intellectual Property (IGWG) from 2006 to 2008, which contributed to making this topic one key element of the EU role in global health.

The EP Working Group aims to promote and develop a meaningful dialogue between MEP, the EC and civil society organizations to ensure that European policies deliver a comprehensive and meaningful response to tackle the need for needs-based innovation, access to medicines and quality healthcare for diseases in low- and middle-income countries. Through a series of public events with experts and the media at the EP, the group has succeeded in addressing the issue of the participation gap between European citizens and European institutions, and in redressing the balance between the EU trade and development agenda. It has also managed to show the implications of a lack of policy coherence between trade and health, within the European continent.[p]

One of the most remarkable results produced by the fruitful interaction between the EP and the CSOs concerning global health matters is the rejection of the Anti-Counterfeiting Trade Agreement (ACTA) by the EP on 4 July 2012. ACTA has been vigorously questioned by an extremely large NGO community, including the NGO constituency dealing with health, on the severe consequences that the treaty might have on access to essential medicines in low- and middle-income countries.[q] ACTA was negotiated by the EU and other countries (the US, Australia, Canada, Japan, Mexico, Morocco,

---

[n] See http://www.epwg.org.

[o] See http://www.msfaccess.org/content/european-parliament-working-group.

[p] It has, for example, organized a large symposium to show the risks of not addressing the patients' rights appropriately in the case of multidrug-resistant TB (MDR-TB) on the doorstep of Europe.

[q] See http://euobserver.com/justice/115846.

New Zealand, Singapore, South Korea and Switzerland) to improve the enforcement of anti-counterfeiting law internationally.[r] While the EP had repeatedly asked the Commission to make ACTA documents available so as to enhance MEPs' role in negotiating the contents, the final version of ACTA was so agreed that the EP could not alter it, but only approve or block it. In the event, the EP declined to give its consent to ACTA, which meant that the entire EU stayed out of the agreement. The EP's vote means that neither the EU nor its individual Member States can join the treaty. While debating whether to give its consent to ACTA, the EP experienced unprecedented direct pressure by thousands of EU citizens, who called on it to reject ACTA, via street demonstrations, e-mails to MEPs and calls to their offices. It also received a petition, signed by 2.8 million citizens worldwide, urging the rejection of the agreement. The July decision marked a historic day in European politics. For the first time, the EP exercised its Lisbon Treaty power to reject an international trade agreement. The Commission and the Council are now more aware that the EP, whose mandate is also to safeguard EU citizens' rights, has a crucial role in granting the democratic exercise in Europe.

Mechanisms and Opportunities for Civil Society to Tackle and Influence EU Policies

The **Transparency Portal** of the European Union is the gateway for citizens to be informed about the EU decision-making process, including legislation, funding and actors involved. Its **Transparency Register** provides citizens with a direct and single access to information about "who is who" in influencing the EU decision making process, which interests are being pursued and what level of resources is invested in these activities. Citizens have the right to claim transparency in EU policy-making, in compliance with the law. Accessible via http://europa.eu/transparency-register/index_en.htm.

Your Voice in Europe is the European Commission's "single access point" to a wide variety of consultations, discussions and other tools which enable citizens to play an active role in the European policy-making process. Accessible via http://ec.europa.eu/yourvoice/index_en.htm.

(*Continued*)

[r] See http://en.wikipedia.org/wiki/Anti-Counterfeiting_Trade_Agreement.

(Continued)

The **European Citizens' Initiative** is a submission to the European Commission to propose legislation on matters where the EU has competence to legislate, for example on the environment, agriculture, transport or public health. A citizens' initiative has to be backed by at least one million EU citizens, coming from at least 7 out of the 27 member states. The Citizens' Initiative right is set out in Article 11(4) of the consolidated version of the Treaty on European Union (a result of the Lisbon Treaty, 2010). Accessible via http://ec.europa.eu/citizens-initiative/public/welcome.

The **Global Health Policy Forum** is the venue where the three EC directorates on Development Cooperation, Health and Consumers, and Research consult with civil society networks, professional organizations, academia and commercial actors on matters related to EU global health. Installed in September 2010, this policy forum uses the Commission Communication on the EU Role in Global Health as its policy framework. Accessible via http://ec.europa.eu/health/eu_world/events/index_en.htm#anchor0.

The **EU Health Policy Forum** brings together pan-European stakeholder organizations in the health sector at EU level to ensure that the EU's health strategy is open, transparent and responds to public concerns. It advises the Commission (and EU countries if appropriate) on health matters. It gathers about three times a year. Accessible via http://ec.europa.eu/health/interest_groups/eu_health_forum/index_en.htm.

The **European Ombudsman** investigates complaints about maladministration in the institutions and bodies of the European Union. If you are a citizen of a Member State of the Union or reside in a Member State, you can make a complaint to the European Ombudsman. Accessible via http://www.ombudsman.europa.eu/en/atyourservice/home.faces.

Civil society actors can submit a **petition** to the European Parliament on matters related to EU competency and legislation, or initiate a **parliamentary hearing** in cooperation with a Member of the European Parliament (MEP). Accessible via http://www.europarl.europa.eu/aboutparliament/en/00b3f21266/At-your-service.html.

Prospects of the EU Role in Global Health and the Role of Civil Society

In times of financial austerity, the EU evidently struggles with health equity within its own borders. In several member countries, health and development budgets are under severe pressure. Also, in February 2013, EU leaders agreed on a budget cut of 3.4% in the upcoming seven-year multi-annual framework, raising a good deal of concerns among civil society actors.[s]

The main challenge for the EU position in global health, though, may not be so much in terms of maintaining its level of financing for activities in this field. Rather, the challenge will be to preserve European institutions' political interest in global health at a time when the EU feels compelled to foster its economic competitiveness globally — at a time, in other words, when its productive superiority is at stake, and "modernization without westernization" is becoming a more likely prospect.[12] The challenge is immense: despite CSOs' engagement in shaping the new financial perspectives of the EU 2014–2020,[t,u,v] the global health horizon is simply not mentioned. Yet, themes such as health innovation, health equity, health security and public–private cooperation will be important issues within EU policy frameworks.

As things stand today, there are several ways in which CSOs can advance the global health agenda in Europe:

(1) Civil society can use the EU Commission Communication and Council Conclusions on the EU Role in Global Health to help develop and monitor national strategies for global health in different European Member States, building on a few pilot projects in countries to

---

[s] See http://www.socialplatform.org/News.asp?DocID=31886.
[t] See http://ec.europa.eu/health/interest_groups/docs/euhpf_contributions_post2013_en.pdf.
[u] See http://ec.europa.eu/europeaid/documents/consultations/5240_eu_external_action_after_2013_funding_en.pdf.
[v] See http://ec.europa.eu/research/horizon2020/pdf/consultation-conference/summary_analysis.pdf#view=fit&pagemode=none.

demonstrate the advantage of a political approach based on the assumption that *good governance for health starts at home.*

(2) Civil society must use the framework based on equity, health in all policies and human rights as "an agreed common *acquis*" when advocating EU policies impacting global health, be it at the WHO or in other multilateral or bilateral negotiations.

(3) Capturing DG DEV's work to develop a "program of action on global health" in 2013,[w] CSOs could suggest and contribute to a practical framework for the topics enshrined in the "EU role in Global health."

(4) Further cooperation needs to be sought with members of the European Parliament to advance EU work on global health. Based on the concept that health is a global common good, this would entail not only addressing health inequities within the European community but also guaranteeing that Europe's external policies are fair and benefitting health equity around the world. While this approach may seem problematic in times of financial crisis, it provides the conditions for security in Europe, a priority goal to be achieved.

(5) Lastly, civil society groups need to promote the conditions for a more democratic decision-making space on health in their own countries, as a precondition for more democratic decision making within the EU. The Lisbon Treaty foresees this possibility through the European Citizens' Initiative.[x] Health is increasingly becoming a key theme for European citizens, but activism in this field requires professional health and development NGOs to raise awareness among European citizens about the linkages between global and national health policies, and about the relevance of the EU institutions in this arena. Health democracy in European countries will enhance the legitimacy of EU activities in global health.

Acknowledgments

The authors like to thank Samantha Battams, a former research fellow of the Global Health Programme of the Graduate Institute, for her reflections and inputs into the original draft of this chapter.

---

[w] See http://ec.europa.eu/health/eu_world/docs/ev_20120322_mi_en.pdf.

[x] See http://www.citizens-initiative.eu.

References

1. Nye J. (2009) Jospeh Nye on Global Power Shifts. TED Talk, July 2010.
2. Morlino L. (2008) Democracy and changes: how research tails reality. *West European Politics* **31(1–2):** 40–59.
3. Kickbusch I, Hein W, *et al.* (2010) Addressing Global Health Governance Challenges Through a New Mechanism: The Proposal for a Committee C of the World Health Assembly. *Journal of Law Medicine & Ethics* **38(3):** 550–563.
4. Sridhar D, Gostin L. (2011) Reforming the World Health Organization. *Journal of the American Medical Association*, online. 29 March 2011.
5. Dentico N. (2009) In Focus: Implementing the WHO global strategy on public health, innovation & IP: an opportunity that should not be squandered by poor implementation. *IQ Sensato* **3(1):** 1–8.
6. Yach D, Khan M, *et al.* (2010) The role and challenges of the food industry in addressing chronic disease. *Globalization and Health* **6(10):** 1–8.
7. Richter J. (2012). WHO reform and public interest safeguards: an historical perspective. *Social Medicine* **6(3):** 141–150.
8. Plehwe D. (2012) Measuring European Relations of Lobby Power: An Analysis of Available Statistical Data on the Development and on the Unequal Status of the Representation of Interests in Brussels (Organisations, Personnel, Finance). Austrian Chamber of Labour, February 2012. Available at http://wien.arbeiterkammer.at/online/page.php?P=68&IP=66235&AD=0&REFP=2842.
9. Riekmann SP. (2007) The cocoon of power: democratic implications of inter-institutional agreements. *European Law Journal* **13(1):** 4–19.
10. Smith S, Dalakiouridou E. (2009) Contextualising public (e) participation in the governance of the European Union. *European Journal of ePractice* **7:** 11.
11. Castel R. (2003) *L'insécurité social. Qu'est-ce qu'être protègé?* Seuil, Paris, pp. 47–50.
12. Bauman Z. (2004) *Europe: An Unfinished Adventure.* Policy Press, Cambridge, Malden.
13. Jachtenfuchs M, Kohler-Koch B. (2003) Governance and institutional development. Nashville, TN: 30.
14. Kaczynski PM, Broin P, *et al.* (2010) The Treaty of Lisbon: A Second Look at the Institutional Innovations. Joint Study: EPC, CEPS, Egmont.
15. Kohler-Koch B. (2010) Civil society and EU democracy: "astroturf" representation? *Journal of European Public Policy* **17(1):** 100–116.

16. European Commission. (2012) The European Citizens' Initiative.
17. Council of the European Union. (2010a) Council Conclusions on the EU Role in Global Health. 3011th Foreign Affairs Council Meeting, Brussels, 10 May 2010.
18. Medico. (2011) Delhi Statement. Time to Untie the Knots: The WHO Reform and the Need to Democratise Global Health.
19. Medicus Mundi International. (2011) Letter by Medicus Mundi International on behalf of the Democratizing Global Health Coalition to the Sixty-First Session of the WHO Regional Committee for Europe on Agenda Item 8: Who Reform for a Healthy Future. Amsterdam, 26 August 2011.
20. Action For Global Health. (2010) A Guide to the EU's Global Health Policies. Available at http://www.globalhealthguide.eu/files/ACTION_AID_WEB_GUIDE.pdf.
21. EuroHealthNet. (2010) European Commission Communication on the EU Role in Global Health Policy Briefing. Available at http://eurohealthnet.eu/sites/eurohealthnet.eu/files/publications/Global-Health-Communication_1. pdf.
22. Health Action International Europe, Oxfam International. (2009) Trading Away Access to Medicines — How the European Union's Trade Agenda Has Taken a Wrong Turn. Available via: http://haieurope.org/wp-content/uploads/2010/12/20-Oct-2009-Report-Oxfam-HAI-Trading-Away-Access-to-Medicines-EN.pdf.
23. Global Health Europe. (2010) EU Event a Starting Point for a New Era in Global Health Governance. Available at http://www.globalhealtheurope.org/index.php?option=com_content&view=article&id=302:eu-event-a-starting-point-for-a-new-era-in-global-health-governance&catid=81:event-reports&Itemid=353.
24. Action For Global Health. (2011) Critical Stories of Change — United Behind the Right to Health. The Story of the Action for Global Health Network Europe. Available at http://www.actionforglobalhealth.eu/fileadmin/AfGH_Intranet/AFGH/Publications/Stories_of_Change_Final_LORES.pdf.

15

The European Union as a Global Health Actor: A Critical View[a]

*Samantha Battams** and *Louise van Schaik*[†]

Introduction

In the previous decade the health policy of EU countries has increasingly been internationalized and Europeanized, despite citizens and national governments considering health a predominantly national issue. This has raised tensions with regard to where, how and by whom health issues should be addressed. In this respect the legitimacy of both the EU and the WHO on international health matters is contested. The EU's role in global health debates surfaced prominently in 2010, when for the first time some common viewpoints and objectives were formulated in the form of EU Council Conclusions, right after the entry into force of the Lisbon Treaty. This prompted a revision of the system of EU external representation with

*Associate Professor and Public Health Programme Director, Torrens University, Australia and Senior Lecturer, Southgate Institute of Health, Society & Equity, Flinders University, South Australia.

†Senior Research Fellow, Clingendael Institute in The Hague, Neetherlands.

[a]This article is based upon conference papers and related research presented at the conference "The European Union in International Affairs 3" (May 2012, Brussels) and the Lisbon workshop "EU External Representation and the Reform of International Contexts: Practices After Lisbon" (February 2012, Clingendael Institute, The Hague). We wish to thank our colleague Remco van der Pas, who conducted interviews for the former paper, and Prof. Ilona Kickbusch, who provided comments on the latter paper, as well as conference participants and discussants who provided feedback on both papers.

an upgraded role for EU foreign policy actors. Differences of opinion emerged with regard to the key objectives of global health policy in relation to internal health objectives, development cooperation and broader foreign policy objectives. In addition, the degree of EU competence on international health questions and what it means for the EU's involvement and role in external representation was and is contested.

The debate on the EU's role in global health runs parallel to major international debates on health, including: the reform of the WHO; the expansion of non-communicable diseases (NCDs), as was discussed *inter alia* in the UN General Assembly; and the need to address social determinants of health (SDOH). Since the 1980s, the WHO has been plagued by insecurity of resources as mandatory assessed financial contributions from Member State countries have been frozen. Since voluntary contributions have increased significantly in the same period, the balance has shifted: from being 80% (1978–1979) to just 24% (in 2010–2013) of the total WHO revenue.[1] Subsequently, debates on WHO core tasks (in relation to the wishes of the Membership and to earmarked contributions of Member States and others), its relationship with other international actors encroaching upon its remit, and possible conflicts of interest when accepting funding provided (either directly or indirectly) by the private sector have emerged.[2] This has culminated in the WHO reform process which started in 2009. In addition, the current global health debate concerns the difficult questions of addressing health system financing, combating the rise of NCDs and addressing the social determinants of health, all of which go beyond the health sector and the traditional remit of national health ministries as well as the WHO. Simultaneously, the question of which multilateral organization(s) should take on what role has emerged. One would expect the EU to take a strong position in such key debates, in line with its objective of "effective multilateralism," and given its commitment to a social-determinants approach.[b] In this chapter, we examine

---

[b]*Cf.* Effective multilateralism was a central objective of the EU's Security Strategy of 2003, which was later articulated in specific EU policy documents (such as a 2006 Commission Communication on the EU's Choice for Effective Multilateralism). The EU's support for the social-determinants-of-health approach was emphasized by the Council of the European Union.[18] Council Conclusions on the EU Role in Global Health, 3011th Foreign Affairs Council meeting (Brussels, 10 May 2010).

whether the EU is a strong supporter of the goals of UN agencies such as the WHO, and whether it seeks to further multilateral action as a key instrument for effectively tackling cross-border (determinants of) health policy problems.[3]

The chapter will build on previous chapters in elaborating and analyzing the role of the EU at the international level. It will look at the interplay between the national, European and international levels, and in particular at whether incoherencies exist across different tracks of policy-making, i.e. those primarily focusing on health, foreign policy or development (horizontal coherence), and between activities of EU Member States and EU institutions (vertical coherence). It questions to what extent the EU operates as an international actor with a single voice and how this influences its effectiveness in discussions on global health in general, and in debates on WHO reform, NCDs and SDOH specifically. To answer this question we will discuss and analyze the EU's coherence on substance and form. With regard to substance we will analyze whether the EU is entitled to speak on global health policies, and whether it has positions, is able to accommodate/balance different perspectives on global health (healthcare, foreign policy, development cooperation, research), and take a coherent social-determinants approach. With regard to form we will analyze whether the EU is able to coordinate effectively and speak with a single voice.

On the question of effectiveness, the key question is whether the EU is perceived to be effective in achieving its positions in key debates. We will look specifically at two key debates, one on WHO reform and the other on NCDs and the SDOH statements made at the WHO and UN.

On the basis of these empirical data we will analyze the relationship between coherence and effectiveness and the inherent limitations of EU action in a Westphalian international system, where states are supposed to be sovereign and equal, which translates into their having seats and votes in the governance bodies of the vast majority of international organizations. Indeed, the EU is a "strange animal" within this system: on many topics the EU has supranational features and it has obtained membership in a few international organizations and treaties, but its construction is far from being a (federal) state and it has not replaced EU Member States, which makes it difficult to place it within the traditional system of international organizations.[1,4]

In the concluding section we will reflect on how the EU's capacity to act on global health matters relates to its effectiveness, and how well it manages to integrate health, foreign policy and development perspectives into one coherent position.

EU Coherence on Global Health Questions

According to Thomas[5] EU foreign policy coherence is best defined by "the adoption of determinate common policies and the pursuit of those policies by EU Member States and institutions." He thus distinguishes between the EU's ability to define policy positions on a given topic (policy determinacy) and the support of EU actors for whatever policy that has been agreed upon (political cohesion). These key concepts can also be found in other literature on EU actorness and EU unity. For instance, Jupille and Caporaso[6] in their seminal article on EU actorness refer to the EU having authority and cohesiveness, Bretherton and Vogler[7] refer to capability, and Van Schaik[6] centers on EU competence and preference homogeneity.[6,8] Although these concepts are certainly not fully interchangeable, they all somehow focus on the EU's ability to agree upon strong policy positions and EU actors working together to bring these forward.[9,10] Usually it is assumed that such ability to act "coherently" or in unity is related to a shared view on what direction to take and to what extent the EU is speaking with a single voice on the matter. Subsequently, literature has linked these "capacity" issues to the EU's actual effectiveness in multilateral negotiations, something we will also do here.

Little research is available on the coherence of the EU in debates on international health questions. Van Schaik[11] in an article on the EU's performance within the WHO, found: (1) a (vertical) coherence challenge between Member States and the EU on the extent to which the EU has the competence to act on health matters, and (2) a (horizontal) coherence challenge between "health" and foreign policy specialists, including those from the recently established European External Action Service (EEAS). In addition, policy coherence across various parts of the European Commission (including parts of the EC, such as health, development and research) and national governments (health, economy, foreign ministries, development agencies and health research institutes) is another potential challenge.[12,13] We will discuss below the issue of coherence by means of identifying first the extent to which the EU has competence and policy positions, and then how the issue of global health is increasingly broadened and related to more policy areas, in line with a social-determinants-of-health approach. Despite the EU adopting a social-determinants approach, which recognizes the importance of non-health sectors to health, this approach leads to a greater risk of incoherent visions on policy debates within the EU. In relation to this, we will raise the EU challenge of speaking with a single voice.

Policy Determinacy: EU Competence and Positions on Health and Global Health

According to Article 6 of the Treaty on the Functioning of the European Union (TFEU), "the protection and improvement of human health" is one area where the EU has only the competence "to support, coordinate or supplement the actions of the Member States" insofar as no common safety questions in public health are concerned for which it has shared competence (Article 4, TFEU). Whilst public health policy and service provision is still primarily seen as the competence of the Member States, "shared sovereignty" has *de facto* emerged over public health issues that cut across borders.[13] The Member States have *de facto* agreed to share their sovereignty on such issues, and thus EU policies can jointly be decided upon — this also applies with regard to the "external dimension" (i.e. interactions with international bodies). The white paper "Together for Health: A Strategic Approach for the EU 2008–2013" outlines the EU's role on cross-border issues (pandemics, bioterrorism) and health in relation to the "free movement of goods, services and people."[14] It includes overseeing areas such as pharmaceutical regulation and food safety standards based on the internal market or the agricultural article, which constitute also shared competence.

According to Mamudu and Studlar,[13] the EU has developed greater authority in public health in an "evolutionary manner." Guigner[15] and, Emmerling and Heydemann[16] explain that EU health-related legislation mainly emerged on the basis of Treaty articles other than public health (e.g. agriculture, environment, internal market). The European Parliament has also been instrumental in strengthening EU health actions, both before and in response to crises such as the BSE crisis they called for legislative reform.[16] The EP has recently been involved in "a high number of discussions dedicated to health-related topics" (e.g. *E. coli* outbreaks, Alzheimer's, antibiotic resistance, tuberculosis vaccines, the EU global response to HIV/AIDs).[17]

The Maastricht and Amsterdam Treaties laid out the legal basis for EU involvement in health protection. The Maastricht Treaty of 1992, for instance, included for the first time an article on public health which focused on disease prevention.[16] This provision further supported the EU work on an anti-tobacco policy, which eventually also allowed it to become involved in international policy discussions on this matter.[13] Over time, disease-specific approaches to programs and activities were replaced by more horizontal approaches,[16] and the EU policy on global health now recommends "systems-based" rather than "disease-specific" solutions to global health and health system strengthening.[18]

The Lisbon Treaty (Council of the EU[19] — in force from 2009) determined that the EU "shares competence with the Member States on common safety concerns in public health matters," whilst health protection is a "complementary competence" and the development aspect of health is a field where the EU and Member States have parallel competence.[16] EU citizens typically indicate (via polls) that they consider health to be a national issue, an area where Brussels' interference should be limited as much as possible. EU competence on health issues is thus a particularly politically sensitive issue, certainly in comparison with other issues, such as environmental policy.[11]

Article 168 of the Treaty outlines the EU's role in public health, and states that "the Union and the Member States shall foster cooperation with third countries and the competent international organizations in the sphere of public health." The Communication of the European Commission on "the EU's role in global health"[20] recognizes challenges in global health governance, the importance of strong leadership and the need to coordinate the broad range of global health actors. It recommends a unified position for the EU on global health when dealing with UN agencies and promotes the participation of a range of stakeholders within governance processes.[20] The EU Member States welcomed its suggestions in the Council

Conclusions,[21] but were somewhat cautious about formulating the role of the EU in global debates. This was formulated in the following way: "Without prejudice to the respective competencies, the EU and its Member States will endeavour to speak with a stronger and coherent voice at the global level and in a dialogue with third countries and global health initiatives".[21]

The Council Conclusions of 2010 form the heart of the EU's current approach to global health, even though they cover only parts of the international debate on international health issues. They recognize challenges in global health governance, the importance of strong leadership and the need to coordinate the broad range of global health actors. A unified position for the EU on global health is recommended when dealing with UN agencies, and also advocated is the participation of a range of stakeholders within governance processes. The EU acknowledges that economic and social conditions are crucial determinants of health. It thereby follows the WHO Commission on the Social Determinants of Health.[22] The EU also underlines that it has a central role to play in accelerating progress on global health challenges, including the health-related Millennium Development Goals, Sustainable Development Goals, and non-communicable diseases.

Based on its own Communication and the Council Conclusions, the European Commission continues to be working out its plan of action following the Communication on global health, including how its various different directorates (e.g. health, development, research) will work together on global health. Health has been a feature of EU development policy; the recent *Increasing the Impact of EU Development Policy*[23] declares that the EU should have a role in health system strengthening, reducing inequalities in access to health services, promoting policy coherence and protecting against global health threats. The EU is also committed to and has promoted access to essential medicines, following the Doha Declaration on the TRIPS agreement.[16] In addition, it has Council Conclusions from the time of the Finnish Presidency on Health in All Policies[24] and HiAP and Equity[18] and requirements for Health Impact Assessments within the European Commission.[25] These policies necessitate "health working with other sectors" (consistent with a social-determinants approach), the WHO working with other intergovernmental agencies, and better coordination within the EU on global health governance and strategy.

The health in all policies and health-impact assessments are based on a social-determinants approach which recognizes that health outcomes can be achieved only through policy and action across many policy areas. It has been acknowledged that a social-determinants approach requires more cross-government, cross-sector, interagency and intergovernmental strategies and resources dedicated to it. This also has repercussions for the involvement of various EU actors and will increase the need to coordinate different viewpoints on health and to balance it with other objectives, such as social protection, freedom of choice and economic growth objectives.

Health has also been increasingly acknowledged as a foreign policy issue, centrally linked to issues like human rights and sustainable development.[26] It is playing an increasing role in foreign affairs, particularly in trade and security affairs.[27] This is well established through agreements related to trade, such as the Doha Declaration on the TRIPS Agreement and Public Health (which enabled countries with insufficient capacity for manufacturing pharmaceuticals to have access to essential generic medicines) and the WHO's Pandemic Influenza Preparedness Framework (leading to sharing of influenza viruses and promotion of access to vaccines).[28] Regional institutions such as ASEAN help facilitate policy coherence between trade and health, for example through the ASEAN Sectoral Protocol for Health Care, which covers among other things free trade in health services and the movement of health professionals, and the EU engages with ASEAN for trade.[28] Conversely, trade interests have the potential to conflict with health interests; for example, Investor State Dispute Settlement provisions in regional free trade agreements have been (unsuccessfully) used by tobacco companies to bring a legal case against the Australian government with the argument that its plain packaging legislation on tobacco contravenes trade policy. It has been argued that the US and Europe are pushing trade agreements that extend patent terms and donor exclusivity, and increase the cost of drugs.[29]

Criticism is mounting against the EEAS with regard to a supposed lack of "integrated vision" for foreign affairs and turf wars between the EEAS and the EC's agency for development cooperation, Europeaid.[c] Member States, specifically some of them, such as the UK, resist "centralization" and cooperation on foreign policy issues, posing problems for the newly established service.[30] As health becomes more of a foreign policy issue, there is potential tension not only in vertical coherence between EU Member States and other EU actors (e.g. EC, EEAS), but also in horizontal coherence between health policy experts and specialists in other areas, such as foreign policy and development.

The EU thus has some competence to act on global health matters and some general guidance on global health through the 2010 Council Conclusions, but the broadening of the agenda continues to pose challenges regarding who is responsible for what part of the international issues being discussed. In addition, there appear to be some challenges pertaining to who is allowed to bring the EU message forward and how different views on global health questions can be reconciled, an issue that we will now discuss.

Political Cohesion between EU Actors and EU Member States: The Single Voice Challenge

One of the greatest challenges for the EU in playing a more prominent role in multilateral fora is that the EU continues to operate within a Westphalian system of international governance, whilst itself transcending Westphalia.[31] The Lisbon Treaty provisions were aimed at paving the way for a more coherent and consolidated role for the EU in foreign policy, including in multilateral fora, such as the WHO and UN General Assembly. Following the Lisbon Treaty's establishment of the High Representative of the Union for Foreign Affairs and Security Policy, assisted by the newly created European External Action Service (EEAS), the EU is supposed to develop stronger representation and coordinated action in external affairs. Through the EEAS, a new foreign policy service has been created which, according to HR Ashton,[32] "brings together economics and politics and creates a new capacity for the European Union to add value to what the Member States do on the ground."[32] For global

[c]http://www.devex.com/en/blogs/the-development-newswire/criticisms-remain-as-eeas-turns-1?g=1.

health affairs, the EEAS works with the EU Presidency of the Council and the European Commission, with the latter two actors driving the content of EU positions. According to the new provisions EU delegations to international organizations shall represent the EU at working level and receive instructions from the EEAS and Commission services.

Through a resolution adopted in May 2011 the EU obtained speaking rights at the United Nations General Assembly.[33] This gives the EU actors the right to speak and participate in debates at the UNGA on behalf of its Member States and to make proposals, amendments and interventions (orally), to have its documents circulated as part of the meeting and to have the right of reply.[34–36] A recent debate has emerged regarding whether and in what way provisions of this resolution will be extended to other parts of the UN family, including the WHO. Within the UNGA, the resolution has already resulted in the EU being represented directly in the High-Level Meeting on the Prevention and Control of Non-communicable Diseases, where the EU was represented by (former) EU Health Commissioner John Dalli.

When it comes to the WHO, the EU currently has only observer status, whilst EU Member States are members of the organization. Nevertheless, the EU, for the vast majority of issues, represents a unified voice and has at least one EU Member State on the WHO Executive Board and at the World Health Assembly representing the EU position. This is a strong voice, given that over 30% of the WHO budget comes from EU Member States. In the European regional office of the WHO, i.e. WHO EURO, EU states already have a majority. The fact that its position is now brought forward by a single voice means that it is even more obvious that the EU is able to dominate policy debates at this level of the organization. This also has repercussions for the position of WHO EURO within the World Health Assembly discussions and has caused some anxiety among non-EU WHO EURO Member States, such as Russia and Turkey. More effort now goes into preparing some EURO positions at the global level with the aim to "keep the region together." EU and non-EU Member States take turns as coordinators of the EURO group.

Emerson *et al.*[37] point out that "while the EU's status as observer is reasonable, the arrangements for it to represent its views in plenary WHO meetings is not yet fully in line with the Lisbon Treaty provisions." In addition, the EU does not yet have similar rights with regard to holding statements, bringing in amendments, etc., as it has in the UNGA. Van Schaik[11] has found the expanded role of the EU in the WHO to be contested immediately after the entry into force of the Lisbon Treaty, both by representatives of the EU Member States and by non-EU states. EU Member States have been reluctant to accept the EU delegation in Geneva taking a greater role in coordinating the EU position and representing it at the WHO, and differed with regard to what new provisions for external representation meant for the EU's status in the WHO.[11] Our recent observations tend to indicate improvements with Member States entrusting to a greater extent the EU delegation in Geneva with taking the lead in EU coordination and external representation at the WHO.[38] Some learning has occurred on both sides and the division of tasks on many topics has been clarified.

We found that, to date, linkages between the Commission based in Brussels and the Delegation of the European Union to the UN in Geneva (part of the EEAS) — when it comes to staff working on health — are well-developed, although there is scope to improve "coordination" between the range of Brussels-based and Geneva-based EU officials working on global health, including EU Member State diplomats such as health attachés. Attempts were made by the Danish Presidency of the Council in the first half of 2012 to improve coordination between Brussels and Geneva through a working group that would better link EU public health policy and WHO reform discussions.[38] There is not only greater scope to link EU WHO positions with ongoing health discussions taking place in Brussels, but also scope to develop EU representation and coordination in other international health fora beyond the WHO, including fora both within and outside the UN system (e.g. UNAIDS, GFATM).[38] For example, opportunities have arisen where recently at UNAIDS EU Member States did not wish to speak — and at the Global Fund Member States that had lost their voice because of reduced contributions are now happy to group around the Commission seat.

A debate emerged in 2012 which concerned a demand by the Secretariat of the EU Council to have all coordination for multilateral fora being prepared in Brussels-based EU Council bodies and not in other capitals. This would mean that the center of gravity of debates on global health would shift from Geneva to Brussels, with those based at the EU delegation and permanent representations in Geneva becoming just the "messengers" with a small role in fine-tuning positions at the spot of WHO negotiations and conducting outreach. Those based in Geneva argue against the centralization at Brussels, since they would be best positioned to judge the negotiating environment, have the most knowledge on issues discussed at the WHO, and would need flexibility and authority to adjust the EU position to what is realistically achievable within the context of WHO negotiations.

Coordination between Member States and the EU on technical matters is relatively smooth, and the EU has played an important role in negotiations on the PIP, IHR and FCTC, as this book demonstrates. However, it is notable that even though the Lisbon Treaty has given the EU a stronger mandate, particularly on foreign policy, there has been tension between the EU and Member States. They quarreled about whether statements could be presented by the EEAS or the Presidency on behalf of the EU on matters where the existence of EU competence could be contested.[38] In 2011 the UK blocked "the EEAS from articulating common EU positions at the UN, the Organization for Security and Co-operation in Europe (OSCE), and in some foreign capitals."[39] The EU statements at the WHO EURO meeting in Baku were also blocked for this reason.[38] Eventually an agreement was reached in the body of permanent representatives of EU Member States to the EU (Coreper), whereby EU representation in matters where competence is shared between the EU and its Member States (as occurs in health matters) was required to include the following words as a prelude: "on behalf of the EU and its 27 Member States."[d]

Nevertheless, and despite these hiccups as to whether statements are to be made on behalf of the EU or on behalf of the EU and its Member States, we generally agree with Emmerling and Heydemann[16] who say that "today, the EU is an important partner in nearly all global health topics: politically, economically and financially — and the implementation of the Lisbon Treaty is expected to strengthen this role." In the next section of this chapter

---

[d]See the Coreper guidelines on external representation: http://register.consilium.europa.eu/pdf/en/11/st15/st15901.en11.pdf.

we will analyze whether the EU has in fact become more effective in key debates: on WHO reform, the NCDs and the social determinants of health.

Effectiveness of the EU in Debates on Gobal Health

According to Thomas[5] EU effectiveness is best defined as "the Union's ability to shape world affairs in accordance with the objectives it adopts on particular issues…. The EU typically pursues its objectives through the use of traditional policy instruments such as sanctions or *démarches*, through the persuasiveness of arguments made by representatives of the Union, its institutions and Member States, and simply through its example as a functioning union of states based on pooled sovereignty".

The EU is famous for its use of soft power. Soft power, which entails getting others to do what you want them to do through the use of persuasion, networks and dominant narratives,[e,40] is increasingly important for global health diplomacy.[41] However, the EU, or at least EU representatives and EEAS/EC staff working in a multilateral context, appear cautious about engaging in soft power strategies at the WHO, due to Member State concerns.[38] There is more scope for development of EU strategy and prioritization on global health issues and positions — and delegation of tasks across Member States in WHO coordination and policy processes. This would require greater Member State trust in EU representation and EU freedom to engage in soft power, trust building and "behind the scene" strategies. These strategies may become more important as other REIOs and blocs, such as the G77, play more of a role in international governance processes.

---

[e]Lee and Gomez[41] explain soft power as: "… the capacity to persuade or attract others to do what one wants through the force of ideas, knowledge and values. Coined by Joseph Nye, the concept of soft power contrasts with 'hard power' whereby coercion (underpinned by military and economic might) is used to influence others to act in ways in which they would not otherwise do. He argues that, in a more interconnected world of accelerating globalization and resultant collective action problems, the currency of global leadership favors soft over hard power. In recent years, world leaders have begun to talk about 'smart power' whereby soft and hard power is combined in ways that are mutually reinforcing." More recently, Nye has employed the concept of "smart power," which is the use of a mix of soft and hard power, particularly in order to bring about global public goods.[42]

In general, it is recognized that "in most cases, measuring effectiveness requires evidence of the situation or outcome that the EU has sought to influence, both before and after the EU has adopted its position, *and* evidence that links change or stability in those conditions to the existence and/or efforts of the EU."[5] The effectiveness of the EU in WHO reform negotiations can for instance only truly be judged by examining EU positions and the EU's role in negotiation processes and comparing these with the outcomes of the WHO reforms — outcomes which have not yet been established due to the reform being a current and ongoing process. Nevertheless, perceptions of well-informed insiders on how effectively the EU is operating within this process are relevant as well, since effectiveness at the end of the day continues to be a relative concept, dependent on perception. This is why we have also explored the perceptions of the EU's effectiveness within WHO negotiations[38] and we base the following discussion on such research. On this basis we will now go on to discuss the EU's effectiveness in the debate on WHO reform and in the UNGA debate on NCDs.

The EU's Effectiveness in the Debate on WHO Reform

The debate on WHO reform began as a discussion concerning WHO financing, commencing with the financial crisis in 2008 and leading to consultations on broader reform in January 2010. Besides financing, discussions soon turned to the role and core business of the WHO, along with the governance and management of the organization.[43] Better coordination and participation of stakeholders and partnerships contributing to global health is also now a topic of the reform,[44] with non-government organizations particularly concerned with managing conflicts of interest in WHO governance processes.[45] The WHO reform debate is contextualized by: the WHO being plagued by accusations of being susceptible to private interests (such as pharmaceutical industry interests); the organization having rather serious financial difficulties; it facing competition from a plethora of private foundations, such as the Gates Foundation; other international organizations, such as the OECD, engaging in health-related activities; and divergence of opinion regarding whether the WHO should engage in health aid/development.

There is a common EU position on the importance of the WHO's normative and global mandate and the need for clear processes on priority setting linked to resources, albeit with some divergence from EU Member States on methods/processes of reform.[38,46] France is generally concerned about the visibility of the WHO, the legitimacy of its governance processes and the effectiveness of decision-making. It is keen on emphasizing that WHO Member States should be the only actors in terms of decision-making. The UK accepts greater involvement of non-state actors in financing WHO activities, but argues that distinctions should be made clearer with regard to who pays what. Conversely, Germany supports the idea of greater involvement of non-state actors in order to increase the transparency of WHO, but argues that agendas should always be set by states and not by big private donors.

Furthermore, within a string of common EU positions and statements, the EU is bringing to the table its experience and current practices, and the EU's authority in reform debates appears to partly derive from the experience and practice of the Commission itself. Whilst the EU appears to be taking a leadership role in WHO reform matters, and there is recognition that the WHO could learn from EU policy practices, the EU is cautious about advocating its own practices, let alone "preaching" certain models This is especially true since the Dalligate scandal — highlighting the role of lobbying interests — has come to light, which has led to a greater need to focus on EU/EC transparency issues.[47]

Another important point when considering EU influence is the plethora of actors now operating within global health. Indeed, this is one important area of concern within the WHO reform — recognition that the WHO needs to take a leadership role and have a normative (standard-setting) role, amidst a sea of actors with various interests and significant resources and activity in global health. It is difficult for the WHO, and also the EU, to have a strong role in this altered environment, although they are continuing to push for the WHO's central role in norm-setting (such as on how states should address outbreaks of infectious diseases). However, on many of these issues, key policy agenda-setting groups have different opinions on the extent of leadership that the WHO should be taking. For example, the NCD alliance, a major influencer leading to the development of the UN Summit on the Prevention and Control of Non-communicable Diseases, is calling for a global platform on NCDs which is an independent stake-holder forum, where the WHO plays a part but is not leading the platform,[48] whilst other NGO stakeholders wish to see the WHO as the major leader in global health governance. The EU seems to share the latter view.

Within the WHO reform process, the EU is thus emphasizing the normative role of the WHO, whilst many developing countries are focusing on the WHO as a development agency which should be effective at a country level or for the WHO to take a "health and sustainable development" approach.[38] Despite the EU Council conclusions on global health[21] also focusing on development aspects of global health policy, the EU is clear that it does not want the WHO to be a "development agency" due to the potential for duplication of resources and overlap with the work of other agencies.[38] However, also within the EU there is some degree of debate between development specialists on the one hand and health and foreign policy specialists on the other (see also above).

Whilst the EU is perceived to have a growing influence on global health, there are mixed opinions about the prominence of health in foreign affairs generally. One view is that those working on global health based in EU Member State, delegations in Geneva are "driving" positions for Member States rather than vice versa.[38] It is notable that the WHO reform is one area where there was no EU *acquis*, but where there was value seen in the EU having a common position, and EU Member States requested such EU involvement. However, in general, it has been claimed that only a small number of people in Member States and NGOs were involved in the discussion on the WHO reform, and hardly any attention was paid to the matter by the recently established EEAS. Despite the EU delegation in Geneva (part of the EEAS) and European Commission taking care of the EU's positioning in this debate, some in the EEAS in Brussels considered that it was not a foreign policy priority.[38]

UN Debate on NCDs and SDOH

Recently, the EU has already played a more prominent role in the UN High-Level Meeting on the Prevention and Control of Non-communicable Diseases. Since 2008, "social determinants" of health have been formally recognized by the UN and WHO as an issue of concern.[22,43] This topic is also of key priority for the EU.

Prior to the UN High-Level Meeting on NCDs, the European Parliament passed a resolution affirming its commitment to the meeting.[49] This recognized NCDs as the major cause of death in Europe, along with major NCD risk factors, the low level of health expenditure on prevention, and the role of social determinants in health inequalities. It called for the EC and EU Member States to have a strong political commitment to address the NCD epidemic, to endorse five key commitments on NCDs and ensure that they were in the Political Declaration on NCDs arising from the High-Level Meeting,[33] and to develop national NCD plans by 2013. Even though EP resolutions are not binding upon the EU, and certainly do not equal EU positions or mandates for international negotiations that are decided upon by the EU Member States convening in the Council, they do indicate a political will to pay more attention to the issue. They also indicate the EP's likely support for EU policies to curb NCDs within the EU. The former Commissioner for Health and Consumer Policy, John Dalli, represented the EU at the UN meeting on NCDs. This was possible due to the new speaking rights on the EU's role in the UNGA.

Despite strong support for the UN High-Level Meeting on the Prevention and Control of Non-Communicable Diseases from all countries and its resolution (adopted at the WHO Executive Board meeting in January 2011), there have been some issues with maintaining the momentum of this meeting and debates about the best way forward for the implementation of its resolution. In particular, at the 65th World Health Assembly, there were debates and a lack of consensus among countries about which NCD targets to adopt as part of an NCD monitoring framework. By the end of the assembly, only one target had been adopted (with the assistance of heavy lobbying by the NCD Alliance): "a global target of a 25% reduction in premature mortality from non-communicable diseases by 2025." The EU was not part of the team of Member States which developed the resolution on NCD targets; however, it expressed support for the resolution. The EU in its statement expressed disappointment with the low participation of Member States in consultation on this topic. It advocated the adoption of voluntary targets in relation to four risk-related lifestyle factors, along with the adoption of other indicators and targets in national NCD control strategies.[4]

At the 65th World Health Assembly, the EU also confirmed its support for the Rio Political Declaration on the Social Determinants of Health and a "health in all policies" approach in its official statement.[50] During this assembly, a debate emerged on the social determinants of health; "the main contentious issue was the extent to which the SDOH were being considered in the WHO's Global Programme of Work (GPW).… During negotiations, Brazil argued for a focus on health and well-being, rather than disease,[f] and quoted the definition of health in the WHO constitution." [29] Brazil strongly argued for "health and development" and "health in all policies" approaches, and for the WHO to take a role in health and sustainable development in order for the burden of disease to be reduced. Conversely, we found one EU perspective arguing that the WHO should not be a "development agency," in the interest of preventing duplication with other UN bodies and NGO activities.[38] In the subsequent WHO Regional Committee for Europe meeting, the EU emphasized the role of national action plans and a revised global action plan for NCDs, along with the need for a preventative, multisectoral, "health in all policies" approach to be adopted in addressing NCDs.[10] A "health in all policies" approach would entail health working closely with other sectors and multilateral agencies. It appears that, at the international level, there is a lack of clear strategies for how to adopt an SDOH approach; however, at the 65th WHA, it was agreed that social determinants should be a priority across all work areas of the GPW.

Relating Coherence and Effectiveness

Having a single voice is not the same as effective having an single voice, as the former, may simply mean a lowest-common-denominator position. This has been recognized by Thomas,[5] who has considered the relationship between coherence and effectiveness, with coherent positions not necessarily leading to influencing other States. Too much of a focus on a

---

[f] Brazilian delegation. (2012) 65th World Health Assembly. WHO Reform — Statement by the Delegation of Brazil. Geneva, May 2012.

single voice, representation and coordination can detract from a focus on EU influence in international negotiations and different methods of influence besides common policy positions. In this respect, following the conceptualization of Kissack, we see a single voice not as an end in itself.[51] It is notable, however, that EU policy and standards on trade and the environment, where the single voice is more firmly established, can strongly affect non-EU Member States that wish to do trade with the EU.

Lack of flexibility/maneuvering space or trust by Member States in EU representation may affect the single voice, since Member States themselves may engage in behind-the-scenes meetings for diplomacy and influence. Member States can vie for influence within the EU, making statements in addition to EU statements and adjustments to EU positions. Larger states can be more influential *within* the EU, with smaller Member States having more potential to benefit from EU coordination due to their lower level of resources.

The case studies above have illustrated that formal established positions on WHO discussions represent only one mode of influence. Trust-building (including informal meetings), soft power diplomacy and flexibility in negotiations are important to global health diplomacy and the perceived effectiveness of EU representation. Lack of EU flexibility in negotiations and EU Member State cautiousness about straying from a common position have previously been recognized in relation to negotiations over the FCTC, with the argument that EU representatives require more space to negotiate.[52] A lack of maneuvering space in EU positions and subsequent negotiations could potentially block or lead to impasses in future negotiations.[38,39] Burke[39] suggests that the EU has failed to foresee opposition to its speaking rights at the UN General Assembly (including from traditional allies), which "exposed the lack of diplomatic capability within the EU, where an overwhelming focus on internal dialogue and coordination prevailed over outreach to external partners and political analysis." Conversely, it has been stated that the EC has brought "vital practical diplomatic and coordinating experience to the negotiation table" when coordinating its position for the FCTC, and has a lot of experience to offer EU Member State staff with health backgrounds in terms of diplomacy and experience with international agreements.[52] However, lengthy coordination processes and other barriers to the EU reaching out to external partners within negotiation processes have also been cited as an issue.[38]

Previously, the EU had a largely undetermined role within intergovernmental agencies, and in 1985 Delors famously feared that in 30 or 40 years the EU could be a UPO — an "unidentified political object."[g] The UN system still has problems with what the EU is as its very nature does not fit the present rules of intergovernmental governance. However, as Zielonka[31] has said, "Westphalian solutions are largely inadequate for coping with an enlarged EU." The EU should perhaps have an interest in a more network-based, plurilateral form of governance based on soft power (i.e. negotiating with other non-EU Member States or blocs with common positions) in order to push its weight Van Langenhove[53] has argued that the EU "could play a central role in transforming the current multilateral system." He describes a future of multistakeholder governance, including at the regional level, which is less about hegemonic power where states are the "star players" and where "one can expect a fluid web of multistakeholder partnerships between different types of actors at different levels of governance including the regional level."[53] Indeed, Nye claims that there are two recent forms of power transition globally, where (1) power has changed amongst States from "West to East" and where (2) there has been power diffusion and greater power amongst non-state actors.[40]

Whilst Member States are already using soft power strategies and meeting with non-EU Member States having common positions, the EU itself is beginning to think about how it works with third countries to gain support for EU positions. Engaging in such negotiations would require strong *acquis*, a high level of Member State trust in EU representation, and greater flexibility and freedom of the EU to act. It should be recognized that the EEAS is a relatively young and emerging service which is still engaging in the processes of trust and confidence-building with its Member States.

---

[g]"It cannot be dismissed that in 30 or 40 years, Europe will form an UPO — a sort of unidentified political object — or an ensemble which, once more, will be able to give to each of our countries the effect of a dimension which will permit it to prosper internally and to hold its place [*tenir son rang*] externally." (Delors, 9 September 1985).

Many political science scholars have suggested that the EU plays different roles with different amounts of leadership/proactivity exhibited across different multilateral governance fora.[54] The EU appears to have more influence in global health and the WHO generally than in other international health fora (aside from the Global Fund) due to different constituencies and the coordination role being played for the development of EU positions on WHO matters. However, it is perceived as being less influential in global health than in other policy areas, such as trade or the environment, due to less clear *acquis* in the health arena and ongoing debates about competences.[38]

Conclusion

Where the EU once had only a "supporting role" in health, it has developed a more prominent role in global health strategy through its role in negotiating the FCTC and IHR as well as the Pandemic Influenza Framework, its Council Conclusions on the EU role in global health, European Parliament statements on NCDs, and its common positions on the WHO reform debate. After the entry into force of the Lisbon Treaty, the EU has appeared to gradually act in a more coordinated fashion and consequently with a single voice in the WHO and other multilateral fora, including the UN General Assembly. The EU has now developed its role in global health and is improving its external representation within UN bodies, including the WHO.[47] It has taken a proactive role in initiatives such as the UN High-Level Meeting on the Prevention and Control of NCDs, it now has a voice in the UNGA, and has established common positions through the WHO reform processes.[47] However, EU influence on global health is relative when we consider: (1) the broader context of global health, where a plethora of organizations with significant resources operate; (2) the global power shift toward emerging economies; (3) the diminishing power and resources of the WHO, where voluntary financial contributions are increasingly tied to the priorities of individual governments — which in turn influences the "business" of the WHO (and the requirement to focus on core activities); and (4) the "social determinants" and "health in all policies" approaches, which require the commitment and cooperation of a range of sectors and international agencies.

There is scope for more integration between the EU global health strategy and the WHO reform, and more horizontal integration between health, foreign policy, development and research actors of the EU and EC. This is consistent with the EU's "health in all policies" approach,[20,24] and with health being one of three key priorities for "inclusiveness" in the EU's Development Policy.[55] The Lisbon Treaty initially led to some tension between EU Member States and the EU, and whilst there are now well-coordinated EU positions when it comes to the WHO reform and some other topics, tensions do still arise between Member States and the EU when it comes to who is allowed to speak on behalf of the EU.

However, having a single voice should not be equated with having an effective voice. Aside from common EU statements, trust-building, soft power diplomacy and behind-the-scenes strategies are important for political influence, as are financial contributions. The EU appears cautious about engaging in such soft diplomacy and the EEAS is still in the process of confidence-building with Member States. Initial EU Member State monitoring and distrust of EU representation are possible factors in such caution. More plurilateral forms of governance and soft power diplomacy strategies may be necessary for greater EU influence; however, this would also require more efficient (internal) coordination processes, greater Member State trust in EU representation, and flexibility in negotiations.

References

1. Laatikainen KV, Smith KE. (2006) *The European Union at the United Nations: Intersecting Multilateralisms*. Palgrave Macmillan, Basingstoke, New York.
2. Battams S. (2014) What can the WHO learn from EU lessons in civil society engagement and participation for health. *International Journal of Health Services* **44(4)**.
3. Battams S., Van Sachik L, van der Pas (2014) The EU as a global health actor: Policy coherence, health diplomacy and WHO reform. *European Foreign Affairs Review* **19(4)**.
4. Jørgensen KE, Laatikainen KV. (2013) *Routledge Handbook on the European Union and International Institutions: Performance, Policy, Power*. Routledge, London, New York.

5. Thomas D. (2012) Still punching below its weight? Coherence and effectiveness in European Union foreign policy. *Journal of Common Market Studies* **50(3):** 457–474.

6. Caporaso J, Jupille J. (1998) States, agency and rules: the European Union in global environmental politics. In *The European Union in the World Community.* Lynee Rienner, Boulder, pp. 213–249.

7. Bretherton C, Vogler J. (2006) *The European Union as a Global Actor.* Routledge, London, New York.

8. Van Schaik L. (2013) *EU Effectiveness and Unity in Multilateral Negotiations: More Than the Sum of Its Parts?* Palgrave Macmillan, Basingstoke.

9. Jørgensen KE, Oberthur S, *et al.* (2011) Introduction: assessing the EU's performance in international institutions — conceptual framework and core findings. *Journal of European Integration* **33(6):** 599–620.

10. Niemann A, Bretherton C. (Forthcoming) EU external policy at the crossroads: the challenge of actorness and effectiveness. *International Relations.*

11. Van Schaik LG. (2011) The EU's performance in the World Health Organization: internal cramps after the "Lisbon cure." *European Integration* **33(6):** 699–713.

12. Princen S. (2007) Advocacy coalitions and the internationalization of public health policies. *Journal of Public Policy* **27(1):** 13–33.

13. Mamudu HM, Studlar DT. (2009) Multilevel governance and shared sovereignty: European Union, Member States, and the FCTC. *Governance* **22(1):** 73–79.

14. European Commission (2007). White Paper. Together for health: A strategic approach for the EU 2008–2013. COM (2007) 630, 23 October 2007.

15. Guigner S. (2009) "The EU and the health dimension of globalization: playing the World Health Orgnization card," Chapter 8. In Orbie J, Tortell L. (eds.), The European Union and the Social Dimension of Globalization: How the EU influences the world, Routledge, Oxon.

16. Emmerling T, Heydemann J. (2012) The EU as an actor in global health diplomacy. In: Kickbusch I, Lister G, Told M, Drager N (eds.), *Global Health Diplomacy: Concepts, Issues, Actors, Instruments, Fora and Cases.* Springer, New York.

17. European Commission. (2012a) General Report on the Activities of the European Union 2011. EC Publications, Brussels.

18. Council of the European Union. (2010b) Council Conclusions on Equity and Health in All Policies: Solidarity in Health. Brussels.

19. Council of the European Union. (2007) Treaty of Lisbon amending the Treaty on European Union and the treaty establishing the European Community. E. Union. Brussels. 13th December 2007.

20. Council of the European Union. (2010a) Council Conclusions on the EU Role in Global Health. 3011th Foreign Affairs Council meeting. Brussels, 10 May 2010.

21. Council of the European Union. (2010) Council conclusions on the EU role in global health. 3011th Foreign Affairs council meeting. Brussels, 10 May 2010.

22. Commission on Social Determinants of Health. (2008) Closing the Gap in a Generation: Health Equity Through Action on the Social Determinants of Health. Final report. World Health Organization, Geneva.

23. European Commission. (2011) Communication from the Commission to the European Parliament, the Council, the European Economic and Social Committee and the Committee of the Regions. Increasing the Impact of EU Development Policy: An Agenda for Change. DEVCO. European Commission, Brussels.

24. Council of the European Union. (2006) Council Conclusions on Health in All Policies.

25. European Commission. (2012b) Health in All Policies.

26. Haines A. *et al.* (2012) "From the Earth Summit to Rio+20: integration of health and sustainable development." *The Lancet*, **379(9832):** 2189–2197.

27. Kickbusch I, Berger C. (2011) Global health diplomacy. In: Parker R, Sommer M, *Routledge Handbook in Global Public Health*. Routledge, London, New York.

28. Helble M, Mok E, *et al.* (2009) International trade and health: loose governance arrangements across sectors. In: Buse K, Hein W, Drager N (eds.), *Making Sense of Global Health Governance: A Policy Perspective*. Palgrave Macmillan, UK, pp. 164–208.

29. Battams S. (2012) The social determinants of health and civil society engagement in the WHO reform and beyond: negotiations at the 65th World Health Assembly. *Health Diplomacy Monitor* **3(4)**.

30. Vanhoonacker S, Reslow N. (2010) The European External Action Service: living forwards by understanding backwards. *European Foreign Affairs Review* **15:** 1–18.

31. Zielonka J. (2006) *Europe as Empire: The Nature of the Enlarged European Union*. Oxford University Press, Oxford.
32. Ashton C. (2012) Address by HR/VP Catherine Ashton at the seminar "The EU and Brazil in the World," in the presence of the Foreign Minister of Brazil, Antonio Pratriota. Diplomatic Academy, 8 February 2012.
33. United Nations General Assembly. (2011a) Political Declaration of the High-Level Meeting of the General Assembly on the Prevention and Control of Non-communicable Diseases. A/66/L.1. UNGA.
34. Laatikainen KV. (2010) Multilateral leadership at the UN after the Lisbon Treaty. *European Foreign Affairs Review* **15(4)**.
35. Grevi G. (2011) *From Lisbon to New York: The EU at the UN General Assembly*. Fride, Madrid.
36. Drieskens E. (2012) What's in a name? Challenges to the creation of EU delegations. *The Hague Journal of Diplomacy* **7(1)**: 51–64.
37. Emerson M. *et al.* (2011) Upgrading the EU's Role as Global Actor-Institutions, Law and the Restructuring of European Diplomacy. Centre for European Policy Studies, Brussels.
38. Battams S, van Schaik L, *et al.* (2012) The European Union's Voice and Influence on Global Health and the Reform of the World Health Organization: The Role of Diplomacy. The European Union in International Affairs 111 Conference, Brussels.
39. Burke E. (2012) What Europe's New Diplomatic Service Can Do for Britain. Centre for European Reform blogspot (accessed on 7 March 2012).
40. Nye J. (2004). *Soft Power: The Means to Success in World Politics*. Public Affairs, US.
41. Lee K, Gomez E. (2012) Brazil's ascendance: the soft power role of global health diplomacy. *The European Business Review*.
42. Nye. (2010) Joseph Nye on Global Power Shifts. TED Talk, July 2010 (if it is not ok to reference a TED talk, you could use this one; Nye, J. (2009). Get smart: Combining hard and soft power. Foreign Affairs. july/August 2009.)
43. World Health Organization. (2010) The Future of Financing for WHO: Report of an Informal Consultation Convened by the Director-General. WHO, Geneva.
44. World Health Organization. (2011) Governance and Promoting Engagement with Other Stakeholders and Involvement with and Oversight of Partnerships. EB130/5 Add. 4.

45. HAI Europe. (2011) Conflicts of Interest and the Future Financing for WHO. HAI Europe Staff Blog, 17 May 2011. Available at http://haieuropestaffblog. blogspot.com/2011/05/conflicts-of-interest-and-future-of.html.

46. Battams S, van der Pas R, *et al.* (2012) The EU's Role in Global Health and the WHO Reform; Between Health and Foreign Policy. Lisboan Erasmus Academic Network workshop "EU External Representation in International Contexts: Reform Practices After Lisbon." Clingendael Institute, The Hague.

47. Battams S. (2014) What can the WHO learn from EU lessionss in civil society engagement and participation for health? *International Journal of Health Services* **44**(4).

48. The NCD Alliance. (2012) Submission to WHO Consultations on NCDs, 19 April 2012. Geneva.

49. European Parliament. (2011) European Parliament resolution of 15 September 2011 on European Union position and commitment in advance to the UN high-level meeting on the prevention and control of non-communicable diseases. P7 TA (2011) 0390.

50. European Union. (2012b) EU Statement on the Social Determinants of Health: Outcome of the World Conference on Social Determinants of Health. World Health Assembly, Geneva.

51. Kissack R. (2011) The Single Voice Problematique: Pragmatic Policy or Intergovernmental Handmaiden? The European Union in International Affairs Conference 111. Brussels, 3–5 May 2012.

52. Faid M, Gleicher D. (2011) Dancing the Tango: The Experience and Roles of the European Union in Relation to the Framework Convention on Tobacco Control. P. f. E. D. Sanco. Global Health Programme, The Graduate Institute of International and Development Studies, Geneva.

53. Van Langenhove L. (2010) *The EU as a Global Actor in a Multipolar World and Multilateral 2.0 Environment.* Academia, Brussels.

54. Basu S, Schunz S. (2008) Pathways for an Interdisciplinary Analysis: Legal and Political Dimensions of the European Union's Position in Multilateral Governance. Working Paper No. 11, February 2008. Leuven Centre for Global Governance Studies, Leuven.

55. Council of the European Union (2012). Council conclusions "Increasing the Impact of EU Development Policy: an Agenda for Change," 3166th Foreign Affairs Council meeting, 14 May 2012, Brussels.

Index

Printed in the United States
By Bookmasters